Ophthalmic Surgery: A Case-Based Approach

Ophthalmic Surgery: A Case-Based Approach

Editor: Lexi Price

AMERICAN
MEDICAL PUBLISHERS
www.americanmedicalpublishers.com

AMERICAN
MEDICAL PUBLISHERS
www.americanmedicalpublishers.com

Cataloging-in-Publication Data

Ophthalmic surgery: a case-based approach / edited by Lexi Price.
p. cm.
Includes bibliographical references and index.
ISBN 979-8-88740-649-7
1. Eye--Surgery. 2. Eye--Diseases--Treatment. 3. Ophthalmology. I. Price, Lexi.
RE80 .H36 2023
617.71--dc23

American Medical Publishers,
41 Flatbush Avenue,
1st Floor, New York,
NY 11217, USA

ISBN 979-8-88740-649-7 (Hardback)

Contents

Preface

The medical specialty that deals with the diagnosis and treatment of eye diseases is known as ophthalmology. The surgical sub-specialty within this field is known as ophthalmic surgery. It involves the surgical procedures performed on the eyes or its surrounding structures to correct various eye conditions and improve visual function. Some of the common types of ophthalmic surgeries are cataract surgery, refractive surgery and retinal surgery. Cataract surgery involves the removal of a cloudy lens, known as the cataract, from the eye and replacing it with an artificial intraocular lens in order to restore clear vision. Refractive surgeries, such as LASIK, photorefractive keratectomy and small incision lenticule extraction, aim to correct vision problems such as nearsightedness, farsightedness, astigmatism and presbyopia. This book is compiled in such a manner, that it will provide in-depth knowledge about the ophthalmic surgery. It includes contributions of experts and scientists which will provide innovative insights into this field of medicine.

This book is a comprehensive compilation of works of different researchers from varied parts of the world. It includes valuable experiences of the researchers with the sole objective of providing the readers (learners) with a proper knowledge of the concerned field. This book will be beneficial in evoking inspiration and enhancing the knowledge of the interested readers.

In the end, I would like to extend my heartiest thanks to the authors who worked with great determination on their chapters. I also appreciate the publisher's support in the course of the book. I would also like to deeply acknowledge my family who stood by me as a source of inspiration during the project.

Editor

1

Cystoid Macular Edema 18 Years after Anterior Chamber Phakic Intraocular Lens Implantation

Elias L. Warrak,[1] Majd S. Haddam,[1] Walid N. Dandan,[1] John E. Warrak,[2] and Fady K. Sammouh[1]

[1]*Department of Ophthalmology and Visual Sciences, University of Balamand, Advanced Eye Care Hospital, Lebanon*
[2]*University of Balamand, Faculty of Medicine and Health Sciences, Lebanon*

Correspondence should be addressed to Elias L. Warrak; advancedeyecare.ew@gmail.com

Academic Editor: Hsin Yi Chen

We report a case of a 54-year-old female patient who underwent PAC-IOL implantation 18 years prior to presentation. The patient had a best corrected visual acuity (BCVA) 20/20 in the right eye (OD) postoperatively with normal eye exam on routine follow-up since then. The patient presented for acute onset decreased visual acuity in the right eye. BCVA was 20/60, and exam showed blunted macular reflex with no evidence of inflammation. Optical coherence tomography (OCT) showed CME. She was started on topical treatment (ketorolac 0.5%) OD four times daily. Three weeks later, the patient had a BCVA of 20/20 OD with a normal macular reflex and an OCT showing the resolution of the CME. To our knowledge, this is the first reported case of a CME 18 years post PAC-IOL implantation. The possible cause of this incidence could be related to subclinical intraocular inflammation. Ophthalmologists should be aware of the possibility of such a latent CME post-PAC-IOL implantation.

1. Introduction

The introduction of phakic anterior chamber IOL (PAC-IOL) by Strampelli and Barraquer in the 1950s has offered an innovative method to treat ametropia with a better and more stable visual acuity and a rapid recovery [1, 2]. The surgery was temporarily abandoned due to high rates of intraocular complications that were overcome in the 1980s with the introduction of new sites of implantation by Fechner and Baikoff [3–5]. The three known sites of phakic IOL implantation include posterior chamber IOL, anterior chamber angle fixated, and anterior chamber iris fixated [3]. The angle-supported PAC-IOL was introduced by Jan Worst in the 1980s with the phakic 6H® IOL introduced around 1998. Cystoid macular edema (CME) post-IOL implantation is one of the common complications causing eyesight deterioration usually within 3 to 12 weeks postoperatively due to vascular retinal disease and inflammatory cascades that particularly targets the macula [6]. The underlying mechanism is based on fluid accumulation in cyst-like spaces located within the neurosensory layers of the retina, mostly involving the outer plexiform layer, the watershed area of the retina [7]. This paper demonstrates a case of latent CME 18 years after the implantation of a PAC-IOL with complete resolution upon topical treatment.

2. Case Presentation

This is the case of a 54-year-old female patient with no prior medical history who presented to our facility with acute onset of blurred vision in her right eye of one-week duration 18 years after anterior chamber phakic intraocular lens (Phakic 6H®) placement. History goes back to November 2003 when the patient presented to our facility with interest in refractive surgery. She had an unremarkable ophthalmological history at that time. The best corrected visual acuity (BCVA) was 20/25 in the right eye (OD) and 20/20 in the left eye (OS) with a manifest refraction of $-11.25 + 1.25 \times 130°$ and $-9.25 + 2.25 \times 110°$, respectively. Slit lamp examination and dilated funduscopy were unremarkable. Intraocular

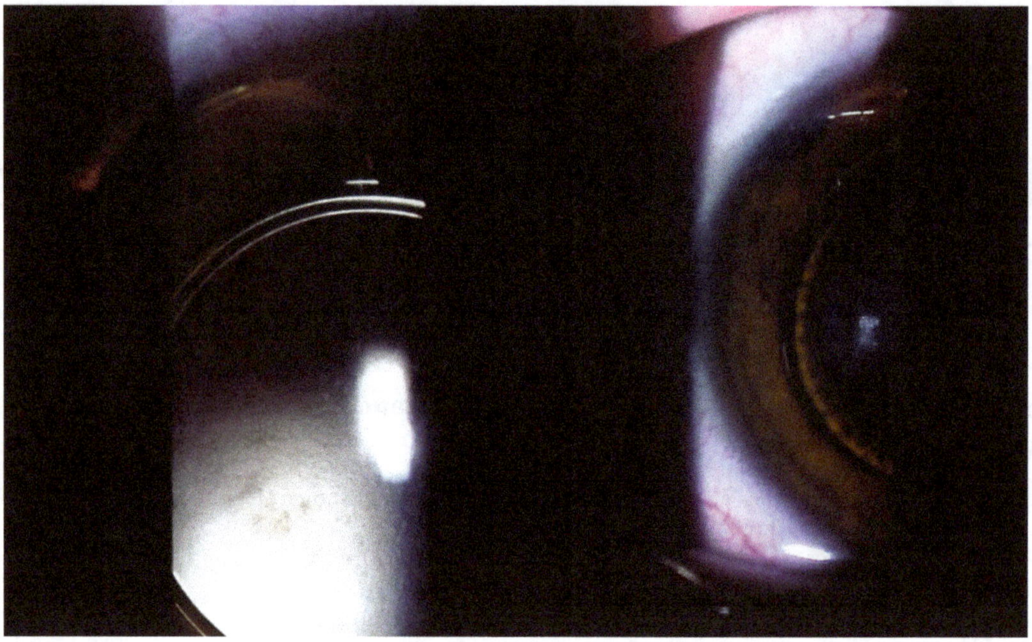

Figure 1: Slit lamp photo showing PAC-IOL with superior haptic migration into the PI.

pressure using Goldmann applanation tonometry was 15 mmHg OD and 16 mmHg OS. Corneal topography showed a central corneal thickness of 504 μm OD and 510 μm OS. The highest keratometry (K_{max}) values were 44.62 D OD and 45.58 D OS. The anterior chamber depth (ACD) was 3.42 mm OD and 3.25 mm OS. Central endothelial cell density by specular microscopy was 2645 cells/mm^2 OD. Accordingly, laser-assisted in situ keratomileusis was performed for the left eye which yielded an uncorrected visual acuity of 20/20 measured two months after the surgery and PAC-IOL implantation was performed for the right eye. The risks and benefits of the procedure were explained to the patient prior to the procedure. PAC-IOL was implanted through a 6.25 mm superior corneal incision, followed by a surgical peripheral iridectomy (PI)superiorly. The nonfoldable Phakic 6H® lens was introduced into the anterior chamber and implanted at 6–12 o'clock orientation, with careful attention to proximity to the crystalline lens, iris, and endothelium. The wound was sutured with 10-0 nylon after verification of an open angle, and suture knots were buried. Antibiotic and steroid eye drops were given for four weeks postoperatively. Uncorrected visual acuity (UCVA) in the right eye was 20/30 at one and six months postoperatively. BCVA was 20/20 OD with a manifest refraction of −0.75 + 0.50 × 125 at the one and six months postoperative follow-ups. The patient was then routinely followed up with no complications and stable vision.

On the day of presentation (March 2021), the patient complained of decreased visual acuity OD. BCVA was found to be 20/60 OD and 20/25 OS. Slit lamp examination for the right eye showed a deep and quiet anterior chamber, a clear cornea, an intact iris without any transillumination defects or synechia, and the PAC-IOL haptic migrated into the PI in the right eye (Figure 1). The sclera was white with no evidence of inflammatory changes. Dilated funduscopy showed clear vitreous, normal optic nerve, and retinal vasculature in both eyes. However, a blunted macular reflex with minimal macular edema was noted OD. Consequently, optical coherence tomography (OCT) was performed showing cystoid macular edema (CME) (Figure 2). The patient was started on topical nonsteroidal anti-inflammatory (NSAID) eye drops (ketorolac 0.5%) OD four times per day. Three weeks later, the BCVA improved to 20/20. The dilated fundus exam and repeat OCT showed the restoration of normal foveal anatomy and complete resolution of the CME in the right (Figure 3). Follow-up examination in one and three months revealed a normal slit lamp examination and funduscopy with a BCVA of 20/20 OD and 20/25 OS.

3. Discussion

Postsurgical cystoid macular edema (Irvine-Gass syndrome) is a major cause of reduced visual acuity secondary to phacoemulsification and other ocular surgeries and pathologies. It commonly occurs after penetrating keratoplasty, vitreoretinal procedures, IOL implantation, diabetes, uveitis, retinitis pigmentosa, and vascular occlusion [8]. Although the etiology is not fully clear, it is suggested that it is mainly mediated by postoperative inflammatory cascades and mediators that promote fluid accumulation in the perifoveal retina secondary to increased permeability of the perifoveal capillaries with possible direct macular traction [9]. In our case, the patient did not have any ocular surgeries or interventions except for the PAC-IOL implantation. Her medical history is negative for any systematic or autoimmune disease. Her biannual routine eye exam and funduscopy were always normal with no evidence of any inflammation.

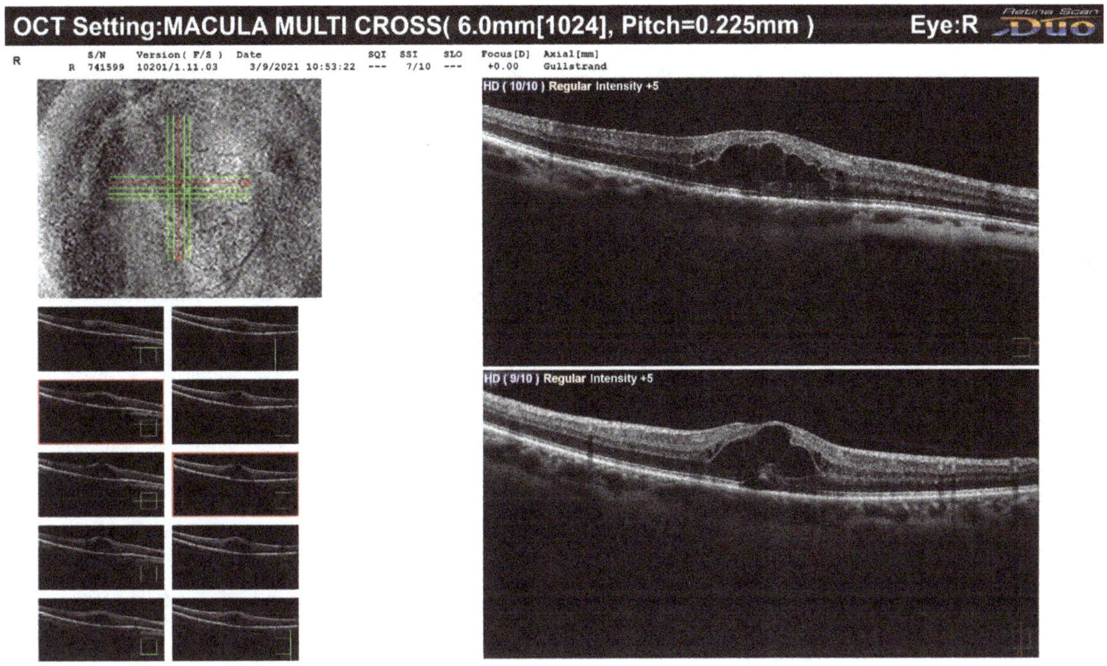

FIGURE 2: OCT scan showing CME 18 years after PAC-IOL implantation.

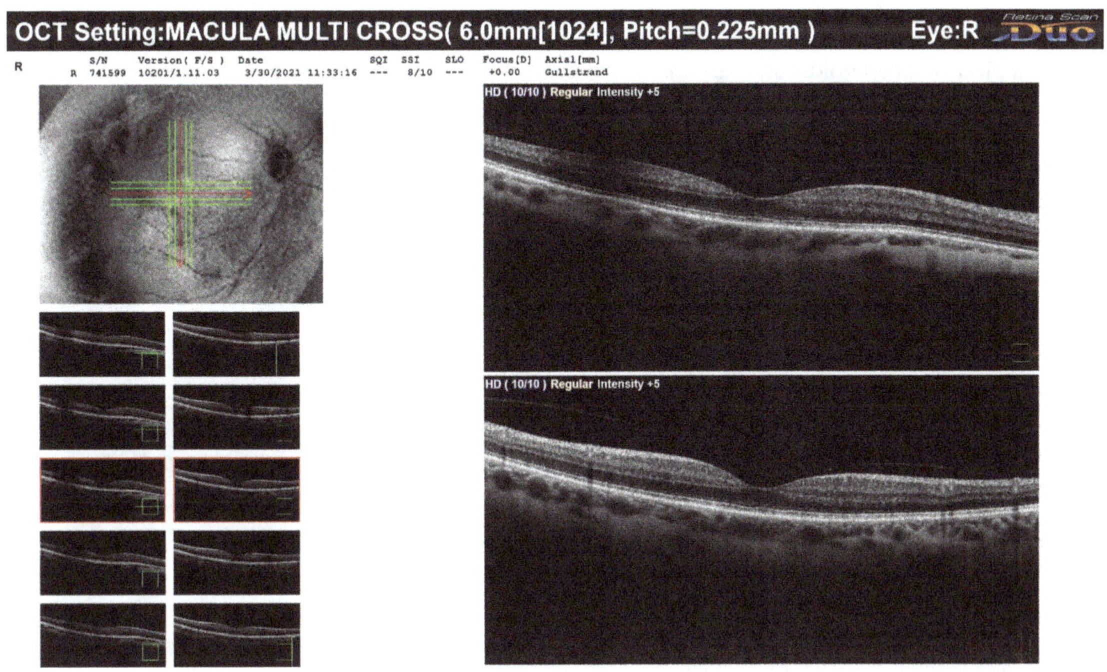

FIGURE 3: OCT scan showing resolution of CME 3 weeks after topical NSAID treatment.

Our patient selection criteria for PAC-IOL implantation procedure included a stable refractive error for more than 6 months, an anterior chamber depth greater than 3.0 mm, an endothelial cell count greater than 2500 cells/mm^2, contact lens intolerance, BCVA of 20/200 or better, no evidence of cataract formation, and a corneal thickness not suitable for laser refractive surgery. Our patient was a good candidate for the Phakic 6H® implantation with all criteria applicable.

To our knowledge, this is the first report of a latent CME, 18 years after an ocular procedure. A previous case report demonstrated a refractory CME after toric ICL placement. The CME resolved 3 months after the explantation of the ICL with topical NSAID (Nepafenac®) treatment [10]. A case series involved six eyes of five patients who had iris fixated intraocular lens who suffered from chronic CME resistant to medical therapy. The visual acuity was severely impaired until the iris fixated intraocular lens was replaced by a scleral sutured IOL (with posterior vitrectomy for some cases) which led to complete resolution of the CME with improved visual acuity reaching 20/20 [11].

In our patient, a possible explanation for the latent CME that resolved completely by topical NSAIDs is that it occurred as a sequel of subclinical low-grade inflammation/uveitis. This subclinical uveitis can be considered since no evidence of anterior chamber inflammatory changes such as cells, flares, or keratic precipitates were observed in any of the follow-up visits. The contributing factors for this subclinical inflammation could be explained by three possibilities. First, the IOL could have minute surface defects rubbing on the iris. Second, the stability of the angle-fixated IOL could be distorted due to haptic migration or gradual iris atrophy secondary to microscopic movement of the PAC-IOL against the iris. Third, the haptics could be triggering microscopic trauma to the peripheral iris with subsequent low-grade inflammation/uveitis. In a case series involving 35 eyes with PAC-IOL followed 8 months to 8.5 years, the incidence of haptic migration into the superior PI was 23% but without any alteration on the BCVA, intraocular structures, or evidence of inflammation [12].

In conclusion, ophthalmologists should be aware about such cases of latent CME with no evident ocular inflammation that might respond well on topical conservative treatment. There are different approaches to CME that include topical NSAIDS, topical corticosteroids, oral carbonic anhydrase inhibitors, periocular and intravitreal corticosteroid injections, anti-VEGF intravitreal injections, and surgery in refractory cases. However, further studies need to be conducted at a larger scale to confirm our findings and construct standardized treatment protocols.

Authors' Contributions

Elias L. Warrak and Majd S. Haddam contributed equally to the work.

References

[1] B. Strampelli, "Tolerance of acrylic lenses in the anterior chamber in aphakia and refraction disorders," *Annali di ottalmologia e clinica oculistica*, vol. 80, pp. 75–82, 1954.

[2] J. Barraquer, "Anterior chamber plastic lenses. Results of and conclusions from five years' experience," *Transactions of the Ophthalmological Societies of the United Kingdom*, vol. 79, pp. 393–424, 1959.

[3] D. Huang, S. C. Schallhorn, A. Sugar et al., "Phakic intraocular lens implantation for the correction of myopia: a report by the American Academy of Ophthalmology," *Ophthalmology*, vol. 116, no. 11, pp. 2244–2258, 2009.

[4] P. U. Fechner, G. L. van der Heijde, and J. G. Worst, "The correction of myopia by lens implantation into phakic eyes," *American Journal of Ophthalmology*, vol. 107, no. 6, pp. 659–663, 1989.

[5] G. Baikoff, "The refractive IOL in a phakic eye," *Ophthalmic Practice*, vol. 9, no. 58–61, p. 80, 1991.

[6] R. F. Spaide, "Retinal vascular cystoid macular edema," *Retina*, vol. 36, no. 10, pp. 1823–1842, 2016.

[7] S. Scholl, A. Augustin, A. Loewenstein, S. Rizzo, and B. D. Kuppermann, "General pathophysiology of macular edema," *European Journal of Ophthalmology*, vol. 21, pp. 10–19, 2011.

[8] G. Coscas, "Postsurgical Cystoid Macular Edema," *Macular Edema*, vol. 47, pp. 148–159, 2010.

[9] K. Miyake and N. Ibaraki, "Prostaglandins and cystoid macular edema," *Survey of ophthalmology*, vol. 47, pp. S203–S218, 2002.

[10] J. C. Umurhan Akkan, K. Tuncer, and A. Elbay, "Postsurgical cystoid macular edema following posterior chamber toric phakic intraocular lens implantation surgery: a case report," *Case Reports in Ophthalmology*, vol. 6, no. 2, pp. 223–227, 2015.

[11] H. F. Massa, I. Gobej, P. Jacquier, C. Jonescu-Cuypers, and O. le Quoy, "Cystoid macular oedema and iris-fixated intraocular lens treated with intraocular lens exchange: a case series and review," *Journal of International Medical Research*, vol. 47, no. 1, pp. 188–195, 2019.

[12] F. K. Sammouh, T. A. Baban, H. M. El Ballouz, and E. L. Warrak, "Asymptomatic haptic migration of phakic anterior chamber intraocular lens through the peripheral iridectomy," *Canadian Journal of Ophthalmology*, vol. 51, no. 2, pp. 83–86, 2016.

2

Ipsilateral Lymphatic and Venous Malformations Affecting the Midface Area

Şükran Bekdemir,[1] Ahmet Kaan Gündüz,[2] and Ömür Ataoğlu[3]

[1]*Ophthalmology Clinic, Polatlı Duatepe State Hospital, Ankara, Turkey*
[2]*Department of Ophthalmology, Ankara University Faculty of Medicine, Ankara, Turkey*
[3]*Private Mikro-Pat Pathology Laboratory, Ankara, Turkey*

Correspondence should be addressed to Ahmet Kaan Gündüz; drkaangunduz@gmail.com

Academic Editor: Stephen G. Schwartz

A 22-year-old woman presented with progressive swelling of the nasal conjunctiva in the left eye. Anterior segment examination revealed a diffuse cystic appearance to the inferonasal bulbar conjunctiva and plica semilunaris. Anterior segment swept-source optical coherence tomography (OCT) revealed clear hyporeflective spaces demarcated by hyperreflective septae in the affected conjunctiva, consistent with the diagnosis of lymphatic malformation (LM). Magnetic resonance imaging revealed a well circumscribed intraconal mass located inferonasally in the left orbit. Systemic examination revealed a lesion similar to LM on the left hard palate. The left conjunctival mass was excised subtotally. Subsequently, a transconjunctival anterior orbitotomy was performed and the left orbital mass was completely removed intact. Histopathologically, the conjunctival mass was diagnosed as LM and the orbital mass as venous malformation (VM). This case represents a rare coexistence of histopathologically proven conjunctival LM and orbital VM as well as a presumed LM of the hard palate, all 3 lesions occurring in the ipsilateral midface area.

1. Introduction

Hemangiomas develop as a result of abnormal changes in angiogenesis that allow overproliferation of vascular tissues. The term "hemangioma" has been superceded by cavernous venous malformation or venous malformation (VM). Several authors have elucidated the interaction between angiogenic and angiostatic forces involved in normal and pathologic processes [1]. Many of the angiogenic markers including fibroblast growth factor (FGF), vascular endothelial growth factor (VEGF), E-selectin, and type IV collagenase are increased during the proliferative growth phase of hemangiomas [2]. It has been speculated that hemodynamic changes cause opening of new channels allowing for budding of the vascular channels into surrounding soft tissues. After sufficient growth of the lesion, cosmetic or visual disturbances arise leading to imaging studies to be performed so that the lesion is diagnosed.

Lymphangiomas (referred to as lymphatic malformations, LM) are collections of lymph vessels filled with serous fluid. The formation of LMs may reflect a failure of lymph ducts to connect with the venous system during embryogenesis, abnormal sequestration of lymphatic structures, or both [3]. Many LMs are initially asymptomatic until an inciting factor causes an increase in the size of the lesion. Growth of the LMs is usually related to upper respiratory tract infections and minor trauma to the periocular region.

We herein report an interesting case demonstrating ipsilateral coexistence of orbital VM, conjunctival LM, and hard palate LM.

2. Case Presentation

A 22-year-old woman presented with progressive nasal conjunctival swelling in the left eye of 2-years duration. The patient had no history of systemic illness, ocular disease, or allergy. Thyroid function tests were within normal limits. Family history was negative for any ocular and cranial vascular malformation. Visual acuities at presentation were 20/20 in the right and 20/40 in the left eye. Intraocular pressures were

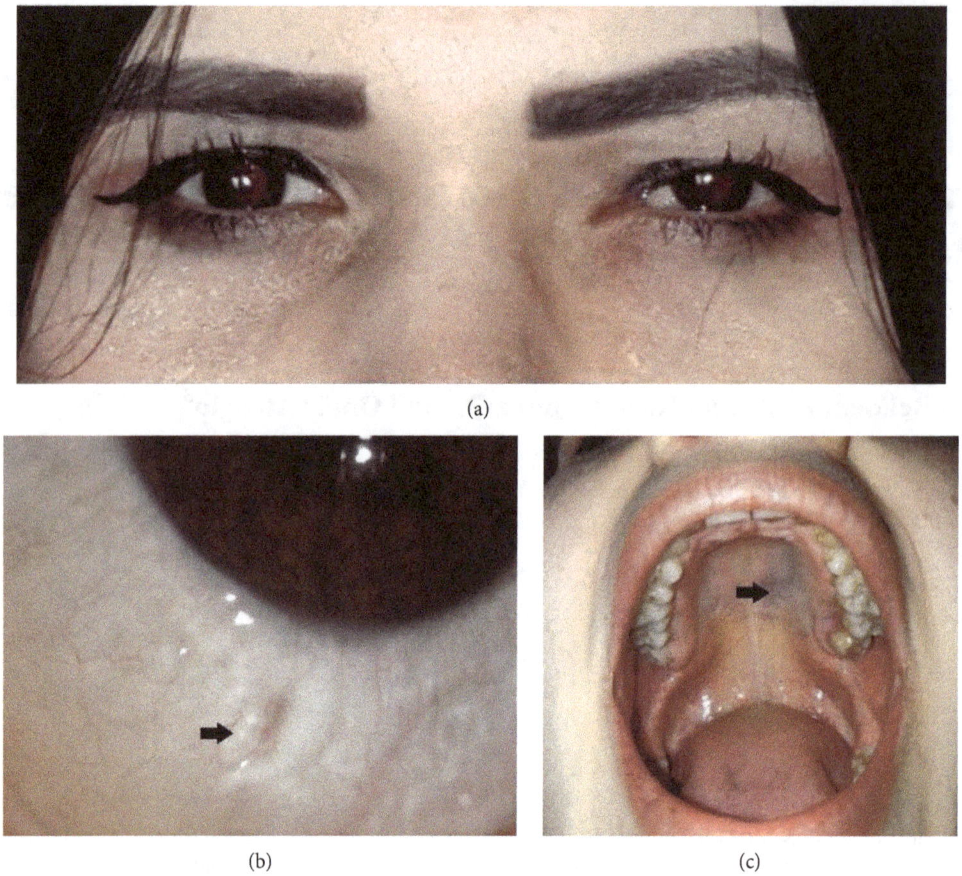

FIGURE 1: (a) Facial appearance of the patient at presentation showing slight lateral displacement of the left eye. (b) Anterior segment photograph shows lymphatic malformation cysts in the inferonasal conjunctiva (arrow). (c) Lesion similar to lymphatic malformation affecting the left hard palate (arrow).

17 mmHg in both eyes. There was no relative afferent pupil defect bilaterally. Ocular motility was full, and there was no proptosis in either eye. The left eye was mildly displaced laterally although the patient did not complain of double vision (Figure 1(a)). Anterior segment biomicroscopic examination of the left eye revealed that the plica semilunaris and inferonasal bulbar conjunctiva had a multicystic appearance (Figure 1(b)). Anterior segment and fundus examination of the right eye were normal. There was a lesion similar to LM on the patient's left hard palate (Figure 1(c)). Anterior segment swept-source optical coherence tomography (AS-SSOCT) (DRI OCT Triton Plus, Topcon, Tokyo, Japan) showed there was elevation of the plica semilunaris and bulbar conjunctiva comprising variable-sized hyporeflective spaces separated by hyperreflective tissue in the left eye (Figure 2(a)). AS-SSOCT of the right eye revealed normal findings. The patient subsequently underwent orbital and brain magnetic resonance imaging (MRI) which revealed an oval-shaped, intraconal mass located inferonasally in the left orbit.The orbital mass was in the same quadrant as the conjunctival LM. The mass was isointense with respect to the extraocular muscles on T1-weighted images, hyperintense on T2-weighted images, and demonstrated contrast enhancement (Figures 2(b) and 2(c)). There was no vascular malformation affecting the brain and meninges.

Surgical intervention was planned to perform conjunctival biopsy and to remove the orbital tumor. Under general anesthesia, the patient first underwent subtotal excisional biopsy of the left conjunctival mass. Subsequently, an anterior orbitotomy was performed via the inferonasal transconjunctival approach and the orbital tumor was removed in toto with the help of a cryoprobe. The basal diameters of the excised reddish, smooth-edged, capsulated orbital mass were approximately 1.5×1.5 cm (Figure 3(a)). Histopathological examination of the orbital mass revealed enlarged vascular channels featuring thick walls with fibrosis, the lumens of which were filled with erythrocytes. The histopathological diagnosis of the orbital mass was established as VM (Figure 3(b)). Histopathological examination of the conjunctival lesion revealed a vascular structure containing lymphatic fluid surrounded by endothelium and conjunctival epithelial cells on the surface, consistent with LM (Figure 3(c)). At 3 months follow-up, visual acuity in the left eye improved to 20/30. The left eye was orthophoric and there was no proptosis. The conjunctiva looked devoid of any major lymphangioma cysts (Figure 4).

3. Discussion

Venous malformations and LMs are common vascular lesions. The Orbital Society created a new classification of

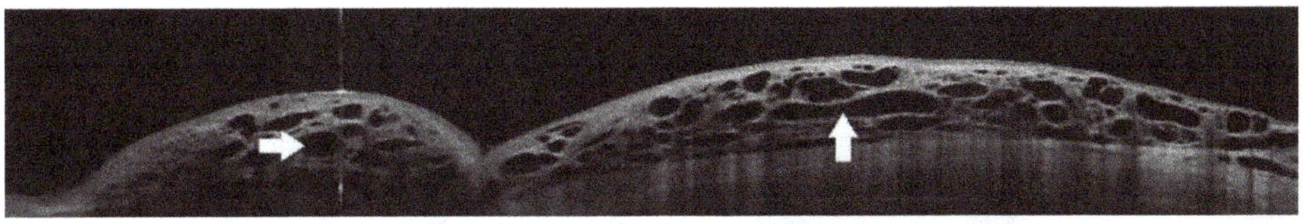

(a)

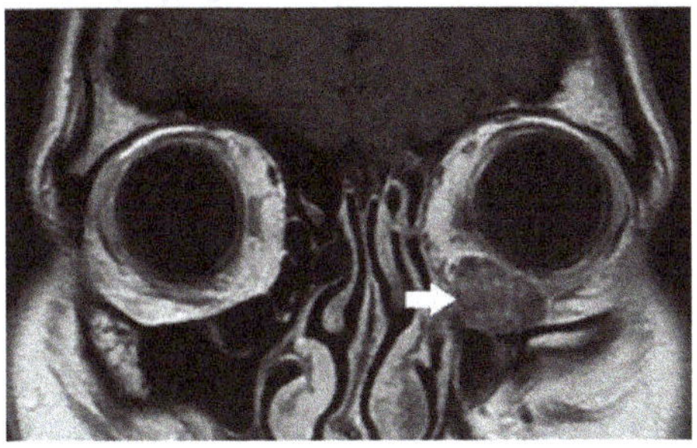

(b)

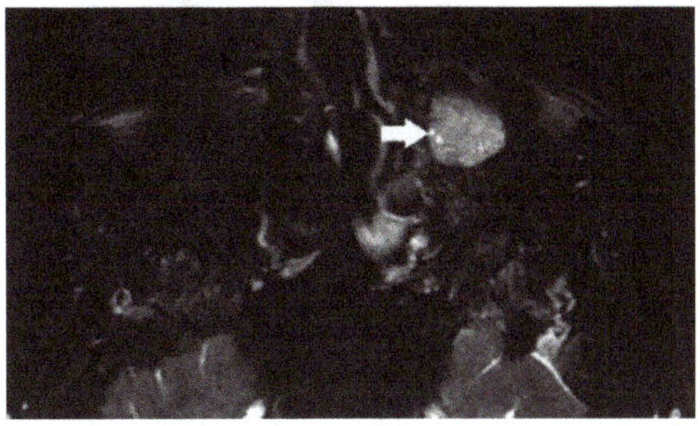

(c)

FIGURE 2: (a) Anterior segment swept source optical coherence tomography of the left eye demonstrates dilated lymphatic channels manifesting as hyporeflective spaces with different sizes demarcated by hyperreflective septae (arrows). (b) T1-weighted coronal MR image shows the inferonasally located intraconal tumor that is isointense with respect to muscle (arrow) in the left orbit. (c) T2-weighted axial MR image shows that the left orbital tumor is hyperintense (arrow).

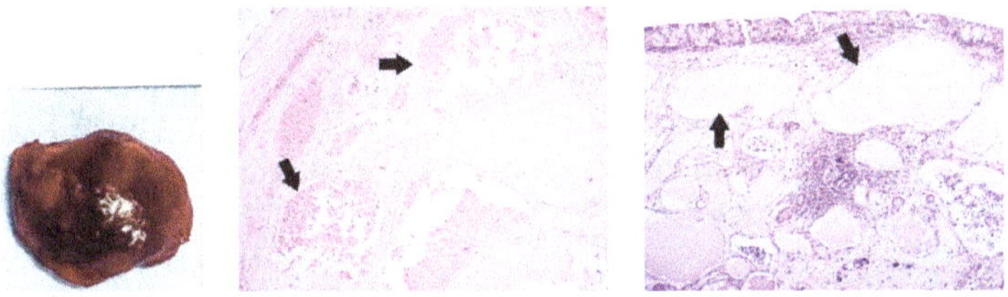

(a) (b) (c)

FIGURE 3: (a) Gross photograph of the excised left orbital tumor showing the reddish well-circumscribed mass measuring approximately 1.5×1.5 cm in base dimensions. (b) Histopathological examination of the orbital tumor reveals enlarged vascular channels with thick walls, the lumens of which are filled with erythrocytes embedded in a fibrous stroma (arrows), consistent with orbital cavernous venous malformation (H.E. ×100). (c) Histopathological examination of the conjunctival lesion shows several ectatic bloodless lymphatic channels, lined with flattened endothelium (arrows). There is prominent lymphoid infiltration and aggregates in the stroma, consistent with the diagnosis of conjunctival lymphatic malformation (H.E. ×100).

vascular lesions based on hemodynamic behavior. The Orbital Society's hemodynamic classification divides vascular malformations into three categories by flow characteristics: no flow (type I), venous flow (type II), and arterial flow (type III) [4]. Capillary hemangiomas and VMs are considered as hamartomas by this classification. Rootman et al. reclassified orbital vascular malformations based on the International Society for the Study of Vascular Anomalies (ISSVA) classification [5]. In this classification, cavernous hemangioma was categorized as a nondistensible cavernous venous malformation. Lymphatic malformations (also known as LMs) were divided into macrocystic, microcystic, or mixed (macrocystic/-microcystic) subtypes. Recently, the ISSVA issued a revised classification of vascular anomalies. In this revised classification scheme, hemangioma is categorically listed as a benign vascular tumor and lymphangioma as a lymphatic malformation (International Society for the Study of Vascular Anomalies (ISSVA) classification available at http://www.issva.org/UserFiles/file/ISSVA-Classification-2018.pdf. May 2018).

Orbital VM is the most common benign tumor of the orbit in adults. It is a benign, slowly progressive vascular tumor composed of endothelial-lined spaces surrounded by a fibrous capsule. It most commonly presents in middle-aged adults (ages 20-40 years) and women are affected more than men. Its location is most often within the muscle cone, lateral to the optic nerve. There is no evidence to suggest a heritance pattern in most cases. In our case, the tumor was located in the inferonasal orbit causing slight lateral displacement of the globe [6].

Orbital VM is generally accepted to be a congenital abnormality although it usually becomes symptomatic later in life. Venous malformations are composed of a network of vascular channels separated by fibrous tissue stroma. Histopathologically, VM is composed of dilated, cavernous vascular spaces separated by connective tissue stroma. Flattened endothelial cells line the vascular spaces, which are filled with blood. Single or multiple layers of smooth muscle cells surround the vascular spaces [6, 7].

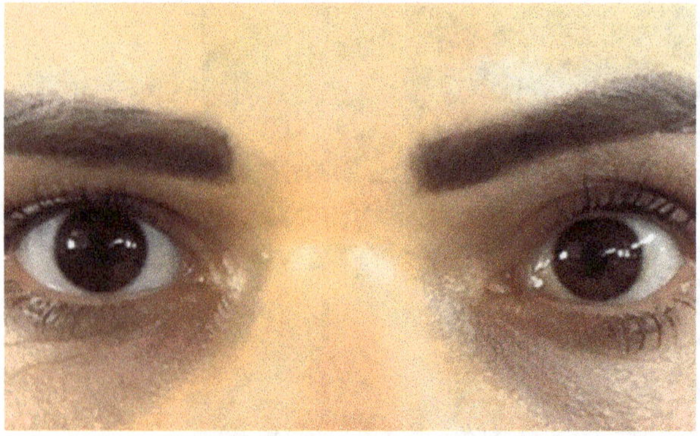

Figure 4: Facial photograph of the patient 3 months after surgery shows excellent outcome with an orthophoric appearance.

Lymphatic malformations are multicystic, localized malformations that involve the lymphatic and vascular systems. Their histology ranges from capillary-sized small vessels to macroscopic fluid-filled vessels. Orbital LMs generally have minimal internal blood flow and an absence of connection to the vascular system (type 1 vascular malformation). They are also believed to be congenital similar to cavernous VM. The exact cause of LM formation is unknown, but most cases are believed to be sporadic. LMs affecting the periocular area are usually seen in the orbit. However, isolated conjunctival LM may also rarely occur, as in the current case [7, 8]. Our case also had a presumed LM on the left hard palate but MRI did not reveal any evidence of LM in the orbit and brain.

Anterior segment optical coherence tomography is a noncontact, noninvasive imaging device that provides high-resolution, real-time, and in situ visualization of tissue microstructure [9]. Although the biomicroscopic findings were suggestive of conjunctival LM in our case, AS-SSOCT was helpful in establishing the tentative diagnosis and in the planning of surgery.

The most important lesion to consider in the differential diagnosis of conjunctival LM is conjunctival lymphangiectasia [10]. Conjunctival lymphangiectasia represents approximately <1% of all conjunctival tumors [11]. Our case had a multicystic septated appearance on AS-SSOCT in contrast to the fewer slit-like, slender, fusiform appearing cysts seen in lymphangiectasia [10]. Further, histopathologic examination revealed multiple prominent lymphatic channels and stromal lymphocytic aggregates, findings that would not be normally expected in conjunctival lymphangiectasia [10]. Conjunctival lymphangiectasia contains only scattered inflammatory cells in the stroma and may feature squamous metaplasia and keratinization of the overlying surface epithelium [10].

Orbital VM can coexist with other tumors including adenoid cystic carcinoma and schwannoma in the same orbit [12, 13]. The occurrence of multiple vascular anomalies in the same orbit has also been reported. Examples include VMs associated with varix, lymhangioma, and arteriovenous malformation [14, 15]. Furthermore, VM and LM have been reported to occur together in other body parts including ulnar nerve and lymph nodes [16, 17].

We postulate that the ipsilateral coexistence of conjunctival LM, hard palate LM, and orbital VM as in our case represents an unusual maldevelopment in vascular embryogenesis. The fact that all 3 lesions occurred ipsilaterally may point out a common pathway in pathogenesis. Our search of the PubMed database using the key words "lymphangioma," "lymphatic malformation," "conjunctiva," "orbit," "cavernous venous malformation," "venous malformation," and "cavernous hemangioma" failed to disclose any previous reports demonstrating ipsilateral coexistence of histopathologically confirmed conjunctival LM and orbital VM as well as a presumed LM on the palate.

References

[1] D. R. Bielenberg, C. D. Bucana, R. Sanchez, J. B. Mulliken, J. Folkman, and I. J. Fidler, "Progressive growth of infantile cutaneous hemangiomas is directly correlated with hyperplasia and angiogenesis of adjacent epidermis and inversely correlated with expression of the endogenous angiogenesis inhibitor, IFN-beta," *International Journal of Oncology*, vol. 14, no. 3, pp. 401–408, 1999.

[2] L. Beck Jr. and P. A. D'Amore, "Vascular development: cellular and molecular regulation," *The FASEB Journal*, vol. 11, no. 5, pp. 365–373, 1997.

[3] J. Rootman, E. Hay, D. Graeb, and R. Miller, "Orbital-adnexal lymphangiomas: a spectrum of hemodynamically isolated vascular hamartomas," *Ophthalmology*, vol. 93, no. 12, pp. 1558–1570, 1986.

[4] G. J. Harris, "Orbital vascular malformations: a consensus statement on terminology and its clinical implications. Orbital Society," *American Journal of Ophthalmology*, vol. 127, no. 4, pp. 453–455, 1999.

[5] J. Rootman, M. K. S. Heran, and D. A. Graeb, "Vascular malformations of the Orbit," *Ophthalmic Plastic and Reconstructive Surgery*, vol. 30, no. 2, pp. 91–104, 2014.

[6] J. Yan and Z. Wu, "Cavernous hemangioma of the orbit: analysis of 214 cases," *Orbit*, vol. 23, no. 1, pp. 33–40, 2009.

[7] A. K. Gündüz, Y. S. Yeşiltaş, and C. L. Shields, "Orbital tumors: a systematic review: part I," *Expert Review of Ophthalmology*, vol. 10, no. 5, pp. 465–483, 2015.

[8] D. M. Meisler, R. A. Eiferman, N. B. Ratliff, and C. D. Burns, "Surgical management of conjunctival lymphangiectasis by conjunctival resection," *American Journal of Ophthalmology*, vol. 136, no. 4, pp. 735-736, 2003.

[9] H. Demirci and D. W. Steen, "Limitations in imaging common conjunctival and corneal pathologies with fourier-domain optical coherence tomography," *Middle East African Journal of Ophthalmology*, vol. 21, no. 3, pp. 220–224, 2014.

[10] J. Welch, S. Srinivasan, D. Lyall, and F. Roberts, "Conjunctival lymphangiectasia: a report of 11 cases and review of literature," *Survey of Ophthalmology*, vol. 57, no. 2, pp. 136–148, 2012.

[11] C. L. Shields, H. Demirci, E. Karatza, and J. A. Shields, "Clinical survey of 1643 melanocytic and nonmelanocytic conjunctival tumors," *Ophthalmology*, vol. 111, no. 9, pp. 1747–1754, 2004.

[12] D. Strianese, M. Ferrara, A. Iuliano, and G. Bonavolonta, "Simultaneous diagnosis of ipsilateral adenoid cystic carcinoma of the lacrimal gland and orbital cavernous hemangioma: case report," *Orbit*, vol. 33, no. 4, pp. 283–285, 2014.

[13] S. Gupta, S. Kaliki, and S. Gowrishankar, "Concomitant orbital cavernous haemangioma and schwannoma in a patient," *BMJ Case Reports*, vol. 2017, article bcr2016218638, 2017.

[14] D. Strianese, M. Napoli, C. Russo et al., "Coexistence of cavernous hemangioma and other vascular malformations of the orbit. A report of three cases," *The Neuroradiology Journal*, vol. 27, no. 2, pp. 223–231, 2014.

[15] G. E. Coll, R. A. Goldberg, H. Krauss, and B. J. Bateman, "Concomitant lymphangioma and arteriovenous malformation of the orbit," *American Journal of Ophthalmology*, vol. 112, no. 2, pp. 200–205, 1991.

[16] M. C. Prater and B. A. Janz, "Mixed lymphangioma and cavernous hemangioma within the ulnar nerve: a case report," *The Hand*, vol. 12, no. 5, pp. NP145–NP147, 2016.

[17] K. Collins and J. A. DiGiuseppe, "Coincidental lymphangioma and hemangioma in a single lymph node," *International Journal of Surgical Pathology*, vol. 27, no. 5, pp. 527-528, 2019.

Hemorrhagic Descemet Membrane Detachment during Ab Interno Canaloplasty

Juan Carlos Izquierdo Villavicencio,[1,2] Josefina A. Mejías Smith,[1] Laura A. Cañola Ramírez,[1] Natalia Agudelo Arbelaez,[1] and Bárbara Rubio Lastra[1]

[1]*Glaucoma Research Department, Instituto de Ojos Oftalmosalud, Lima, Peru*
[2]*Glaucoma Department, Instituto de Ojos Oftalmosalud, Lima, Peru*

Correspondence should be addressed to Bárbara Rubio Lastra; rubio.barbara@gmail.com

Academic Editor: Nicola Rosa

Purpose. To describe a Descemet membrane detachment in peripheral cornea after canaloplasty with ab interno approach in glaucoma. *Case Report.* A 60-year-old male with uncontrolled primary open-angle glaucoma (POAG) underwent ab interno canaloplasty in the left eye. The previous corrected visual acuity was 20/400 and intraocular pressure 26 mmHg with maximum medical therapy. There was evidence of minor intrastromal bleeding and limited Descemet membrane detachment during the introduction of intracanalicular viscoelastic. Speculate that the Descemet detachment occurred owing to the excessive pressure while injecting the viscoelastic. A conservative management was decided due to the size of the detachment outside the visual axis. On the first postsurgical day, the slit lamp biomicroscopy confirmed that the paralimbal extension of the pre-Descemet hemorrhage was 3mm and the radial extension was 2mm. Moreover the initial thickness of the pre-Descemet hemorrhage measurement with anterior segment OCT was 0.6mm. The follow-up was done weekly. At 3 months postoperatively, cornea recovered its transparency and morphology and intraocular pressure was 18mmHg with maximum medical therapy. *Conclusion.* Descemet membrane detachment by viscoelastic with partial intrastromal hematoma is a rare complication of the ab interno canaloplasty, which can be managed conservatively if it has not compromised the visual axis and has a limited extension.

1. Introduction

Ab interno canaloplasty is a nonpenetrating glaucoma surgery which increases the drainage of aqueous humor from the anterior chamber through the trabecular meshwork to the Schlemm canal [1]; it is safe and effective and it may be conducted with other surgeries [2, 3]. Its purpose is to renew entire drainage system in a more physiological way which differs from the conventional glaucoma surgeries [4, 5].

The ab interno canaloplasty was discussed because according to Lewis et al., some patients undergoing ab external canaloplasty could only have viscodilation, and during the monitoring process to these patients after 3 years, it was evidenced that the results obtained were successful despite the fact that the technique was not complete [4]. This new approach was described when the Schlemm canal is dilated through viscoelastic and the trabecular meshwork is extended, thus creating microfractures in 360° circumferential direction to the canal [2, 6].

This article is the first report related to hemorrhagic Descemet membrane detachment due to viscoelastic in ab interno approach and we opted for observative management due to the extent of the injury, evidencing favorable results for the patient during 3-month monitoring process.

2. Case Report

A 60-year-old man with advanced bilateral open-angle glaucoma for 3 years, not controlled with maximum medical therapy in the left eye, underwent phacoemulsification in the left eye in 2014. The medical records did not register coagulation disorders and the patient denied to have taken antiplatelet medicine or anticoagulants.

Table 1: Monitoring of Visual acuity, intraocular pressure and number of medications.

Periods	UCVA(LogMAR)	IOP (mmHg)	Medications
Preoperative	1.30	26	3
Day 1	2.30	40	4
Week 1	2.10	14	3
Month 1	0.80	14	3
Month 2	0.80	8	2
Month 3	0.80	18	3

Before the surgery, the uncorrected visual acuity (UCVA) was 2.5 and 1.3 LogMAR in the right and left eye, respectively. The intraocular pressure was 12mmHg in the right eye and 26mmHg in the left eye with maximum medical therapy. On Humphrey Field Analyzer (HFA) 24-2 automated perimetry mean deviation (MD) was -16.92 in the left eye, pachymetry was 517 microns in the right eye and 492 microns in the left eye, and the number of central endothelial cells was 2127 cells/mm2 in the right eye and 1312 cells/mm^2 in the left eye.

Ab interno canaloplasty was performed routinely in the left eye by a glaucoma specialist. The temporary corneal incision was made at hour 9 and another lateral incision was made at hour 2 to introduce the iTrack catheter (iTrack-250A; iScience Interventional, Menlo Park, CA, USA). Sodium hyaluronate was injected (Healon GV; Abbott Medical Optics, Santa Ana, CA, USA) in the anterior chamber. Gonioscopy was used (AVG; Surgical Gonio Lens, Volk Alcon, Mentor, OH, USA) for goniotomy with Kahook dual blade (KDB; New World Medical, Rancho Cucamonga, CA, USA), and by using tying forceps (Intraocular Tying Forceps, 23G 4-1891, Rumex, USA) the catheter was pushed circumferentially through 360°, by applying two viscoelastic clicks per hour when removing it.

The procedure was performed correctly; however, during the viscodilation of the Schlemm canal with sodium hyaluronate, a small hemorrhage was observed with viscoelastic related to the Descemet membrane detachment. The paralumbar extension was 3.0 mm and radial extension was 2.0 mm between hours 4 and6 in peripheral inferonasal quadrant. At first we opted for observation because the injury did not compromise the visual axis and the size of the detachment was not large enough to indicate a surgical procedure immediately (Figure 1(A)).

A serial control with anterior segment OCT (Visante, Model 1000, Carl Zeiss Meditec, Dublin CA, USA) has been done to follow the thickness; the initial thickness of intrastromal hemorrhage was 0.6mm, and at the first week it was 0.51mm, at the first month 0.42mm, and at the second month 0.28 mm and third month 0.03 mm. The examination evidenced presence of blood in the peripheral inferonasal quadrant of the pre-Descemet area at hours 4-6 (Figures 1(D), 1(E), 1(F), 1(G), and 1(H)).

Considering the extension of the detachment, a conservative management was decided, monitoring the progressive reabsorption of the hemorrhage and viscoelastic, which progressively occurred (Figures 1(B) and 1(C)).

The intraocular pressure levels remained lower than 21mmHg in the early postoperative period with glaucoma medications; 3 months after the surgery the intraocular pressure was 18mmHg with 3 antiglaucoma medications. The uncorrected visual acuity (UCVA) showed a significant improvement from 1.30 in the preoperative period to 0.8 LogMAR in the left eye after 3 months of monitoring (Table 1). Final BCVA was 0.6 LogMAR.

The number of central endothelial cells registered a small decrease from 2,127 to 1,809 cells/mm^2 in the third month with a 14.9% loss. Final pachymetry was 553 microns in the left eye, showing an increase of corneal thickness of 12.39% in the third month.

According to Hodapp classification, the visual field defect 10-2, stimulus III, and white-on-white of the left eye indicated a stable advanced stage glaucoma with a MD of -31.4.

Three months after the surgery, the Descemet membrane detachment with intrastromal hematoma completely recovered; the membrane was reattached correctly (Figure 1(H)) and remained that way during the monitoring with the transparent cornea along with no visual consequences.

3. Discussion

The hemorrhagic Descemet membrane detachment with viscoelastic is a rare complication reported in the canaloplasty with external approach during the catheterization of Schlemm canal when injecting high-molecular-weight viscoelastic substances [5, 7]. Yalvac et al. reported one Descemet detachment followed by hemorrhage from the episcleral vessels or by blood reflux from the Schlemm canal [8]. This complication may cause a significant reduction of visual acuity if compromising the visual axis, according to the size and location of detachment.

The incidence related to the Descemet membrane detachment has been reported up to 7.4%, and in most cases, it is related to excessive viscoelastic during its injection [9]. Alobeidan et al. reported an incidence of 6.7% in most external phacocanaloplasty procedure [1].

The Descemet detachment may occur during the viscoelastic abundant injection or when the microcatheter does not move to the exit continuously; thus viscoelastic may enter to the cornea at Schwalbe's line and blood may flow back from collector canals [10]. To reduce the risk of overexpanding the Schlemm canal during canaloplasty, two clicks must be injected per hour, always considering that there is a delay between the click and the viscoelastic flow in the catheter. It is

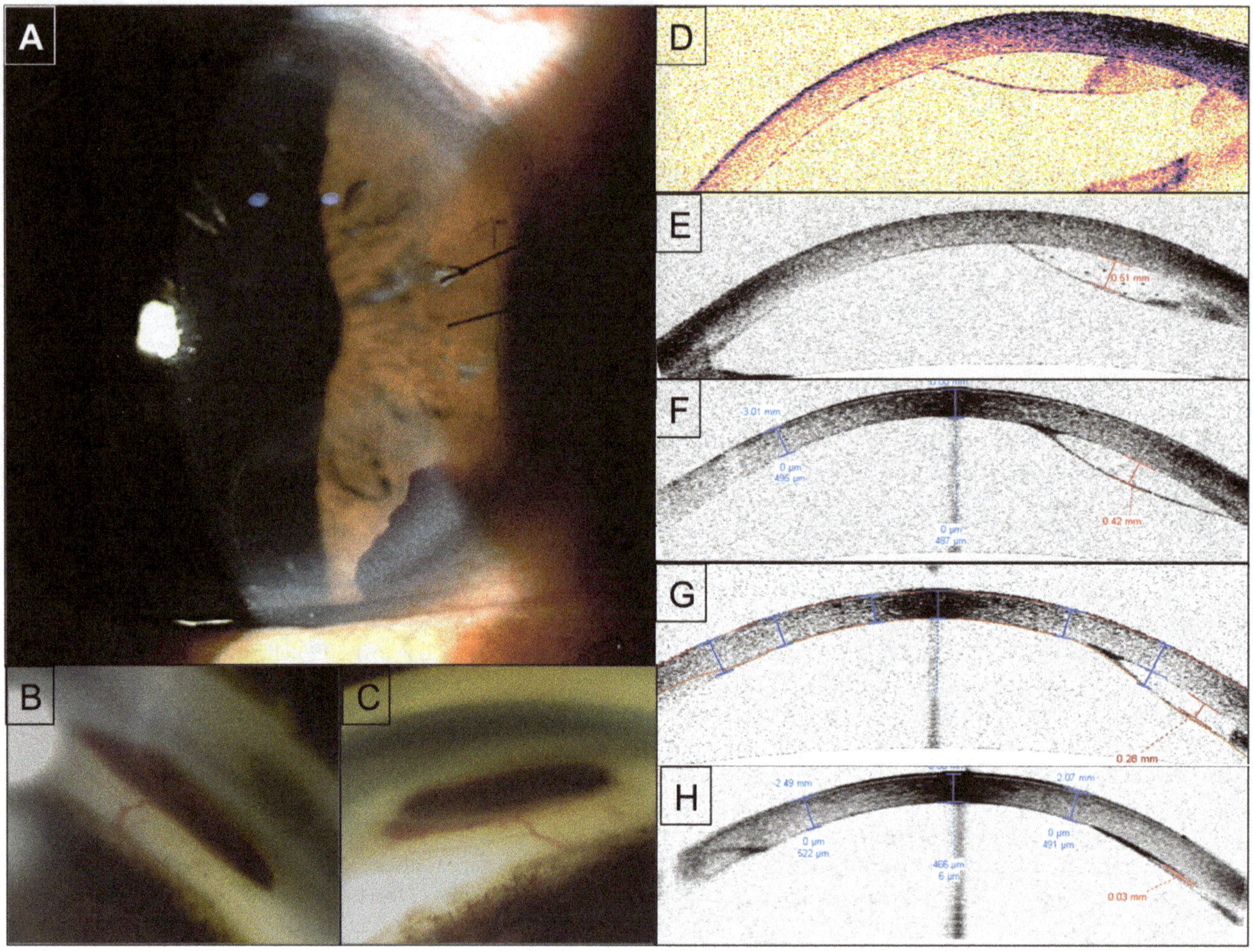

Figure 1: (A) First day after the surgery. Picture of the slit lamp showing a Descemet membrane detachment with partial intrastromal hemorrhage. (B) Gonioscopy evidencing Descemet detachment with intrastromal hemorrhage, 1st day after the surgery. (C) Gonioscopy evidencing Descemet detachment with intrastromal hemorrhage 1st month after the surgery with a reduction of the extent of the injury. (D) OCT of anterior segment (Visante, Model 1000, Carl Zeiss Meditec, *Dublin CA, USA), showing* intrastromal hemorrhage. (E) OCT Anterior Section, second week after the surgery (4 January 2018). (F) OCT Anterior Section, sixth week after the surgery (2 February 2018). (G) OCT Anterior Section, tenth week after the surgery (1 March 2018). (H) OCT Anterior Section, twelfth week after the surgery (19 March 2018).

important to hear the injector click [2]. Most of the reported Descemet membrane detachments [11] with intrastromal hemorrhage after ab externo canaloplasty were located in the inferonasal quadrant [1, 2, 5].

Jaramillo et al. [12] suggested performing surgery in this complication in case the hemorrhage is over 3mm and close to the visual axis, so based on previous experience and reported cases, we decided a conservative management despite the fact that there are reports where the spontaneous resolution may take from 6 months to 2.5 years [10, 13].

Lewis et al. presented a 2-year follow-up of patients after ab externo canaloplasty, finding a 30% decrease in IOP [12]. In our patient the complication did not alter the expected outcome of the procedure, because after three months about 30% IOP decrease was recorded with the same number of glaucoma medications. Interestingly according to a study no significant IOP lowering difference was found after ab externo and ab interno canaloplasty in a series of twelve patients who underwent ab interno in one eye and ab externo canaloplasty in the other eye [14].

The ab interno canaloplasty is effective and less traumatic than ab externo canaloplasty. It requires no two scleral flap dissections to expose Schlemm canal and Descemet window and no placement of tensioning suture, as in ab externo procedure, and allows the expansion of both Schlemm canal and collector canals. However, also in ab interno canaloplasty, maneuvers that could lead to the Descemet membrane detachment should be avoided [3]. Quite recently in a consecutive series of 20 ab interno canaloplasties one limited descemetolysis near the limbus by the viscoelastic during the dilation of Schlemm canal was reported [15]. In our case observation proved to be a wise decision regarding the hemorrhagic Descemet membrane detachment following ab interno canaloplasty. The expectant management is a feasible option when the extension and thickness of intrastromal hemorrhage are limited and do not involve the visual axis.

The Descemet detachment with intrastromal hemorrhage is a rare complication after ab externo canaloplasty. The non-conservative management options include partial thickness paracentesis [5], intracameral SF6 [1], and intracorneal blood with balanced saline solution following deep corneal incision and air bubble injection of the shallow anterior chamber [13].

Consent

The study was approved by the Institutional Review Board Statement. The patient consented to the publication of the case in writing. This report does not contain any personal information that could lead to the identification of the patient.

Disclosure

All authors attest that they meet the current ICMJE criteria for authorship.

Acknowledgments

Thanks are due to Jose Chauca and Carmen Maldonado for statistical analysis and technical support.

References

[1] S. A. Alobeidan and F. A. Almobarak, "Incidence and management of haemorrhagic Descemet membrane detachment in canaloplasty and phacocanaloplasty," *Acta Ophthalmologica*, vol. 94, no. 5, pp. e298–e304, 2016.

[2] L. M. Brandao, S. Orgul, and M. C. Grieshaber, "Hemorrhagic descemet membrane detachment after classic canaloplasty," *Klinische Monatsblätter für Augenheilkunde*, vol. 231, no. 4, pp. 348–350, 2014.

[3] M. A. Khaimi, "Canaloplasty: a minimally invasive and maximally effective glaucoma treatment," *Journal of Ophthalmology*, vol. 2015, Article ID 485065, 5 pages, 2015.

[4] T. Ichihashi, Y. Suzuki, M. Nagahara, and K. Kawai, "A case of open-angle glaucoma successfully treated using canaloplasty," *The Tokai Journal of Experimental and Clinical Medicine*, vol. 40, no. 4, pp. 157–160, 2015.

[5] M. Gismondi and P. Brusini, "Intracorneal hematoma after canaloplasty in glaucoma," *Cornea*, vol. 30, no. 6, pp. 718-719, 2011.

[6] B. A. Francis, H. Akil, and B. B. Bert, "Ab interno Schlemm's Canal Surgery," in *Glaucoma Surgery*, vol. 59, pp. 127–146, 2017.

[7] M. Hamid, P. Thompson, and P. Harasymowycz, "Novel treatment for hemorrhagic descemet detachment after canaloplasty," *Cornea*, vol. 34, no. 12, pp. 1611-1612, 2015.

[8] I. S. Yalvac, M. Sahin, U. Eksioglu, K. Budak, B. S. Aslan, and S. Duman, "Hemorrhagic Descemet's membrane detachment after viscocanalostomy," *Journal of Cataract & Refractive Surgery*, vol. 29, no. 7, pp. 1440–1442, 2003.

[9] A. Jaramillo, J. Foreman, and R. S. Ayyala, "Descemet membrane detachment after canaloplasty: incidence and management," *Journal of Glaucoma*, vol. 23, no. 6, pp. 351–354, 2014.

[10] H. Fujimoto, T. Mizoguchi, S. Kuroda, and M. Nagata, "Intracorneal hematoma with Descemet membrane detachment after viscocanalostomy," *American Journal of Ophthalmology*, vol. 137, no. 1, pp. 195-196, 2004.

[11] M. C. Grieshaber, "Viscocanalostomy and canaloplasty: ab externo schlemm's canal surgery," in *Glaucoma Surgery*, vol. 59, pp. 113–126, 2017.

[12] R. A. Lewis, K. von Wolff, M. Tetz et al., "Canaloplasty: circumferential viscodilation and tensioning of Schlemm's canal using a flexible microcatheter for the treatment of open-angle glaucoma in adults: interim clinical study analysis," *Journal of Cataract & Refractive Surgery*, vol. 33, no. 7, pp. 1217–1226, 2007.

[13] A. Rossetti, D. Doro, and N. Koerber, "Intracorneal blood removal six weeks after canaloplasty," *Indian Journal of Ophthalmology*, vol. 61, no. 5, p. 232, 2013.

[14] M. Gallardo, R. Supnet, and I. I. Ahmed, "Circumferential viscodilation of Schlemm's canal for open-angle glaucoma: ab-interno vs ab-externo canaloplasty with tensioning suture," *Clinical Ophthalmology*, vol. 12, pp. 2493–2498, 2018.

[15] N. Körber, "Ab interno canaloplasty for the treatment of glaucoma: a case series study," *Spektrum der Augenheilkunde*, vol. 32, no. 6, pp. 223–227, 2018.

4

Taenia solium in the Anterior Chamber: Surgical Management of a Rare Case of Live Free-Floating Parasite

Amrit Banstola,[1] Sweta Singh,[1] Sarita Maharjan,[1] Gyanendra Lamichhane,[1] and Anadi Khatri[2,3]

[1]*Lumbini Eye Institute and Research Center, Lumbini, Nepal*
[2]*Birat Eye Hospital, Biratnagar, Nepal*
[3]*Department of Ophthalmology, Birat Medical College and Teaching Hospital, Biratnagar, Nepal*

Correspondence should be addressed to Anadi Khatri; anadikc@gmail.com

Academic Editor: Alexander A. Bialasiewicz

Ocular cysticercosis is a preventable cause of blindness. It is a parasitic infestation caused by Cysticercus cellulosae—which is the larval form of Taenia solium. In 1829, Soemmering reported the first case of a live anterior chamber cysticercosis. In the following, we report a rare case of a 13-year-old male who presented with a live adult Taenia solium in the anterior chamber without any systemic features and its successful management.

1. Introduction

Ocular parasitosis continues to intrigue ophthalmologists with a variety of presentations [1]. They can remain obscure and continue to manifest as a "masquerade" until specifically searched for. Even when identified, it provides a challenge to the treating physician to decide on how to proceed further [2–4]. One of such similar parasitic infestations is cysticercosis.

Cysticercosis parasitic infection/infestation of human tissue is caused by the cystic form of the larvae of Taenia solium [5]. It gains entry into the human body via a faeco-oral route as a result of consumption of contaminated food/-water [6]. While adult worms are mainly responsible for inducing malnutrition and intestinal obstructions, the larvae (cysticerci) can produce more life-threatening conditions. It has the potential to invade muscles, subcutaneous tissues, and central nervous system and is in fact one of the major causes of adult-onset seizures in low-income countries [1, 5, 7, 8]. Eyes and adnexal structures such as eyelids, orbit, extraocular muscles, subconjunctival space, anterior chamber, vitreous, and subretinal space are affected in 13-46% of infected individuals [8]. Ocular manifestations can be devastating if the cysticercoses increase in size or die releasing toxic products leading to profound inflammatory reaction causing blindness in 3-5 years [9]. We here report an extremely rare case of a live adult Taenia solium in the anterior chamber and also discuss on how it was successfully managed.

2. Case Report

A 13-year-old boy presented with complaints of progressive diminution of vision associated with redness in the left eye for 9 days. The episode was not associated with pain and discharge. The patient denied seeing floaters or shadows. Otherwise healthy, the patient also denies history of trauma, similar history in the past, or use of any topical medication. He was a student by profession but occasionally helped in feeding the livestock of the family—which involved cows and buffalos. The patient gives no history of consumption of undercooked meat. The patient and his party also denied any history of abnormal body movement or seizure till date. The rest of the history was found to be insignificant. Visual acuity and intraocular pressure of the affected eye were hand movements close to face and 21 mmHg, respectively. The findings of the unaffected eye were found to be normal.

On slit-lamp examination, the conjunctiva was found to be congested with circumciliary congestion and hazy cornea (Figure 1). On evaluation of the anterior chamber, exudative infiltrates with the presence of a mobile and slender tubular worm-like intraocular foreign body were visible at 6 o'clock. The entity responded to increased intensity of the light from the slit lamp with increased mobility—episodic elongation and curling. Right eye examination was within normal limits.

Detail fundus examination could not be done due to hazy cornea and the presence of dense exudates in the anterior segment chamber. Ultrasonography (USG) of the left eye was done, and the posterior segment was found to be radiologically normal.

Routine blood counts with differential/absolute eosinophil counts were unremarkable. Stool examinations revealed no ova, cysts, or adult worm. USG of abdomen and pelvis were unremarkable. The patient was also advised for non-contrast-enhanced computerized tomography (NECT) of the head and orbit which yielded normal reports. The patient was planned for surgery to remove the worm via viscoexpulsion and parasitological examination.

2.1. Surgical Procedure and Postoperative Management. The patient was prepared for surgery under peribulbar anesthesia. After painting and draping, two 2.8 mm clear corneal incisions were made at 9 o'clock and at 2 o'clock positions (Figures 2(a)–2(c)). Pilocarpine nitrate 0.5% was injected into the anterior chamber (Figure 2(d)). This helps in constricting the pupil and is also a chemoparalyzing agent which can help in decreasing the movement of the worm [3, 10].

Once the worm was observed to be hypomobile, the anterior chamber was injected with viscoelastic surgical device (VSD) from the corneal port created at 2 o'clock to push the worm and the exudates away from the pupil (Figure 2(e)). The port at 9 o'clock was opened using angled plain forceps (Figure 2(f)). The worm was viscoexpulsed in toto using the no-touch technique. The worm was then transferred into a bottle containing normal saline and transferred to the microbiology and parasitology department for identification.

2.2. Postoperative Management and Follow-Up. The patient was started on oral prednisolone 1 mg/kg/day and also given a single dose of 400 mg albendazole. On the first postoperative day, the VA of the patient was still hand movement with intraocular pressure of 14 mmHg. The anterior chamber still had signs of inflammation while the posterior segment looked normal echogenically. The patient was started on topical moxifloxacin 0.5% and prednisolone acetate 1%—both 2 hourly—and tropicamide 1% thrice daily. He was advised to follow up in a week. At the first follow-up, the patient had best-corrected visual acuity of 6/36 and the anterior chamber inflammation had subsided. The patient was advised to continue the same medications with steroids being tapered on weekly basis. The patient was advised to follow up after 4 weeks. At the second follow-up, the patient presented with the best visual acuity of 6/18. Anterior segment examination revealed iris pigmentary patches over the pupillary axis secondary to medical synecholysis and anterior synechiae at 6 o'clock but without inflammation (Figure 3(a)). Due to media opacity, the posterior segment findings looked hazy but retinal and optic disc structures could be appreciated and appeared normal (Figure 3(b)). All his medications were stopped, and he was kept under regular follow-ups for observation.

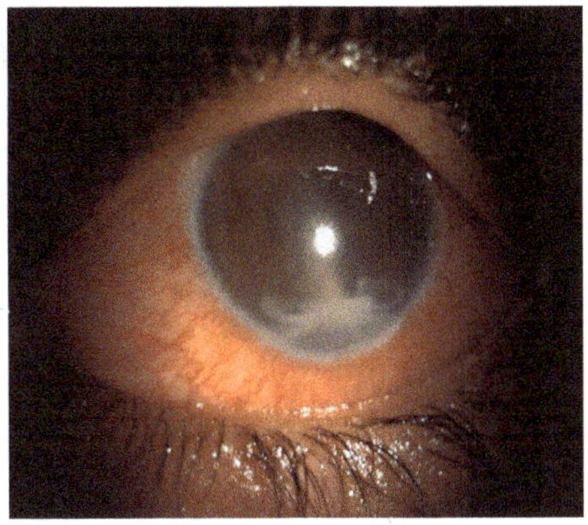

Figure 1: Clinical picture of the affected eye. Note the hazy cornea, circumciliary congestion, and the worm along with exudates in the inferior angle.

2.3. Microbiological and Parasitological Findings. On histopathological examination using hematoxylin and eosin stain, a translucent flexible worm measuring 11×1.5 mm was observed. There was presence of an outer refractile cuticle with reticular tissue. The subcuticular layer consisted of aggregated subcuticular cells, small myofiber bundles with scolex, two suckers, and birefringent four hooklets consistent with Taenia solium (Figure 4).

3. Discussion

Taeniasis, the condition caused by infection with adult worm, Taenia solium, is worldwide in distribution, but endemic in some parts of the world [7]. While taeniasis is rarely seen in those who do not eat pork, cysticercosis occurs in all ethnic groups regardless of dietary habits. In the normal life cycle of T. solium, man is the definitive host and pig is the intermediate host. Cysticercosis is known to involve ocular tissues—mainly intraocular structures (anterior and posterior segment) and extraocular tissues (extraocular muscles, orbit, subconjunctival space, eyelids, optic nerve, and lacrimal gland) [1]. Table 1 enlists the findings from the relevant existing literature regarding its manifestations in the eye when present in the anterior chamber.

Anterior chamber cysticercosis is an unusual presentation, and the occurrence of a live mobile parasite in the anterior chamber is a rarer occurrence. The route entry of the cyst in the anterior chamber is inconclusive so far, but it has been suspected to enter the anterior chamber from the

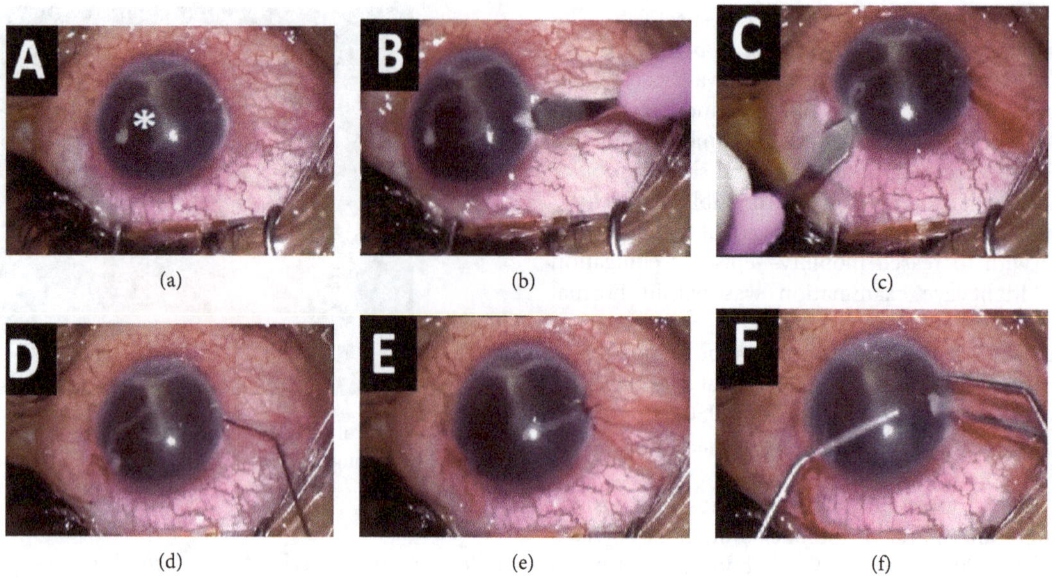

FIGURE 2: (a) Worm in the anterior chamber (marked with asterisk ∗). (b, c) Clear corneal incisions made at 9 and 2 o'clock. (d) Injecting pilocarpine 0.5% intracamerally. (e) Paralyzed worm which has coiled up. (f) Worm removed in toto with the use of a viscoelastic device from 2 o'clock port and expression from 9 o'clock port.

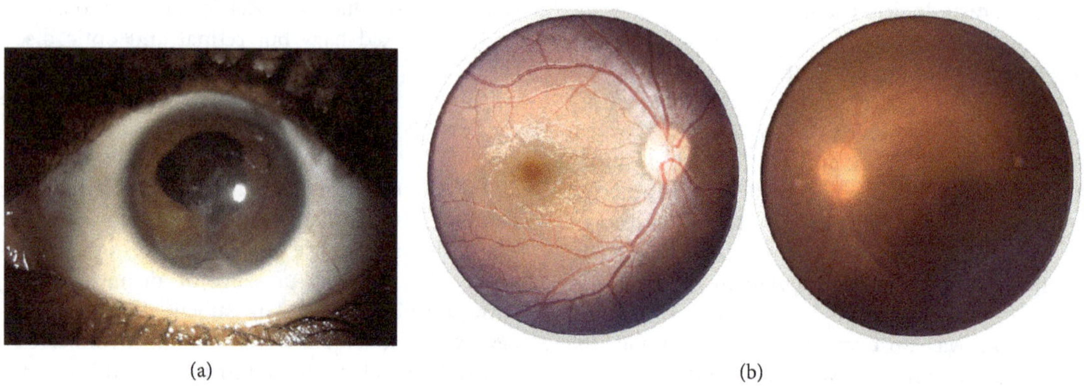

FIGURE 3: (a) Anterior segment photograph at 4th postoperative week. A large patch of iris pigment can be observed over the pupillary axis over the anterior capsule. Posterior synechia remained from 2 to 7 clock hours. Opacification of the anterior capsule was also present on the central region. Also, note an anterior synechia at 6 o'clock—where the worm was residing presurgically. (b) Fundus photo of the right eye (normal) and the left eye (affected) at 4th week of follow-up. No obvious vitreous or chorioretinal lesions were seen. Note the hazy fundus picture due to media opacity over the anterior lens capsule.

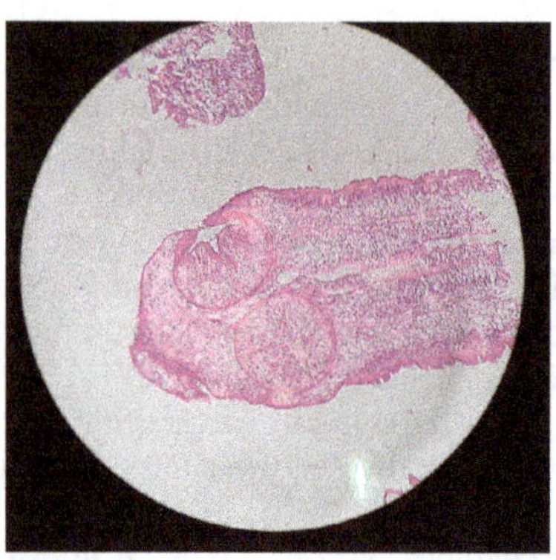

FIGURE 4: Microbiological assessment of the parasite. Note the refractile cuticle with reticular tissue. The subcuticular layer consisted of aggregated subcuticular cells, small myofiber bundles with scolex, two suckers, and birefringent four hooklets.

posterior segment through the pupil in aphakes, through vessels supplying the ciliary body, or through the anterior chamber angle. [17].

As with any other parasitic infestation in the ocular tissues, the inflammation is usually very intense. There may be pain and redness with associated iridocyclitis or glaucoma [16]. Glaucoma may be inflammatory in the presence of iridocyclitis or due to pupillary block caused by the cyst. Surgical management by removal of the parasite is the treatment of choice for all live cases. The most commonly adopted method is the "no-touch technique with viscoexpression" [2, 3, 18]. For a mobile worm, there is often a risk of migration to the posterior chamber via the pupil during the surgical procedure. Various chemoparalytic agents like pilocarpine and carbachols that also have miotic properties can be of great advantage in such cases [3, 10].

TABLE 1: Review of relevant published articles on anterior segment cysticercosis along with their common findings, management, and outcome.

Authors	Findings	Management	Outcome
Soemmerring et al. (1829) [11]	—	Surgical removal	—
Mathur (1962) [12]	Cystic form in anterior chamber, with scolex buried in the iris. Plastic iridocyclitis with hypopyon.	The cyst was removed from the anterior chamber by an ab extemo incision of the cornea from 2-5 o'clock.	Iridocyclitis cleared up early, and the patient's vision improved to 6/12 from counting of fingers at 1 meter.
Welsh and Proctor (1978) [13]	Anterior and intermediate uveitis with inferior exudate in the anterior chamber. Worm was observed within the exudate.	Removal via corneal incision and placement of curette. Oral and topical steroids.	Hypotonic eye with vascularization of the iris and the lens.
Das et al. (2002) [14]	Extension of taenia cellulosae into both ant and post segment of the eye.	Surgical management using viscoexpression and suturing of the corneal incision. Coverage with systemic steroids and albendazole.	6/12 at the time of presentation. 6/18 at the time of follow-up after the surgery.
Chandra et al. (2007) [15]	Cyst in the anterior chamber with occasional protrusion and retraction of the head/scolex by the organism.	Viscoexpression followed by topical steroid coverage.	6/36 at the time of presentation. No relatable complications at follow-ups after the surgery.
Mahendradas et al. (2007) [16]	Multiple cysts of T. cellulosae in the anterior chamber. Plastic uveitis with ocular hypertension.	Viscoexpression followed by treatment with topical antibiotics, steroids, and antiocular hypertensive agents.	6/12 at the time of presentation. 6/6 after treatment.

However, it must be noted that parasites, if dead, may not elicit any inflammation [4]. Such cases have been reported to be well managed simply by observation. It may be advisable to approach such cases as per surgeons' preference. In case of a decision for surgical removal, care must be taken not to disrupt the capsule or the outer coating of these worms which may lead to anaphylaxis-like reaction.

It is of utmost importance that we enlist the possibility of intraocular parasites and specially cysticercosis as a case presenting with atypical uveitis. The clinical suspicion and diagnosis of live intraocular cysticercosis are based on the morphology of the parasite and hence removal in toto followed by proper storage, transportation, and microbiological examination which remains critical for correct diagnosis [6].

For every intraocular parasitosis, systemic treatment with antihelminthic and steroids is often always recommended. But more importantly, systemic manifestations must always be ruled out. Stool examination, high-resolution ultrasonography (USG), computed tomography (CT), and magnetic resonance imaging (MRI) can help in the identification and management of such cases [19].

4. Conclusion

Surgical removal of the live parasite is the mainstay of treatment. Medical therapy is recommended for a duration of at least 1 month with albendazole and steroids given the complexity of route of migration for the organism to reach the eye. A high level of suspicion for probable involvement of other systemic tissues, such as the central nervous system, must always be considered, and systemic treatment is considered to alleviate the benefit of doubt.

References

[1] C. S. Ament and L. H. Young, "Ocular manifestations of helminthic infections: onchocersiasis, cysticercosis, toxocariasis, and diffuse unilateral subacute neuroretinitis," *International Ophthalmology Clinics*, vol. 46, no. 2, pp. 1–10, 2006.

[2] A. Khatri and B. K. Khatri, "Live Ascaris in anterior chamber causing hypertensive uveitis," *International Journal of Case Reports and Images*, vol. 8, no. 5, p. 390, 2017.

[3] A. Khatri, B. Khatri, and S. Singh, "Surgical management of live intraocular parasite in the anterior chamber," *Nepalese Journal of Ophthalmology*, vol. 10, no. 2, pp. 203–205, 2019.

[4] R. Sah, A. Khatri, R. Kharel et al., "Case report: management of dead intraocular helminth parasites in asymptomatic patients," *The American Journal of Tropical Medicine and Hygiene*, vol. 103, no. 2, pp. 719–722, 2020.

[5] H. H. Garcia, A. E. Gonzalez, C. A. W. Evans, and R. H. Gilman, "_Taenia solium_ cysticercosis," *The Lancet*, vol. 362, no. 9383, pp. 547–556, 2003.

[6] O. H. Del Brutto, J. Sotelo, and G. Roman, *Neurocysticercosis: A Clinical Handbook*, Swets & Zeitlinger, Lisse, The Netherlands, 1998.

[7] L. Zammarchi, M. Strohmeyer, F. Bartalesi et al., "Epidemiology and management of cysticercosis and Taenia solium taeniasis in Europe, systematic review 1990-2011," *PLoS One*, vol. 8, no. 7, article e69537, 2013.

[8] R. Dhiman, S. Devi, K. Duraipandi et al., "Cysticercosis of the eye," *International Journal of Ophthalmology*, vol. 10, no. 8, pp. 1319–1324, 2017.

[9] S. J. Ryan, *Helmnthic Disease*5th edition, ch. 86,v. 2.

[10] D. K. Mehta, R. Arora, D. Chauhan, D. Shroff, and R. Narula, "Chemo-paralysis for the removal of a live intraocular worm in ocular angiostrongyliasis," *Clinical & Experimental Ophthalmology*, vol. 34, no. 5, pp. 493–495, 2006.

[11] S. Duke-Elder and E. S. Perkins, "System of Ophthalmology, Vol. IX, Diseases of the Uveal Tract," Henry Kimpton, London, 1966.

[12] R. N. Mathur, "Cysticercosis of the eye," *Archives of Ophthalmology*, vol. 67, no. 5, p. 562, 1962.

[13] N. H. Welsh and E. M. Proctor, "Taenia solium in the anterior chamber," *Australian Journal of Opthalmology*, vol. 6, no. 2, pp. 73–76, 1978.

[14] J. C. Das, Z. Chaudhuri, R. L. Bansal, S. Bhomaj, P. Sharma, and D. Chauhan, "Viscoexpression of anterior chamber cysticercus cellulosae," *Indian Journal of Ophthalmology*, vol. 50, pp. 133–135, 2002.

[15] A. Chandra, M. K. Singh, V. P. Singh, A. K. Rai, S. Chakraborty, and O. P. S. Maurya, "A live cysticercosis in anterior chamber leading to glaucoma secondary to pupilary block," *Journal of Glaucoma*, vol. 16, no. 2, pp. 271–273, 2007.

[16] P. Mahendradas, J. Biswas, and V. Khetan, "Fibrinous anterior uveitis due to cysticercus cellulosae," *Ocular Immunology and Inflammation*, vol. 15, no. 6, pp. 451–454, 2007.

[17] N. Pushker, M. S. Bajaj, M. Chandra, and Neena, "Ocular and orbital cysticercosis," *Acta Ophthalmologica Scandinavica*, vol. 79, no. 4, pp. 408–413, 2001.

[18] N. Venugopal, G. Kummararaj, S. Kummararaj, and B. Bharathi, "Chemoparalysis for removal of anterior chamber motile parasite," *Indian Journal of Ophthalmology*, vol. 62, no. 5, pp. 661–661, 2014.

[19] A. R. Nimir, A. Saliem, and I. A. Ibrahim, "Ophthalmic parasitosis: a review article," *Interdisciplinary Perspectives on Infectious Diseases*, vol. 2012, Article ID 587402, 12 pages, 2012.

5

The New Face of the Switch Flap in the Reconstruction of a Large Upper Eyelid Defect

Biljana Kuzmanović Elabjer[1,2,3] **Mladen Bušić**[1,2,3] **Daliborka Miletić**[1,2,3] **Andrej Pleše**[1,2,3] **and Mirjana Bjeloš**[1,2,3]

[1]*Faculty of Dental Medicine and Health Care Osijek, University Josip Juraj Strossmayer in Osijek, Croatia*
[2]*Faculty of Medicine Osijek, University Josip Juraj Strossmayer in Osijek, Croatia*
[3]*University Eye Clinic-WHO Collaborating Center, University Hospital "Sveti Duh", Zagreb, Croatia*

Correspondence should be addressed to Daliborka Miletić; dada.miletic@gmail.com

Academic Editor: Cristiano Giusti

Reconstruction of a large defect after the removal of a massive malignant upper lid tumor is still a challenge in oculoplastic surgery. Our method of choice is Mustardé switch flap. Due to the lack of Mohs micrographic surgery and frozen section technique as well as waiting time of two weeks for histopathological results, we made modifications enabling us to reexcise in case of positive margins: the width of the pedicle of the flap was 7 mm allowing the length of the flap to be increased if needed, the lids were closed with temporary lateral tarsorrhaphy to protect the eye, and the lower lid is finally reconstructed in the second stage of the procedure. In three patients with malignant upper lid tumors, this method of reconstruction proved to be safe and effective with favorable long-term results.

1. Introduction

Mustardé switch flap for the upper lid defects, described in 1971, is still a state-of-the-art technique for achieving upper lid architecture, curve, eyelashes, and function, all in one [1, 2]. The major advantage to the other two-stage lid-sharing technique (Cutler-Beard procedure) is that the flap is divided in just two weeks as recommended by the author himself or as soon as seven days [1, 3]. The donor site of the lower lid is reconstructed either during the primary or secondary procedure [2–5]. Mohs micrographic surgery is unavailable in our institution, and histopathological results are obtained as late as two weeks. The upper lid defects are closed with Mustardé switch flap combined with temporary tarsorrhaphy and without any additional reconstruction until the histopathological report of either clear or infiltrating edges indicates further procedures. Thus, the final reconstruction of the upper and the lower eyelid is executed in the second stage of the procedure.

We present three patients with extensive upper lid tumors, reconstructed with our modified Mustardé switch flap achieving satisfactory functional and cosmetic results.

2. Case Presentation

2.1. Case No. 1. A 53-year-old male patient was referred to our Oculoplastic Unit for a large tumor involving the lateral half of the right upper lid (Figure 1(a)).

The procedure was performed under local anesthesia. According to the guidelines for well-defined lid tumors of our clinic and the literature [6], the tumor was removed with two millimeters of safety margins, creating a larger than half but not more than three-quarters full-thickness defect of the upper lid (Figure 1(b)). The flap with a nasally oriented vascular pedicle, 7 mm high, and half the length of the lower lid was turned up into the upper lid and hinged at the medial edge of the defect with 6/0 absorbable sutures and one 7/0 nylon suture for the grey line [7]. The aponeurosis of the levator muscle was sutured at the upper border of the flipped

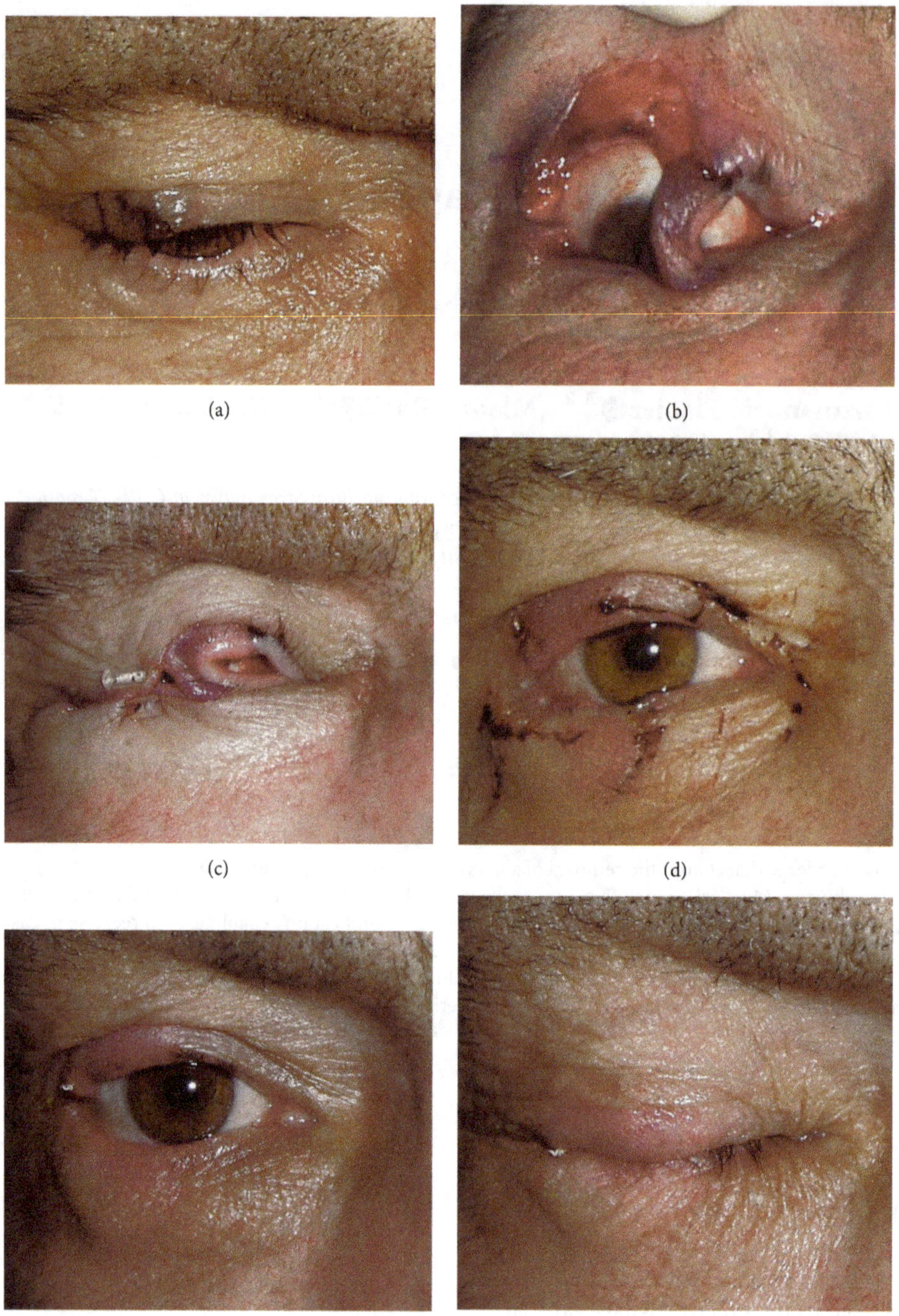

FIGURE 1: (a) A large nodular tumor with telangiectatic surface vessels involving the lateral half of the right upper lid. (b) The flap with a nasally oriented vascular pedicle. (c) The bolster of the lateral temporary tarsorrhaphy in place. (d) The reconstruction of the lower lid at the second stage of the procedure. (e) A satisfactory cosmetic appearance of both lids. (f) The full lid closure.

tarsal plate. Laterally, the lids were closed with temporary tarsorrhaphy (Figure 1(c)). After marking the adequate size of the tarsorrhaphy, a 6-0 single prolene suture was passed through the lids in a horizontal mattress fashion, 4 mm from the lid margin through the skin and muscle staying above the tarsal plate and through the grey line. To protect the skin, we used a bolster made of a vitrectomy cutter tube. The margins of the excised tumor were marked with different vital dyes before it was sent to histopathology. The second stage of the procedure was done two weeks after histopathological confirmation of a basal cell carcinoma with clear margins. The vascular pedicle was divided, and the lower lid was reconstructed using a tarso-conjunctival graft from the contralateral upper lid and a local advancement skin-muscle flap (Figure 1(d)) [8]. Good function and satisfactory cosmetic appearance of both lids were achieved (Figures 1(e) and 1(f)).

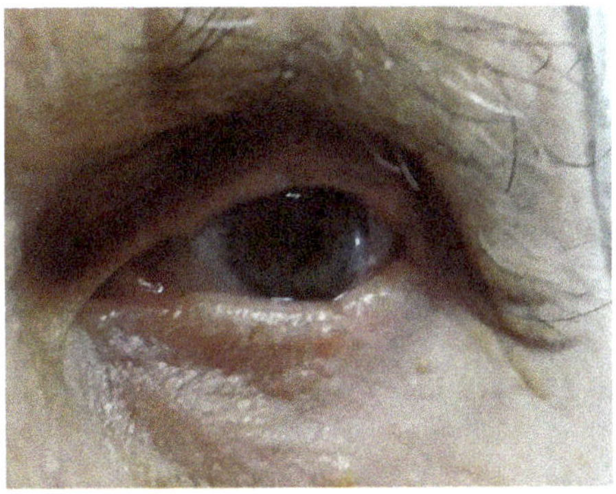

FIGURE 2: Clinical outcome 6 months after the surgery in Case No. 2.

2.2. Case No. 2. Years-long history of a recurrent chalazion in the 70-year-old male patient with a lobular lesion involving one-quarter of the left upper lid were the reasons for the referral to our clinic. Due to the clinical aspect of the tumor suspicious of sebaceous cell carcinoma, the surgical excision included four-millimeter safety margins [9]. The primary surgery was performed in the same manner as in Case No. 1. Unfortunately, the sebaceous cell carcinoma was confirmed on histopathology 10 days after the surgery, with the tumor cells found at the medial edge, that is, the hinge side. Immediately, additional resection was carried out. The lids were divided as well as the hinge of the flap, and three millimeters of tissue at the medial edge of the primary defect was excised. The length of the flap was increased accordingly and sutured in the same fashion as in the primary surgery. The secondary surgery ended up with yet another temporary lateral tarsorrhaphy. Only when the excised tissue from the second surgery came free of the tumor after 9 days, the flap was divided, and the reconstruction of the lids was carried out and resulted in satisfactory function and cosmesis (Figure 2).

2.3. Case No. 3. An 80-year-old male patient presented with an ulcerated tumor of the lateral half of the upper lid (Figure 3(a)). The tumor removal and the first stage of reconstruction were conducted the same as in Case 1, except for setting the pedicle at the lateral end of the flap (Figure 3(b)).

After ten days, the histopathology proved squamous cell carcinoma with the margins free of the tumor, and the pedicle was divided. Lateral canthotomy and direct closure were sufficient for the lower lid reconstruction.

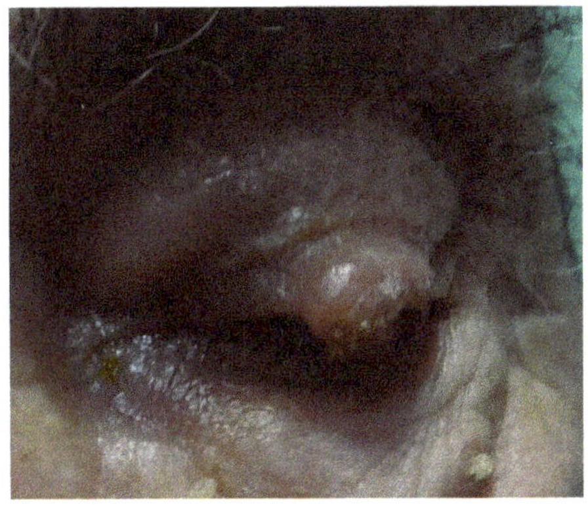

(a)

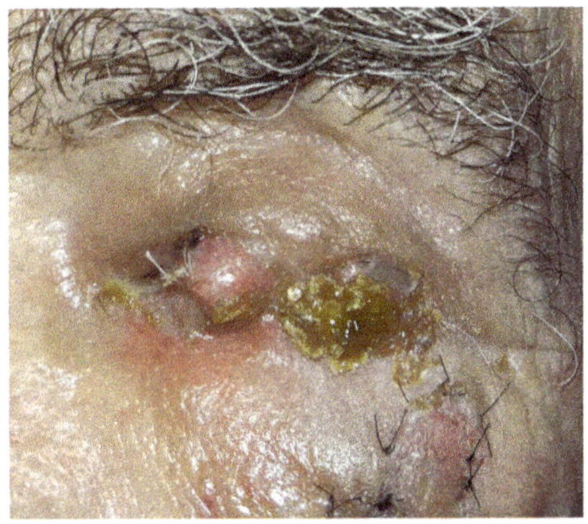

(b)

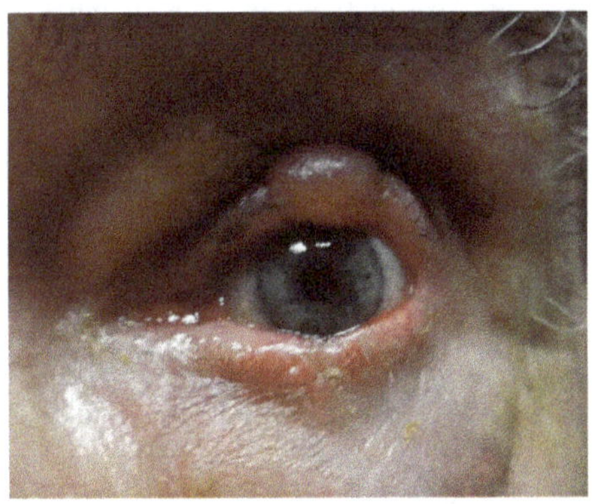

(c)

FIGURE 3: (a) An ulcerated tumor of the lateral half of the upper lid. Note the keratotic plaque at the right bottom of the photo. (b) The flap just before the pedicle separation. The nylon sutures of the modified rhomboid flap used for the reconstruction after the keratosis removal still in place. (c) A prolonged Mustardé switch flap edema.

3. Discussion

Defects of the upper lid after excision of a malignant tumor, without the possibility of Mohs micrographic surgery, require creativity in combining the tissue to cover the eye and to still keep an open possibility to re-excise the edges in up to two weeks postoperatively. Our modification of the Mustardé switch flap enables exactly that the eye is covered and protected, and the lids are not primarily reconstructed so that the flap can be enlarged if needed. The length of the flap may be increased due to the width of the pedicle of the flap being 7 mm, that is, larger than originally recommended 6 mm for large defects [1]. Following the rule of Tyers and Collin, in a large medial remnant of the lid, the pedicle was sited medially; otherwise, it was hinged at the lateral edge of the flap [10]. The only issue we had with the traditional Mustardé switch flap was the risk of histopathological confirmation of the residual tumor and the necessity to cut out the pedicle of the flap. That was the scenario of our Case No. 2: we needed to start the flap all over again. In our opinion, the 7 mm-width-pedicle of the flap enables adjustments of the flap length and buys the time to wait for clear edges. Complications in healing after the lower lid reconstruction were not encountered even three weeks after the primary flap creation. Temporary lateral tarsorrhaphy was used to prevent corneal exposure for up to two weeks before the pedicle was cut. We used our modification of Collin's technique [7]: there was no incision of the grey line nor excision of the conjunctiva from the lid margin posterior to the grey line. This was particularly important in our modification of the Mustardé switch flap because after the tarsorrhaphy was undone the lids were easily separated with undamaged lid margin. Nevertheless, the lids were tightly closed for the period of the flap healing that lasted up to 19 days in our patients without any corneal problems.

The only complication we experienced was a prolonged Mustardé switch flap edema in Case No. 3 (Figure 3(c)) that resolved in four weeks. Mustardé emphasized that it may take several weeks for the eyelid swelling to subside following the flap [1]. The technique involves intense modification in the eyelid tissue's direction, with rotation from inferior to the superior eyelid, disfavoring lymphatic drainage. As oppose to the other two patients, Case No. 3 had the pedicle hinged at the lateral end of the flap where the outer canthus branch of a lymph-collecting vessel could have been surgically altered.

In his paper describing the switch flap in the treatment of malignant tumors of the upper lid, Mustardé always reconstructed the lower lid in the primary stage of the procedure [1]. Our modification thus opens the possibility of increasing the size of the Mustardé switch flap in case of need for additional excision following the findings on the histopathologic specimen. This serves well in settings where neither Mohs micrographic surgery nor frozen section is available and if histopathological results are not feasible in time.

References

[1] J. C. Mustardé, "Surgical treatment of malignant tumours of the upper lid," *Chirurgia Plastica*, vol. 1, no. 1, pp. 25–33, 1971.

[2] J. C. Mustardé, "Major reconstruction of the eyelids: functional and aesthetic considerations," *Clinics in Plastic Surgery*, vol. 8, no. 2, pp. 227–236, 1981.

[3] T. Uemura, T. Yanai, M. Yasuta, H. Kawano, Y. Ishihara, and M. Kikuchi, "Switch flap for upper eyelid reconstruction-how soon should the flap be divided?," *Plastic and Reconstructive Surgery. Global Open*, vol. 4, no. 4, article e695, 2016.

[4] K. Yamashita, T. Yotsuyanagi, A. Sugai et al., "Full-thickness total upper eyelid reconstruction with a lid switch flap and a reverse superficial temporal artery flap," *Journal of Plastic, Reconstructive & Aesthetic Surgery*, vol. 73, no. 7, pp. 1312–1317, 2020.

[5] S. N. Stafanous, "The switch flap in eyelid reconstruction," *Orbit*, vol. 26, no. 4, pp. 255–262, 2007.

[6] S. J. Quazi, N. Aslam, H. Saleem, J. Rahman, and S. Khan, "Surgical margin of excision in basal cell carcinoma: a systematic review of literature: A Systematic Review of Literature," *Cureus*, vol. 12, no. 7, p. e9211, 2020.

[7] J. R. O. Collin, *A Manual of Systematic Eyelid Surgery*, Churchill Livingstone, Edinburgh London Melbourne and New York, 2nd edition edition, 1989.

[8] B. Kuzmanović Elabjer, J. Petrinović-Dorešić, M. Bušić, E. Elabjer, and S. Kaštelan, "Retrospective analysis of reconstruction techniques after periocular basalioma excision," *Collegium Antropologicum*, vol. 31, Suppl. 1, pp. 91–96, 2007.

[9] T. Yunoki, Y. Nakamura, C. Fuchizawa, and A. Hayashi, "Reconstructive surgery of the upper eyelid using the residual tarsus after excision of sebaceous gland carcinoma," *Case Reports in Ophthalmology*, vol. 7, pp. 586–592, 2017.

[10] A. G. Tyers and J. R. O. Collin, *Colour Atlas of Ophthalmic Plastic Surgery*, Elsevier Butterworth Heinemann, 2nd ed. edition, 2001.

6

Rhino-Orbito-Cerebral Mucormycosis: Two Cases with Amaurosis as Presentation, Medical Surgical Management and Follow-Up

Carmen Navarro-Perea [1], Ignacio Cañas-Zamarra,[1] Enrique Mencía-Gutiérrez,[1] Enrique Revilla-Sánchez,[2] María-Dolores Lago-Llinás,[1] Silvia Pérez-Trigo,[1] and Álvaro Bengoa-González[1]

[1]*Ophthalmology Department, 12 de Octubre Hospital, Complutense University, 28041 Madrid, Spain*
[2]*Pathology Department, 12 de Octubre Hospital, Complutense University, 28041 Madrid, Spain*

Correspondence should be addressed to Carmen Navarro-Perea; carmennavarroperea@gmail.com

Academic Editor: Alexander A. Bialasiewicz

Purpose: Mucormycosis is an infection caused by fungi to the class Zygomycetes that usually appears in immunosuppressed patients. Diagnostic confirmation is often delayed, with fatal prognosis in cases in which treatment is not rapidly established. *Case report:* We present two clinical cases of rhino-orbito-cerebral mucormycosis with an atypical presentation form, consisting of a unilateral complete sudden vision loss. Intravenous treatment with liposomal amphotericin B was started and total orbital exenteration surgery was performed. The removed surgical area was filled with gauze impregnated with liposomal amphotericin B and was left open for cures every 12 hours. Due to the good clinical evolution, a reconstruction of the orbital exenteration defect was performed in Case 1 with a temporal muscle flap and a skin island pedicled flap. In Case 2, reconstruction was not performed due to the poor evolution of the patient. *Discussion:* As it is a very aggressive surgery, the aesthetic and functional sequelae are very important. When the survival of the patient is achieved, we should offer reconstructive solutions that improve their quality of life. The reconstruction carried out using a flap of the temporal muscle can be made in a single act without requiring microvascular surgery.

1. Introduction

Mucormycosis is an opportunistic and severe infection caused by fungi of the order of Mucormycetes and class Mucorales that usually appears in immunosuppressed patients. The most common agents of mucormycosis are Rhizopus spp., Mucor spp. and Lichtheimia (formerly Absidia and Mycocladus) spp. Genera of other Mucorales, such as Rhizomucor, Sakseanea, Cunninghamell, and Apophysomyces, are less common [1, 2]. It is infrequent, although it is difficult to know its exact incidence because it is not a notifiable disease. However, the current trend reveals an increase in the incidence of fungal infections. Mucormycosis is the third most common fungal infection after those produced by *Candida* spp. and *Aspergillus* spp. [3]. The most commonly associated comorbidities include: diabetes mellitus, hematologic processes (hematologic malignancies, severe neutropenia, graft-versus-host disease, hematopoietic stem cell transplantation), solid organ transplant, injection drug use, malnutrition, treatment with corticosteroids, burns, severe traumatisms and renal failure [4]. Mucormycosis is classified in six categories: rhino-orbito-cerebral (ROC), pulmonary, cutaneous, gastrointestinal, disseminated and other unusual presentations as [5], with ROC being the presentation in 40% of the cases [6]. A new category has recently been described: isolated renal mucormycosis, but it is rare and has been described mainly in developing countries like India and China. It is rarer still to find this entity in immunocompetent young males without any risk factors [7].

Diagnosis of mucormycosis is based on the identification of the microorganisms in the pathological study with a microbiological culture (although it is usual to find no growth). The endoscopic evaluation of the sinuses with presence of necrosis, incisional biopsy and radiological image are very important for diagnosis. Diagnostic confirmation is often delayed, an important fact considering the fatal prognosis in the cases in which treatment is not rapidly established [3].

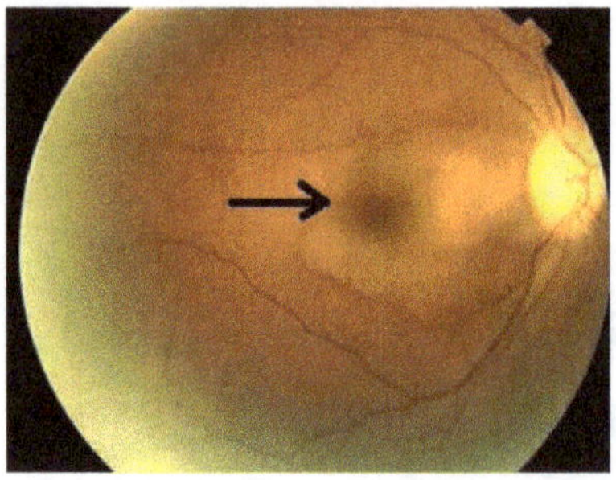

FIGURE 1: Case 1, fundus photography showed obstruction of the central artery of the retina (cherry red spot (arrow)) and posterior pole edema affecting right eye.

We present two clinical cases of ROC mucormycosis with an atypical presentation form, consisting of a unilateral sudden vision loss. In a review of the literature we have found only one case with a similar presentation [8].

2. Case 1

A 50-year-old female, with a renal transplantation the previous year due to chronic renal failure of unknown etiology, arrives at Emergency due to a sudden loss of vision in the right eye (RE) and a right hemicranial headache focused in the temporal area. In the ophthalmological assessment visual acuity of the RE was nonperception of light (NPL); in the fundus there was macular and posterior pole edema with cherry red spot, and reduction of the vascular caliber with sharp arteries and segmentation of blood flow (Figure 1). In the analytical study we observed a slightly increased erythrocyte sedimentation rate and normal C-reactive protein. A computed tomography (CT) was requested in which a partial occupation of right ethmoidal cells and right sphenoid sinus was observed (Figure 2). Nasofibroscopy was normal despite the CT findings. The initial diagnosis was a central retinal artery obstruction. The patient was reassessed 24 hours later due to the lack of any clinical improvement. A magnetic resonance (MR) was performed, which showed right ethmoid and sphenoid occupation with increased density compared to the previous CT, but with no signs of invasion (Figures 3(a) and 3(b)). A new nasofibroscopy demonstrated necrosis of the middle turbinates with purulent discharge, necrosis and sloughing in the uncinate process and in the right middle meatus and on the inferior turbinates. Samples were taken for bacterial and fungal culture and for direct examination and Gram stain, as well as for pathological study. In the direct examination structures of a nonseptate filamentous fungus were observed, compatible with mucormycosis.

Given these findings, intravenous (iv) treatment with liposomal amphotericin B was started at 5 mg/kg dose, anidulafungin and meropenem 1 g/8 h. Urgent surgery was performed for exeresis of the affected tissues; it consisted of: medium meatotomy, uncinectomy, ethmoidal bulla resection, anterior and posterior sphenoid sinus with necrotic and friable mucosa, resection of papyracea lamina mucosa, middle turbinate resection, transnasal sphenoidectomy and inferior turbinate resection. All the tissues were sent for microbiological and pathological study. Suspecting ROC mucormycosis, total orbital exenteration was performed, including the skin of the eyelids, in which necrosis of the medial wall and orbital floor was found, so a broad debridement was performed (Figures 4(a)–4(d)).

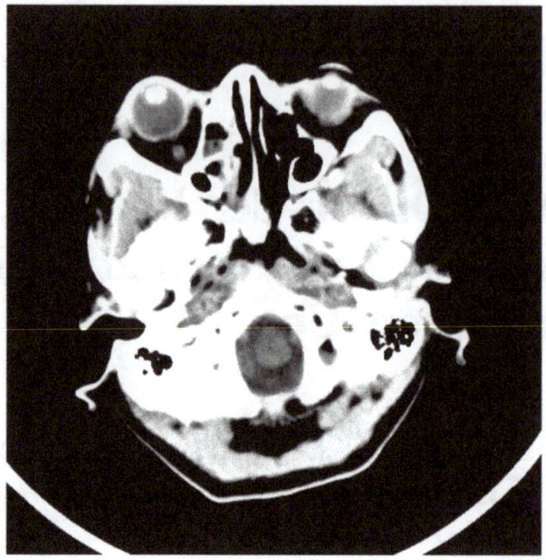

FIGURE 2: Case 1, computed tomography (CT) with partial occupation of right ethmoidal cells and right sphenoid sinus.

The removed surgical area was filled with gauze impregnated with liposomal amphotericin B and the wound was left open for cures (replacement of gauzes) and exploration every 12 hours. The Nephrology service modified the treatment in order to reverse the immunosuppression to which she was subjected due to the kidney transplant: the administration of mycophenolate was suspended and the dose of tacrolimus was reduced until reaching an objective level of 5 mg/ml. On the fourth postoperative day, necrotic tissue in the roof of the orbit and upper area of choana was debrided. One week after the surgery, due to the good evolution, the cures were scheduled every 24 hours. Pathological examination showed abundant wide mycelia (arrow), nonseptate, some of them partitioned, that were arranged angiocentrically, destroying and invading the vascular walls. There were fungal microabscesses with necrotic center in periphery (asterisk) (Figures 5(a) and 5(b)). The culture confirmed *Rhizopus oryzae*. At the first postoperative month, thanks to the recovery of immunosuppression of the patient and the good clinical evolution, the reconstruction of the orbital exenteration defect was performed with a temporal muscle flap and a skin island pedicled flap, and a titanium mesh implant in medial and lower region (Figures 6(a)–6(d) and 7(a)–7(d)). Postoperative images two weeks after the reconstruction (Figures 8(a) and 8(b)) and after 6 months (Figures 9(a) and 9(b)) are shown.

Two years later, there are still no signs of infection or necrosis, and the reconstructed area looks alright.

3. Case 2

A 54-year-old female with diabetes mellitus type 2, arterial hypertension and chronic pancreatitis presented at Emergency

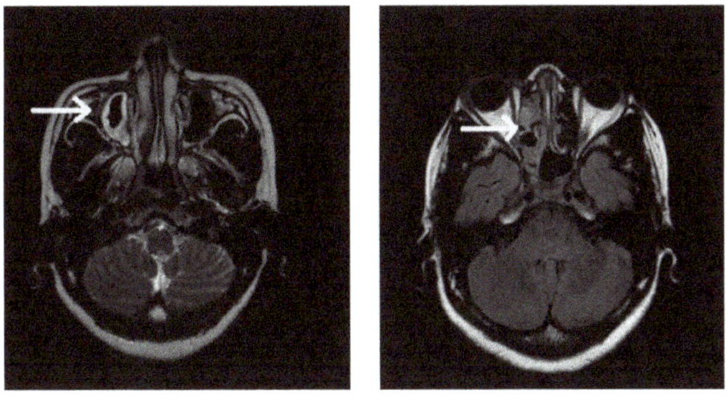

(a) (b)

FIGURE 3: Case 1, magnetic resonance with right ethmoid and sphenoid occupation with increased compared to previous CT (Figure 2).

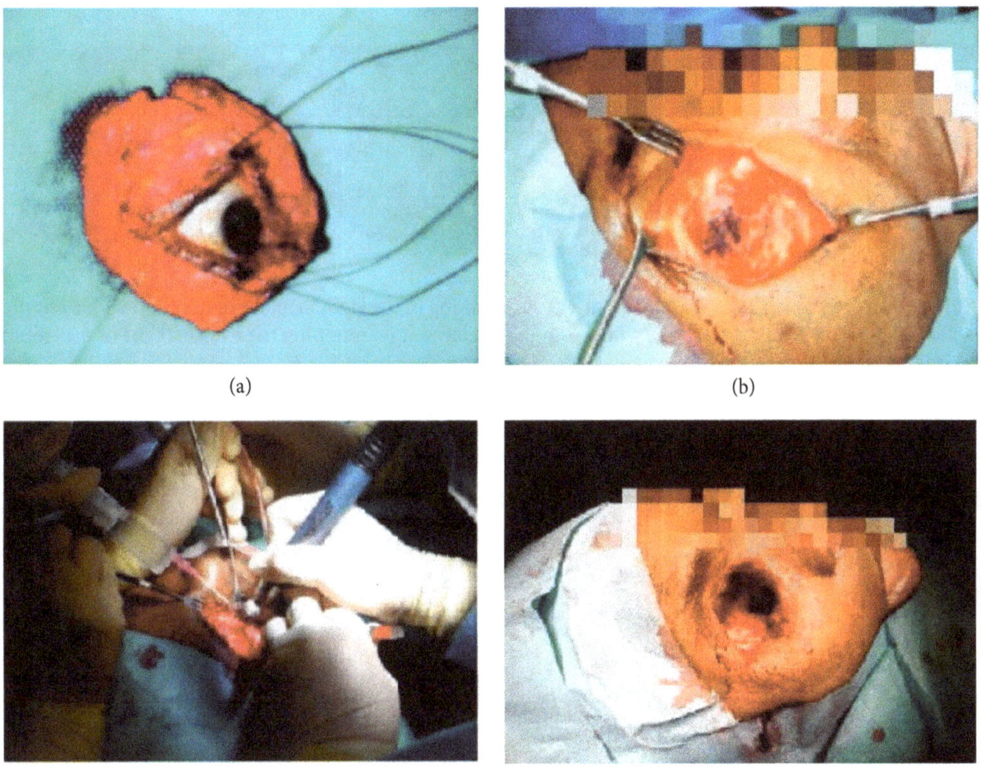

(a) (b) (c) (d)

FIGURE 4: Case 1 (a) urgent surgical intervention with total exenteration of the right orbit (b) (c) (d) orbital cavity exenteration what the surgical bed shows.

due to unilateral loss of vision of the RE. In the ophthalmological examination, visual acuity was NPL. Six hours later there were palpebral ptosis and a complete oculomotor paralysis of the RE. Those signs had not been present in the first examination.

An orbital CT showed right orbital cellulitis, with limited frontoethmoidal occupation and optic ischemic neuritis (apex orbitary syndrome (AOS)). Antibiotic treatment was started with no response. 24 hours later, endoscopic nasosinusal surgery was performed and signs of nasal mycosis were found. Given the poorly controlled diabetes mellitus, a fungal orbital cellulitis was suspected, and an MR was performed 48 hours after the beginning of the symptoms; there was a strong suspicion of invasive fungal sinusitis with orbital involvement. Samples of hard palate were taken and sent to microbiology and histopathology study, reaching the diagnosis of mucormycosis by direct examination with the presence of wide nonseptate mycelia. Immediate intravenous treatment was established, following the same pattern as in the previous case, and total orbital exenteration with maxillectomy was performed (Figures 10(a) and 10(b)), keeping part of the orbital floor, complete ethmoidectomy and sphenoidectomy with opening of lateral recess, frontal sinus opening by external approach and resection of hard hemipaladar. The removed surgical area was washed with liposomal amphotericin B and filled with gauze impregnated with it, and the surgical wound

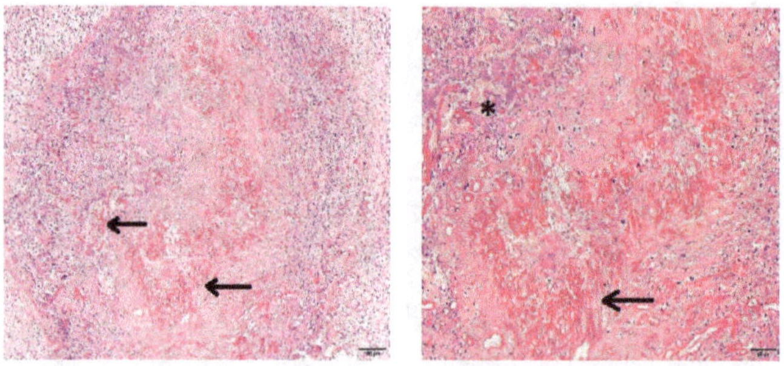

(a) (b)

FIGURE 5: Case 1 pathological study (a) and (b), pathological examination showed abundant wide mycelia (arrow), nonseptate, some of them partitioned, that were arranged angiocentrically, destroying and invading the vascular walls. (a) Hematoxylin&Eosin stain, original magnification × 10, 100 μm scale lower right. (b) Hematoxylin&Eosin stain, original magnification × 20, 50 μm scale lower right. There were fungal microabscesses with necrotic center in periphery (b) (asterisk).

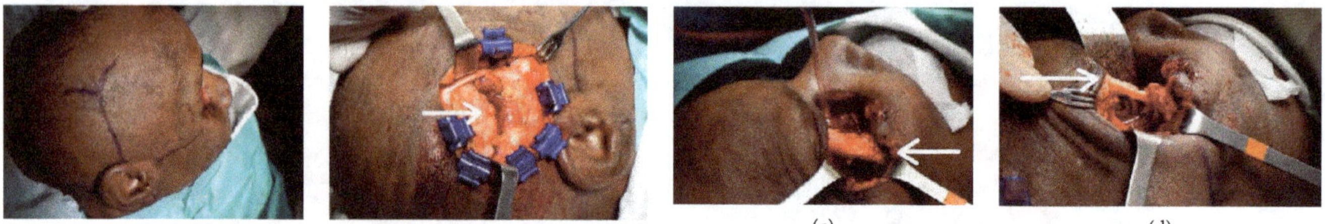

(a) (b) (c) (d)

FIGURE 6: Case 1 (a) reconstructive surgery, (a) temporal cutaneous marking of the right orbital exenteration with a temporal muscle flap (b) (arrow) through a modified lateral orbitotomy (bone window in the lateral wall maintaining the external part of the frontal malar apophysis (c) and (d) (arrow). Initial to mid-stage surgery.

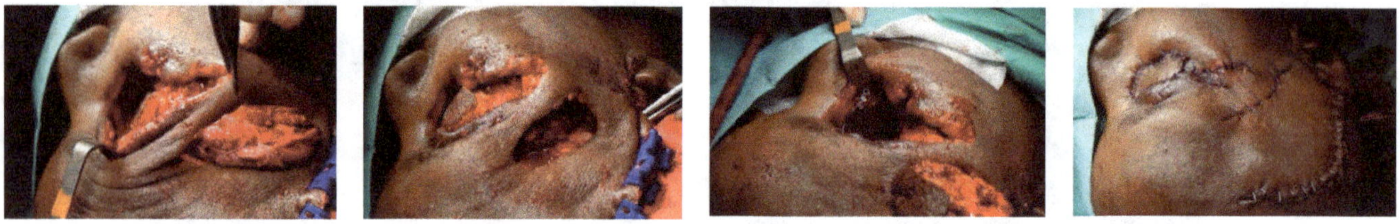

(a) (b) (c) (d)

FIGURE 7: Case 1, (a)–(d) reconstructive surgery of the right orbital exenteration with a pedicle muscle temporal through a modified lateral orbitotomy (bone window in the lateral wall maintaining the external part of the frontal malar apophysis) and a skin pedicle flap. Final stage of surgery.

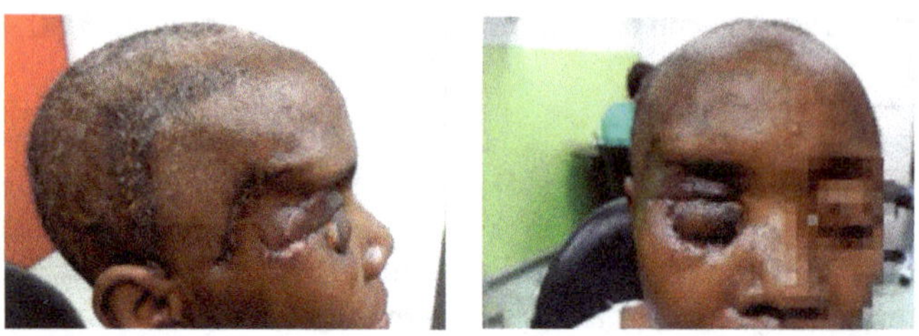

(a) (b)

FIGURE 8: Case 1 (a) and (b) clinical aspect of the patient 2-weeks after reconstruction surgery.

was left open for cures and exploration every 12 hours. One week after surgery, due to good evolution, cures were scheduled every 24 hours. Pathological study showed a respiratory epithelium (pseudostratified ciliated) (arrow). In the underlying chorion, nonseptate hyphae associated with an acute -neutrophilic infiltrate were identified (Figure 11(a)). In (Figure 11(b)) associated nonseptate hyphae (arrow) and a neutrophilic inflammatory infiltrate appear around a nerve (asterisk). And in (Figure 11(c)) there are also nonseptate hyphae (arrow), cellular debris and a neutrophilic infiltrate

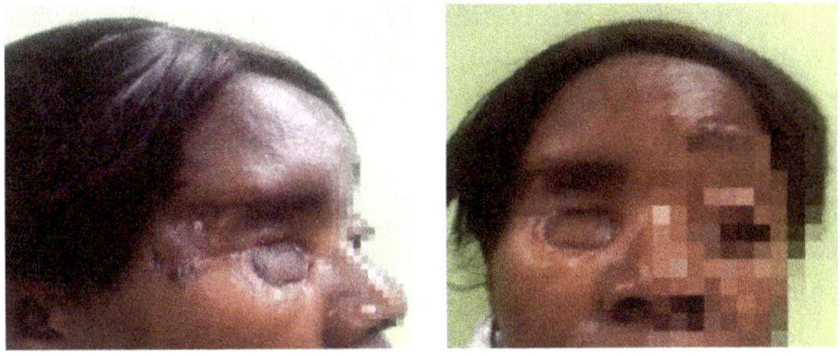

(a) (b)

FIGURE 9: Case 1 (a) and (b) clinical aspect of the patient 6-months after reconstructive surgery.

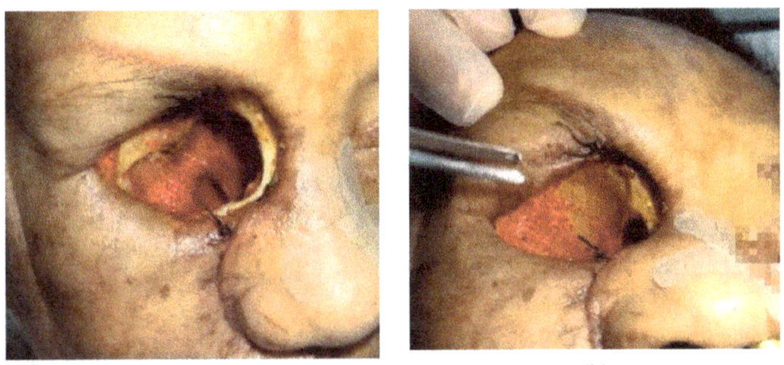

(a) (b)

FIGURE 10: Case 2 (a) and (b) 7-days after postsurgery of right orbital total exenteration.

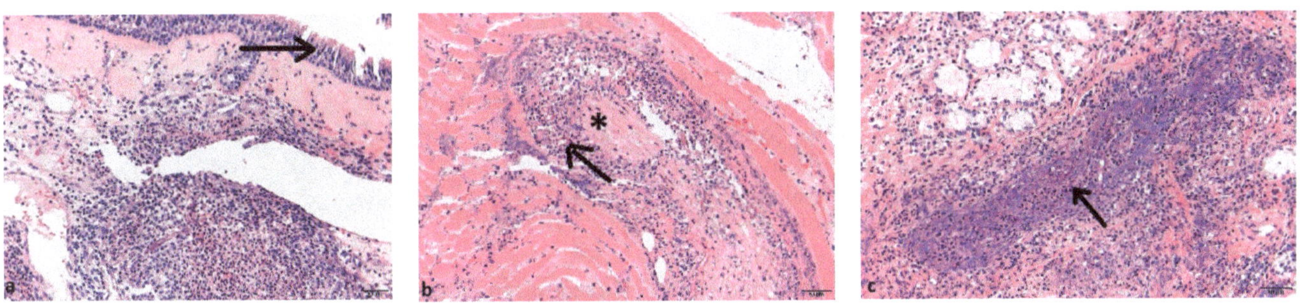

(a) (b) (c)

FIGURE 11: Case 2 (a) pathological study showed a respiratory epithelium (pseudostratified ciliated) (arrow). In the underlying chorionnonseptate hyphae associated with an acute neutrophilic infiltrate were identified, Hematoxilin&Eosin, original magnification × 20 (50 μm scale lower right). In (b) associated nonseptate hyphae (arrow) and a neutrophilic inflammatory infiltrate appear around a nerve (asterisk) Hematoxylin&Eosin, original magnification × 20 (50 μm scale lower right) and in (c) there are also nonseptate hyphae (arrow), cellular debris and a neutrophilic infiltrate that destroys the wall of a blood vessel, Hematoxylin&Eosin stain, original magnification × 20 (50 μm scale lower right).

that destroys the wall of a blood vessel. Microbiological culture showed *Rhizopus oryzae* and sequencing 18S ARNr: PCR confirmed it.

During follow-up, the patient was diagnosed with pulmonary epidermoid carcinoma in the left upper lobe with mediastinal invasion. For this reason, the reconstruction of the orbital defect was not performed.

4. Discussion

Rhizopus is the most common genera and is predominantly observed in patients with ROC mucormycosis [9]. It is a species of ubiquitous and saprophytic fungus that may be found in decomposing organic matter and forms spores that are easily inhaled by humans. In immunosuppressed hosts, the fungus can easily invade blood vessels, which causes thrombosis, hemorrhage and necrosis, which are the characteristic pathological findings found in this type of infection [10]. Mucorales generally affects immunosuppressed people, with diabetes mellitus being the most important risk factor [11]. The reason is that diabetic patients show a decrease in the phagocytic function of neutrophils, myeloperoxidase activity and adherence of neutrophils to the endothelial wall. In addition, the states of acidosis and hyperglycemia suppose a perfect environment for the growth of fungi [12].

Although infection by Mucorales can appear in different locations, the most frequent is the ROC presentation (40%). In ROC mucormycosis, the infection progressively spreads from the nasal mucosa to the facial sinuses, palate, orbits and brain. The nasal and sinus involvement is usually asymptomatic or paucisymptomatic, so it can easily go unnoticed. Patients usually consult when the infection extends, reaching the orbital region. The most frequent symptoms and signs are palpebral edema, ptosis, decreased visual acuity and headache [3].

Early diagnosis and the combination of surgical and pharmacological treatment established in the first 5 days improve prognosis, showing a reduction in the 3-month mortality rate of 48.6% [12]. Patients treated in the first 5 days have a survival rate of 76–81%, while in those treated after the first 12 days the survival rate is reduced to 36–42% [13, 14].

We report two cases of ROC mucormycosis that started with sudden unilateral amaurosis. In the literature we found that the appearance of this symptom is histologically related to the occlusion of the central artery of the retina, necrosis of the ophthalmic artery, with infarction and necrosis of the optic nerve or with direct infection of the optic nerve by Rhizopus [15].

In Case 1, an obstruction of the central artery of the retina was diagnosed, with the nasofibroscopy with sampling providing the diagnostic confirmation of mucormycosis. Case 2 presented with unilateral amaurosis and, several hours later, with a compatible clinical image with OAS. OAS is a rare syndrome that presents with ophthalmoplegia, vision loss and retro-orbital pain [16]. In the literature, it is widely shown that OAS can be the first symptom of mucormycosis [3], but in these cases the first symptom was amaurosis.

Success in the treatment of mucormycosis depends on the following factors: early diagnosis, urgent debridement of the necrotic tissues and resection of infected tissues, parenteral medical treatment and the correction of the predisposing factors in cases where it is possible, with the reversal of immunosuppression being one of the most important factors [17]. Surgery with exeresis of all infected tissues reduces mortality by 49% according to the study published by Tedder et al. [18]. This percentage rises to 71% when the treatment with liposomal amphotericin B, the gold standard treatment in mucormycosis, is added [3, 19]. Mucormycosis produces vascular obstructions, which can hinder the penetration of iv amphotericin into tissues invaded by the fungus. For this reason, the surgical wound is left exposed, in order to be able to irrigate it with liposomal amphotericin B, in combination with the systemic treatment [13, 18]. This also allows the daily assessment of the wound and the resection of any new necrotic tissue that may appear. The therapeutic approach taken, together with the improvement of the patient's immune status, achieved complete healing in both cases, so multidisciplinary management is essential for successfully treating infection. In a period of approximately one month, the complete resolution of the process was achieved, allowing subsequent reconstruction.

As it is a very aggressive surgery, the aesthetic and functional sequelae are very important for the patient. In the cases in which the survival of the patient is achieved, such as those we have presented previously, it is fundamental to offer reconstructive solutions that improve their quality of life once the infection is resolved. The orbital reconstruction carried out using a flap of the temporal muscle, allows the realization of the technique in a single surgical act, without the need for microvascular surgery. In addition, this flap presents adequate vascularization and the healing time is shorter than in other techniques [20, 21]. This procedure is completed with a skin island pedicled flap, avoiding the need to take skin grafts from other locations and reducing the risk of necrosis; with the implant of a titanium mesh in the medial and lower regions, the aesthetic result is very satisfactory for the patient, as in Case 1. We did not find any description of the island pedicled skin flap for reconstruction in the literature.

5. Conclusions

In conclusion, mucormycosis is an uncommon but highly lethal infection, and it is very important to keep this diagnosis in mind, in order to begin treatment early and increase the chances for survival. In addition, a multidisciplinary approach is essential to achieve these objectives. We consider the communication of these clinical cases essential in order to continue improving the therapeutic approach to this infection, to reduce the mortality rate and, in those patients in which survival is achieved, to improve their quality of life.

Consent

Informed consent was obtained from all individual participants included in the study.

References

[1] G. Petrikkos, A. Skiada, O. Lortholary, E. Roilides, T. J. Walsh, and D. P. Kontoyiannis, "Epidemiology and clinical manifestations of mucormycosis," *Clinical Infectious Diseases*, vol. 54, no. 1, pp. S23–S34, 2012.

[2] L. Wagner, S. de Hoog, A. Alastruey-Izquierdo, K. Voigt, and O. Kurzai, G. Walther, "A revised species concept for opportunistic mucor species reveals species-specific antifungal susceptibility profiles," *Antimicrobial Agents and Chemotherapy*, vol. 63, no. 8, e00653 pages, 2019.

[3] N. Jiang, G. Zhao, S. Yang et al., "A retrospective analysis of eleven cases of invasive rhino-orbito-cerebral mucormycosis presented with orbital apex syndrome initially," *BMC Ophthalmology*, vol. 16, no. 1, 2016.

[4] Z. D. Pana, D. Seidel, A. Skiada et al., "Invasive mucormycosis in children: an epidemiologic study in european and non-european countries based on two registries," *BMC Infectious Diseases*, vol. 16, no. 1, 667 pages, 2016.

[5] Y. Kawahara, S. Wada, H. Nijima et al., "Rhinocerebral mucormycosis with temporal artery thrombosis in an adolescent following HLA-haploidentical stem cell transplantation," *Journal of Pediatric Hematology/Oncology*, vol. 40, no. 7, pp. e401–e463, 2018.

[6] J. S. McNulty, "Rhinocerebral mucormycosis: predisposing factors," *Laryngoscope*, vol. 92, no. 10, pp. 1140–1143, 1982.

[7] R. Sriranga, S. Pawar, W. Khot et al., "Isolated renal mucormycosis," *The Journal of the Association of Physicians of India*, vol. 65, no. 4, pp. 77–81, 2017.

[8] C. I. Doty and M. Lucchesi, "Mucormycosis manifesting as proptosis and unilateral blindness," *Academic Emergency Medicine*, vol. 7, no. 8, pp. 944–946, 2000.

[9] W. Jeong, C. Keighley, R. Wolfe et al., "The epidemiology and clinical manifestations of mucormycosis: a systemic review and meta-analysis of case reports," *Clinical Microbiology and Infection*, vol. 25, no. 1, pp. 26–34, 2019.

[10] S. Narayanan, G. Panarkandy, G. Subramaniam et al., "The black evil affecting patients with diabetes: a case of rhino orbito cerebral mucormycosis causing garcin syndrome," *Infection and Drug Resistance*, vol. 28, no. 10, pp. 103–108, 2017.

[11] A. M. Sugar, "Agents of mucormycosis and related species. principles and practice of infectious," *Diseases*, pp. 1962–1971, 1990.

[12] U. Wali, A. Balkhair, and A. Al-Mujaini, "Cerebro-rhino orbital mucormycosis: an update," *Journal of Infection and Public Health*, vol. 5, no. 2, pp. 116–126, 2012.

[13] R. G. Hendrickson, J. Olshaker, and O. Duckett, "Rhinocerebral mucormycosis: a case of a rare, but deadly disease," *The Journal of Emergency Medicine*, vol. 17, no. 4, pp. 641–645, 1999.

[14] Ş. Karadeniz Uğurlu, S. Selim, A. Kopar, and M. Songu, "Rhino-orbital mucormycosis: clinical findings and treatment outcomes of four cases," *Turkish Journal of Ophthalmology*, vol. 45, no. 4, pp. 169–174, 2015.

[15] S. Mathur, A. Karimi, and M. F. Mafee, "Acute optic nerve infarction demonstrated by diffusion-weighted imaging in a case of rhinocerebral mucormycosis," *AJNR American Journal of Neuroradiology*, vol. 28, no. 3, pp. 489–90, 2007.

[16] S. Yeh and R. Foroozan, "Orbital apex syndrome," *Current Opinion in Ophthalmology*, vol. 15, no. 6, pp. 490–498, 2004.

[17] F. Danion, C. Aguilar, E. Catherinot et al., "Mucormycosis: new developments into a persistently devastating infection," *Seminars in Respiratory Critical Care Medicine*, vol. 36, no. 5, pp. 692–705, 2015.

[18] M. Tedder, J. A. Spratt, M. P. Anstadt, S. S. Hegde, S. D. Tedder, and J. E. Lowe, "Pulmonary mucormycosis: results of medical and surgical therapy," *The Annals of Thoracic Surgery*, vol. 57, no. 4, pp. 1044–1050, 1994.

[19] S. R. Seiff, P. H. Choo, and S. R. Carter, "Role of local amphotericin B therapy for sino-orbital fungal infections," *Ophthalmic Plastic and Reconstructive Surgery*, vol. 15, no. 1, pp. 28–31, 1999.

[20] Y. Uyar, T. L. Kumral, G. Yıldırım et al., "Reconstruction of the orbit with a temporalis muscle flap after orbital exenteration," *Clinical and Experimental Otorhinolaryngology*, vol. 8, no. 1, pp. 52–56, 2015.

[21] N. G. Menon, J. A. Girotto, N. H. Goldberg, and R. P. Silverman, "Orbital reconstruction after exenteration: use of a transorbital temporal muscle flap," *Annals of Plastic Surgery*, vol. 50, no. 1, pp. 38–42, 2003.

7

Merkel Cell Carcinoma of the Left Eyelid with Metastasis to the Left Submandibular Lymph Nodes: A Case Report and Brief Review

Caroline Casey,[1] **Nina Gallo**,[1] **and Samuel Gallo**[2]

[1]*University of Central Florida College of Medicine, Orlando, FL, USA*
[2]*Gallo Eye and Facial Plastic Surgery, Dublin, OH, USA*

Correspondence should be addressed to Caroline Casey; caroline.casey@knights.ucf.edu

Academic Editor: Stephen G. Schwartz

Merkel cell carcinoma (MCC) is a cutaneous cancer often found on sun-exposed areas. MCC is rare but very often lethal making early diagnosis challenging although critical. There are only a few cases that have reported MCC of the eyelid making it often hard to identify in clinic. A 52-year-old woman with a firm nodule on the left eyelid was diagnosed with MCC that had also metastasized to a left submandibular lymph node. She underwent surgical excision of the mass and lymph node as well as parotid gland and neck dissection to rule out other metastases and then underwent radiation therapy. The aim of this study is to report a case of eyelid MCC with metastasis to a local lymph node to provide another example of the rare cancer in hopes that diagnosis and treatment options for MCC are more thoroughly studied and understood.

1. Background

Merkel cell carcinoma (MCC) is a rare but aggressive skin cancer, with around 1500 new cases in the United States per year and a mortality rate of up to 40% [1]. It is a cancer with neuroendocrine features that was first described as a "trabecular carcinoma of the skin" in 1972; however, the cancer cell of origin is still debated [2–5]. MCC is associated with either Merkel cell polyomavirus or chronic ultraviolet (UV) light exposure, both of which cause DNA mutations that are characteristic for the condition [1]. Most cases of MCC are found as painless, expanding lesions on sun-exposed areas, and it is more commonly found in Caucasians, males, and the elderly [1]. Immunosuppression is another key risk factor that is more commonly associated with MCC found in younger patients [1]. Eyelid MCC tumors make up around 2.5% of all cases, and women are around two times more likely to have eyelid MCC compared to men [1]. MCC on eyelids is more commonly found on the upper eyelid; this is also where Merkel cells in healthy eyelids are typically found [1, 6, 7]. MCC of the eyelid is often misdiagnosed as cysts, chalazion, or basal cell carcinomas as it is a rare tumor; therefore, an accurate diagnosis is often delayed [1].

2. Case Presentation

A 52-year-old white female presented upon referral in June of 2013 with a recurrent lesion of the left eyelid that was previously diagnosed as a chalazion. Her past medical history was significant for hypertension, measles, mumps, scarlet fever, ruptured lumbar disk, and arthritis, among a few other conditions. She had a family history of stomach cancer with metastases to the rectum in her mother; prostate cancer in her father; breast cancer in her sister, maternal aunt, and cousin; and pancreatic cancer in her grandfather.

Her ophthalmic history was unremarkable, and she had no reports of growths in the past aside from what was believed to be a recurrent chalazion. The lesion was initially excised by her general ophthalmologist. No pathology was sent. Upon recurrence, the patient was sent for a second opinion. The lesion (Figure 1) was biopsied, and histopathology was performed. A

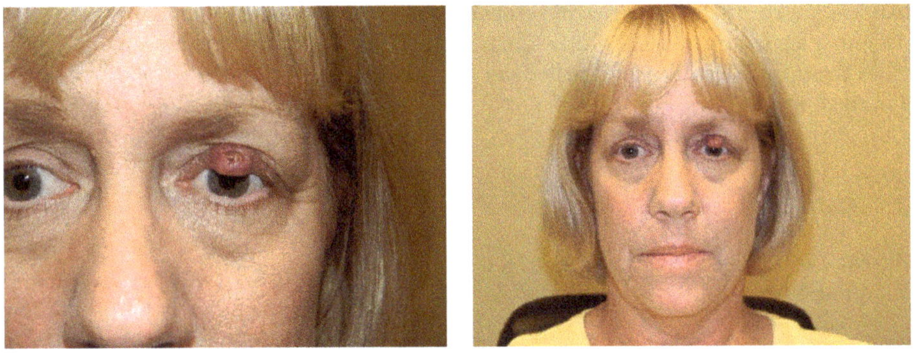

(a) (b)

FIGURE 1: Merkel cell carcinoma (MCC) of the left eyelid in this patient. (a) Closeup image of tumor and (b) head-shot of the patient depicting the size of the tumor in comparison to facial structures.

malignant neoplasm was found extending to the base of the biopsied specimen. The diagnosis was found to be MCC.

Positron emission tomography (PET) and computed tomography (CT) scans revealed an enlarged left submandibular lymph node measuring 1.8 × 1.4 cm with a standardized uptake value (SUV) of 8.5. A fine needle aspiration of the lymph node revealed neuroendocrine carcinoma indicating metastatic MCC.

A wide excision of the tumor and the left submandibular neck contents was completed in July, and one out of two lymph nodes was positive for metastatic MCC. In August, a further neck dissection was completed. The skin excision site was negative for carcinoma. The left lateral parotid lobe was excised, and the salivary gland was found to be without abnormalities. A left cervical lymphadenectomy was also performed. Level I neck contents along with left neck contents in levels II-IV were negative for metastases. All lymph nodes were negative for metastatic carcinoma in levels II-V.

Left eyelid radiation (50.4Gy) was started in October and definitively completed in November of 2013. There has been no evidence of disease since 2013. The patient has since been counseled on UV light protection and self-checks of nevi and other suspicious skin lesions. She has attended regular follow-ups with labs, CXR, and exams of nevi that revealed no evidence of disease.

In 2014, the patient had biopsy-confirmed basal cell carcinoma (BCC) removed from her right upper arm and back. Both lesions were fully excised. In 2014, the patient also had shingles in her right temple/forehead.

Since those incidents, the patient has had no significant skin findings or concerns and is being followed biannually.

3. Discussion

MCC is an aggressive cancer with a high rate of metastases and a high mortality rate, and the number of cases has been on the rise over the past few years [8]. Lesions often first appear as red, firm nodules with overlying telangiectasias possible; however, 5% of MCC are found in the lymph nodes without any skin findings [8, 9]. Diagnosis of MCC is via biopsy, which can reveal small, round, blue cells with a high nucleus to cytoplasm ratio, many mitoses, and dense granules found in the cytoplasm [10]. After diagnosis, appropriate staging is necessary in order to develop a treatment course and effectively counsel patients [8]. With a high propensity to metastasize, full-body PET scans have been found to be most effective at evaluating for distant metastases [8].

MCC has a high rate of local recurrence; so, early diagnosis, rapid treatment, and consistent follow-ups are important to ensure disease remission [11]. Additionally, MCC has a high rate of early metastases to regional lymph nodes, and metastases are more common with a tumor size greater than 2 cm [11]. It is rare for MCC to be found in the area of the eye or eyelid—there are only around 200 reported cases [1]. However, when it is seen, it is often misdiagnosed, as it was initially in this case. There have been previous reports of metastases from the eyelid to regional lymph nodes, parotid lymph nodes, preauricular nodes, submandibular nodes, and distant sites with larger tumors—such as the lungs [12, 13]. However, MCC of the eyelid/eye still remains a very rare finding.

Surgical resection is the mainstay of treatment for localized MCC tumors and with a high rate of recurrence, and immediate excision with clear margins is indicated [14]. Management of metastatic disease; however, involves a multidisciplinary approach. Radiation therapy has been long debated, but is used for MCC involving the lymph nodes or where there is extrascapular extension and has been shown, when combined with surgery, to reduce the risk of local recurrence [14]. Hyperthermic isolated limb perfusion, where high doses of chemotherapy are injected under hyperthermic conditions, is another method that has been shown to provide some clinical benefit [14]. Recently, an immunotherapy agent, Avelumab, in clinical trials has shown some efficacy in treating chemotherapy-resistant MCC [15]. The JAVELIN trial has shown positive results for the treatment of metastatic MCC, and Avelumab is FDA-approved as of June 2020 for treatment of disseminated MCC [16]. MCC is an aggressive cancer, and there continues to be development of treatment options for metastatic disease.

4. Conclusion

In conclusion, this is one of few reports documenting MCC of the eyelid with metastasis to the left submandibular lymph node. Given MCC's high mortality rate, risk of recurrence, and propensity to metastasize, documenting these cases remains critical as treatment strategies and early diagnostic strategies are needed.

Consent

Informed written consent was obtained from the patient for publication of this report and provided to the editors of the journal.

References

[1] V. S. North, L. A. Habib, and M. K. Yoon, "Merkel cell carcinoma of the eyelid: a review," *Survey of Ophthalmology*, vol. 64, no. 5, pp. 659–667, 2019.

[2] J. C. Becker, A. Stang, D. C. JA et al., "Merkel cell carcinoma," *Nature Reviews Disease Primers*, vol. 3, no. 1, article 17077, 2017.

[3] C. Toker, "Trabecular carcinoma of the skin," *Archives of Dermatology*, vol. 105, no. 1, pp. 107–110, 1972.

[4] T. Tilling, E. Wladykowski, A. V. Failla, P. Houdek, J. M. Brandner, and I. Moll, "Immunohistochemical analyses point to epidermal origin of human Merkel cells," *Histochemistry and Cell Biology*, vol. 141, no. 4, pp. 407–421, 2014.

[5] B. Lemos and P. Nghiem, "Merkel cell carcinoma: more deaths but still no pathway to blame," *The Journal of Investigative Dermatology*, vol. 127, no. 9, pp. 2100–2103, 2007.

[6] C. A. May and I. Osterland, "Merkel cell distribution in the human eyelid," *European Journal of Histochemistry*, vol. 57, no. 4, 2013.

[7] G. S. Missotten, D. de Wolff-Rouendaal, and R. J. de Keizer, "Merkel Cell Carcinoma of the Eyelid: Review of the Literature and Report of Patients with Merkel Cell Carcinoma Showing Spontaneous Regression," *Ophthalmology*, vol. 115, no. 1, pp. 195–201, 2008.

[8] C. Cornejo and C. J. Miller, "Merkel cell carcinoma: updates on staging and management," *Dermatologic Clinics*, vol. 37, no. 3, pp. 269–277, 2019.

[9] K. L. Harms, M. A. Healy, P. Nghiem et al., "Analysis of prognostic factors from 9387 Merkel cell carcinoma cases forms the basis for the new 8th edition AJCC staging system," *Annals of Surgical Oncology*, vol. 23, no. 11, pp. 3564–3571, 2016.

[10] M. T. Tetzlaff and P. Nagarajan, "Update on Merkel cell carcinoma," *Head and Neck Pathology*, vol. 12, no. 1, pp. 31–43, 2018.

[11] A. Furdová, M. Michalková, and L. Javorská, "Merkel cell carcinoma of the eyelid and orbit," *Ceská a Slovenská Oftalmologie*, vol. 74, no. 1, pp. 37–43, 2018.

[12] H. M. Herbert, M. T. Sun, D. Selva et al., "Merkel cell carcinoma of the eyelid," *JAMA Ophthalmology*, vol. 132, no. 2, pp. 197–204, 2014.

[13] L. Chen, L. Zhu, J. Wu, T. Lin, B. Sun, and Y. He, "Giant Merkel cell carcinoma of the eyelid: a case report and review of the literature," *World Journal of Surgical Oncology*, vol. 9, no. 1, 2011.

[14] A. N. Abbasi, S. M. Ahmed, and B. M. Qureshi, "Recent updates in the management of Merkel cell Carcinoma," *Journal of the Pakistan Medical Association*, vol. 69, no. 11, pp. 1693–1699, 2019.

[15] H. L. Kaufman, J. Russell, O. Hamid et al., "Avelumab in patients with chemotherapy-refractory metastatic Merkel cell carcinoma: a multicentre, single-group, open-label, phase 2 trial," *The Lancet Oncology*, vol. 17, no. 10, pp. 1374–1385, 2016.

[16] S. P. D'Angelo, S. Bhatia, A. S. Brohl et al., "Avelumab in patients with previously treated metastatic Merkel cell carcinoma: long-term data and biomarker analyses from the single-arm phase 2 JAVELIN Merkel 200 trial," *Journal for Immunotherapy of Cancer*, vol. 8, no. 1, article e000674, 2020.

8

Surgical Management of Complications after Dexamethasone Implant

Giancarlo Sborgia,[1] Alfredo Niro,[2] Francesco D'Oria,[1] Alessandra Galeone,[1] Luigi Sborgia,[1] Francesco Boscia,[3] Alessandra Sborgia,[2] and Giovanni Alessio[1]

[1]*Department of Medical Science, Neuroscience and Sense Organs, Eye Clinic, University of Bari, Bari, Italy*
[2]*Eye Clinic, Hospital "S. G. MOSCATI, " ASL TA, Taranto, Italy*
[3]*Department of Surgical, Microsurgical and Medical Sciences, Eye Clinic, University of Sassari, Sassari, Italy*

Correspondence should be addressed to Alfredo Niro; alfred.nir@tiscali.it

Academic Editor: Nicola Rosa

Purpose. To report surgical management of ocular complications occurred after dexamethasone (DEX) implant (Ozurdex®) injection. *Methods.* Retrospective interventional case series. *Results.* Different surgical procedures including viscoexpression to manage the migration of the implant into the anterior chamber, "phaco-rolling" technique for the intralenticular injection, and vitrectomy with implant removal for an acute endophthalmitis were performed. Successful management of different complications after DEX implant by using individualized surgical approaches was observed. *Conclusions.* Early and targeted surgical management is required in selected cases of ocular complications after DEX implant. The implant removal was needed to preserve ocular anatomy and function.

1. Introduction

The Ozurdex® (Allergan, Irvine, CA, USA) is a 700 mcg dexamethasone (DEX) biodegradable ocular implant, formulated in a solid polymer drug delivery system, designed to be injected into the vitreous using a 22-gauge applicator device. It is used to treat macular oedema (ME) related to diabetic retinopathy, noninfectious uveitis, and retinal vein occlusion [1]. Major complications of this steroid implant include conjunctival haemorrhage, induction or worsening of cataract, glaucoma, retinal detachment, and endophthalmitis [2]. Desegmentation of the implant, lenticular injury during implantation, and migration of the implant into the anterior chamber have been described as rare but known complications [3–7]. We reported a case series of rare ocular complications related to DEX implant, successfully managed by individualized surgical approaches.

2. Report of Cases

This retrospective interventional case series was conducted in the Eye Clinic of University of Bari, Bari, Italy. A total of 1066 cases underwent DEX implant between October 2015 and October 2018 were reviewed. Implant was performed to treat ME secondary to Irvine-Gass syndrome, central or branch retinal vein occlusion, noninfectious uveitis, and diabetic retinopathy. Mayor ocular complications occurred in only four eyes (4/1066; 0.37%). We identified two patients who experienced the migration of the implant into the anterior chamber, one patient with intralenticular implant and one patient with acute endophthalmitis. Patient's age ranged from 60 to 81 years. All these patients underwent a comprehensive ophthalmic examination that included best-corrected visual acuity (BCVA) measurement, slit-lamp examination, intraocular pressure (IOP) measurement, spectral

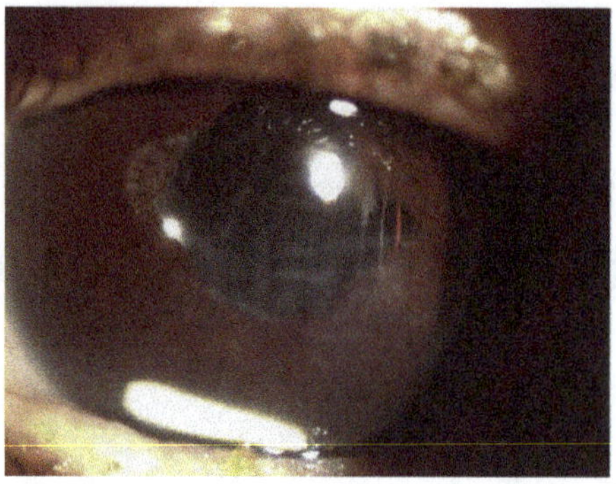

Figure 1: Slit-lamp photograph showing dexamethasone implant migration into the anterior chamber, corneal oedema, and Descemet's membrane folds.

domain optical coherence tomography (SD-OCT), and fundus examination. Ocular ultrasonography was performed when ocular fundus cannot be examined by ophthalmoscopy. We reported targeted surgical management of three patients that experienced ocular complications after DEX implant. The study adhered to the Tenets of the Declaration of Helsinki.

2.1. Case 1. An 81-year-old Caucasian woman underwent a complicated cataract surgery with posterior capsule rupture and sulcus intraocular lens (IOL) implantation. Three months after surgery, a central retinal vein occlusion with ME occurred in the same eye and five consecutive intravitreal injection of anti-Vascular Endothelial Growth Factor (VEGF) were delivered monthly. Due to a poor therapeutic response, she was planned to perform an intravitreal DEX implant. Three weeks following the implant, she complained decreased vision. Visual acuity was limited to 20/200, and IOP was 25 mmHg. We found implant migration into the anterior chamber, and corneal oedema and Descemet's membrane folds were observed (Figure 1). After the informed consent was obtained, the patient underwent surgery by the "viscoexpression" technique, as described by Rahimy et al. [8]. Under topical anesthesia, a clear corneal incision of 2.75 mm opposite from the implant localization was performed. Intracameral injection of acetylcholine chloride was performed to constrict the pupil and avoid the migration of the implant back into the posterior chamber. A dispersive/adhesive ocular viscoelastic device (OVD) was inserted into the anterior chamber to avoid damaging adjacent structures and to facilitate the extrusion of the implant through the paracentesis. Viscoelastic was injected initially through the tunnel in the space between the implant and corneal endothelium. The continuous injection behind the implant maintains the chamber under pressure and pushes the implant toward the incision. Simultaneously, a pressure was posteriorly directed over the corneal incision by the cannula, opening the tunnel and engaging the implant into the tunnel. The OVD was then removed from the anterior chamber using irrigation with balanced salt solution. After two weeks, BCVA was 20/63. Slit-lamp examination revealed the resolution of Descemet's folds and corneal oedema, without any other signs of inflammation in the anterior chamber. Patient required to switch to intravitreal anti-VEGF to treat ME.

2.2. Case 2. A 67-year-old diabetic Caucasian man underwent DEX implant to treat diabetic ME, as the first treatment. At 1-week follow-up, we observed DEX rod impeded into the lens. BCVA was 20/200. IOP was 30 mmHg unresponsive to topical therapy. After the informed consent was obtained, phacoemulsification was performed. The nucleus and the implant were removed using a variation of "phaco-rolling" technique firstly described by Güell et al. [9]. A temporal clear corneal incision of 2.75 mm was performed. The anterior chamber was filled with a viscosurgical device. A 6.0 mm continuous curvilinear capsulorhexis was made, after which hydrodissection and hydrodelamination were performed. A complete rotation of the lens within the capsular bag was performed. A 15-degree phaco tip was placed on the lens beside the capsulorhexis edge and in contact with the nucleus-epinucleus surface, so phacoemulsification was started. Then, we modified the inclination of the tip to 45 degree, directing it toward the lens center. High aspiration was used to keep the probe tip occluded. We used a peristaltic pump for phaco rolling. The lens began to rotate, and phacoemulsification was performed from the periphery toward the center so the nucleus and the implant in the capsular bag were emulsified. No posterior capsular defect was observed intraoperatively. A single-piece intraocular lens (IOL) was placed into the capsular bag, followed by an intravitreal DEX implant (Video 1). At one-month follow-up, ME was reduced, BCVA significantly improved up to 20/32, and IOP was 18 mmHg.

2.3. Case 3. A 60-year-old male patient underwent combined phacoemulsification with in-the-bag hydrophilic acrylic IOL implantation followed by DEX implant for cataract and diabetic ME in the left eye. Five days after surgery, the patient complained pain, redness, and vision loss in the treated eye. Visual acuity was limited to light perception. Slit-lamp examination revealed ciliary injection and 2+ anterior chamber cells. The retinal reflex was poor. B-scan ultrasonography showed high iperecogenous echi with mobile membranes in the vitreous chamber (Figure 2). The diagnosis of acute endophthalmitis was made. After the informed consent was obtained, surgery was performed. Aqueous sample was collected for microbiological evaluation. Then, we performed a standard 3-port 25 Gauge pars plana vitrectomy. Vitreous was aspirated before starting the infusion to get an undiluted sample. The machine was set with an initial aspiration of 0 mmHg moving linearly to 650 mmHg when the foot pedal was fully depressed. A "core" vitrectomy was performed followed by induction of posterior vitreous detachment. The implant was settled peripherally in the vitreous chamber. Vitreous adhesions were removed from the implant with low aspiration and high cut rate. Perfluorocarbon liquid was injected in order to protect the macula. The implant was easily engaged and anteriorized lowering the cut at 0 cut/min and aspiration at 550 mmHg. The IOL was subluxated using a hook introduced through a 1.4 mm superior sclero-lumbar access and the implant was moved to anterior chamber

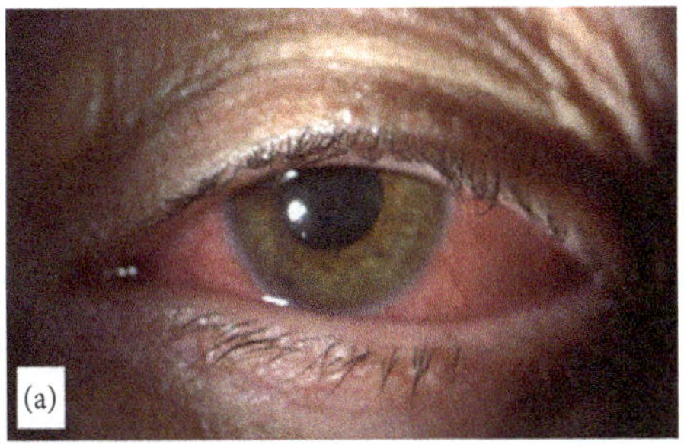

(a)

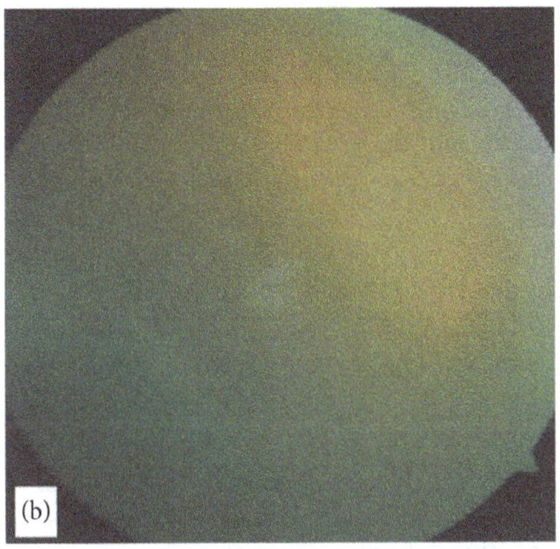

(b)

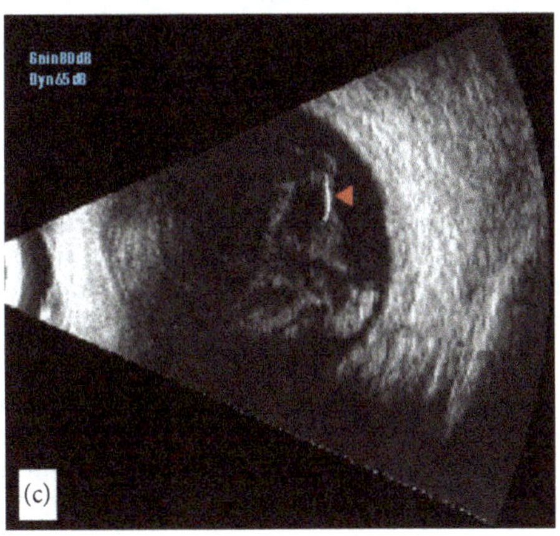

(c)

Figure 2: (a) Slit-lamp photograph showing anterior segment reaction. (b) Vitreous cells and severe vitreous haze hinder funduscopy. (c, d) Ocular ultrasonography B-scan reveals the device as a hyperreflective area (arrowhead) surrounded by dense hyperreflective opacities as dots and membranes in the vitreous cavity.

through a posterior capsule tear observed intraoperatively. The sclero-lumbar access was enlarged to 2.4 mm, and the implant was extracted by applying a gentle pressure on the edge of the tunnel. After an extensive vitrectomy, the patient received an intravitreal injection of vancomycin (1 mg/0.1 mL) and amikacin (0.4 mg/0.1 mL) followed by silicone oil injection (Video 2). The patient was placed on topical Tetracycline 1% six times a day, Dexamethasone 0.1% four times a day, and intravenous Imipenem and Cilastatina Hikma 500 mg four times a day. Vitreous cultures were negative, but aqueous tap yielded Kocuria Rhizophila and Staphylococcus Epidermidis that were sensible to all the antibiotics tested at the antibiogram. After 5 days, ocular inflammation significantly decreased and the patient was discharged with topical antibiotic and a tapering regimen of steroid eye drops. At two-month follow-up, no signs of infections were detected and BCVA improved to 20/63.

3. Discussion

In a retrospective review of 924 DEX implantations performed, Kang et al. reported four cases of anterior chamber migration in the presence of a compromised posterior capsule, [10] as we observed. In another previous report, corneal oedema was observed when anterior migration occurred over 3 weeks after implant. Authors suggested that corneal oedema was due to mechanical trauma of the implant on corneal endothelial layer rather than chemical toxicity. So the earlier removal of the implant was performed to reduce the risk of irreversible corneal endothelial damage [6]. In our patients who experienced anterior chamber migration, ocular symptoms occurred from 3 to 4 weeks after injection when corneal oedema was observed.

Various procedures to remove the implant from anterior chamber such as the aspiration of the disintegrated implant, the use of forceps, viscoelastic material, or IOL injector when the implant is still stiff were reported [6–8]. We performed viscoexpression using OVD without any contact with the implant. This approach ensures that no vehicle particles are left behind after the intervention [8]. We did not perform a repositioning of the implant due to the severe corneal oedema and the risk of migration recurrence. However, the repositioning of the implant into the vitreous cavity may be firstly attempted in the absence of severe corneal decompensation [11]. The accidental injection into the lens is an unexpected complication that occurs rarely. Coca-Rabinot et al. reported a case series of two patients with accidental injection into the lens associated with raised IOP responsive to the topical therapy. Only when cataract occurred after several weeks, authors performed cataract surgery [6]. In our case, we detected an increased IOP not responsive to topical therapy, so we decided to perform phacoemulsification. We decided to perform the "phaco-rolling" technique that allows to reduce phaco time and phaco energy compared to divide-and-conquer technique, as our standard technique, maintaining a constant irrigation/aspiration [9]. To our knowledge, for the first time, "phaco-rolling" technique was used to remove DEX implant embedded into the lens. We tried to reduce the risk of damage to the corneal endothelium and posterior capsule, accidental fragmentation and dispersion of the implant during lens sculpture and removal, and postoperative complications as cystoid macular oedema. Moreover, the implant localized into the lens does not work because of the altered location [5]. The incidence of endophthalmitis after intravitreal implant is low, ranging from 0.019% to 1.4% [12], and no cases of endophthalmitis had been reported in the GENEVA study, one of the main study trials about DEX implant [13]. A study by VanderBeek et al.

concluded that the incidence of endophthalmitis was higher with intravitreal injection of steroids than anti-VEGF. They stated that this could be due to the larger wound outlined by the 22-gauge needle used in steroid injection which could allow an easy bacterial penetration into the vitreous. Furthermore, since steroids have an immunosuppressive action, they might contribute to the growth of infectious agents [14]. In our last case, despite all prophylactic procedures were performed, five days after surgery, endophthalmitis occurred. The diabetic status of patient is a known risk factor for developing infections due to a deficiency of the immune system related to diabetes [15]. Moreover, the rupture of the posterior capsule, that we found, is associated with an increase of the risk of endophthalmitis [16]. The use of vitrectomy is recommended for severe and sight-threatening endophthalmitis, and in particular, early vitrectomy has been associated with better prognosis [17]. We decided to remove the implant moving it from the posterior chamber to the anterior chamber through a rupture of the posterior capsule without damaging the IOL. So we avoided to loss some fragments of the implant as a vehicle of infection if we had used the vitrectome. Oil tamponade limiting the movements of aqueous humor and, as an inert material, the penetration of microorganisms can favor better outcomes [18]. The opportunity of removing instead of repositioning the implant should be considered in case of corneal oedema endophthalmitis or when implant does not work. We performed different surgical maneuvers, of which two were never used before in the management of DEX implant complications to avoid implant fragmentation and damages of intraocular structures.

Consent

Informed consent was obtained from the individual participant included in the case.

Disclosure

The authors alone are responsible for the content and writing of the paper.

References

[1] N. J. London, A. Chiang, and J. A. Haller, "The dexamethasone drug delivery system: indications and evidence," *Advances in Therapy*, vol. 28, no. 5, pp. 351–366, 2011.

[2] K. Schmitz, German Retinal Vein Occlusion Group, M. Maier et al., "Zuverlässigkeit und Sicherheit von intravitrealen Ozurdex-Injektionen," *Der Ophthalmologe*, vol. 111, no. 1, pp. 44–52, 2014.

[3] R. Agrawal, G. Fernandez-Sanz, S. Bala, and P. K. Addison, "Desegmentation of Ozurdex implant in vitreous cavity: report of two cases," *The British Journal of Ophthalmology*, vol. 98, no. 7, pp. 961–963, 2014.

[4] C. S. Cheung, A. W. Wong, A. Lui, P. J. Kertes, R. G. Devenyi, and W. C. Lam, "Incidence of endophthalmitis and use of antibiotic prophylaxis after intravitreal injections," *Ophthalmology*, vol. 119, no. 8, pp. 1609–1614, 2012.

[5] J. Coca-Robinot, B. Casco-Silva, F. Armadá-Maresca, and J. García-Martínez, "Accidental injections of dexamethasone intravitreal implant (Ozurdex) into the crystalline lens," *European Journal of Ophthalmology*, vol. 24, no. 4, pp. 633–636, 2014.

[6] R. N. Khurana, S. N. Appa, C. A. McCannel et al., "Dexamethasone implant anterior chamber migration: risk factors, complications, and management strategies," *Ophthalmology*, vol. 121, no. 1, pp. 67–71, 2014.

[7] M. B. Gonçalves, B. de Queiroz Alves, R. Moura et al., "Intravitreal dexamethasone implant migration into the anterior chamber: a multicenter study from the Pan-American Collaborative Retina Study Group," *Retina*, vol. 14, 2019.

[8] E. Rahimy, J. D. Pitcher III, A. M. Abbey, B. R. Garretson, and J. A. Haller, "No-touch removal of anterior segment-migrated dexamethasone implant," *Retina*, vol. 35, no. 11, pp. 2414–2416, 2015.

[9] J. L. Güell, M. Vázquez, J. Lucena, F. Velasco, and F. Manero, "Phaco rolling technique," *Journal of Cataract and Refractive Surgery*, vol. 30, no. 10, pp. 2043–2045, 2004.

[10] H. Kang, M. W. Lee, S. H. Byeon, H. J. Koh, S. C. Lee, and M. Kim, "The clinical outcomes of surgical management of anterior chamber migration of a dexamethasone implant (Ozurdex®)," *Graefe's Archive for Clinical and Experimental Ophthalmology*, vol. 255, no. 9, pp. 1819–1825, 2017.

[11] D. Pardo-Lopez, E. Frances-Munoz, R. Gallego-Pinazo, and M. Diaz-Llopis, "Anterior chamber migration of dexametasone intravitreal implant (Ozurdex®)," *Graefe's Archive for Clinical and Experimental Ophthalmology*, vol. 250, no. 11, pp. 1703-1704, 2012.

[12] D. S. Boyer, Y. H. Yoon, Belfort RJr. et al., "Three-year, randomized, sham-controlled trial of dexamethasone intravitreal implant in patients with diabetic macular edema," *Ophthalmology*, vol. 121, no. 10, pp. 1904–1914, 2014.

[13] J. A. Haller, F. Bandello, Belfort RJr. et al., "Randomized, sham-controlled trial of dexamethasone intravitreal implant in patients with macular edema due to retinal vein occlusion," *Ophthalmology*, vol. 117, no. 6, pp. 1134–1146.e3, 2010.

[14] B. L. VanderBeek, S. G. Bonaffini, and L. Ma, "The association between intravitreal steroids and post-injection endophthalmitis rates," *Ophthalmology*, vol. 122, no. 11, pp. 2311–2315.e1, 2015.

[15] A. Gupta, J. K. Sun, and P. S. Silva, "Complications of intravitreous injections in patients with diabetes," *Seminars in Ophthalmology*, vol. 33, no. 1, pp. 42–50, 2018.

[16] H. Cao, L. Zhang, L. Li, and S. Lo, "Risk factors for acute endophthalmitis following cataract surgery: a systematic review and meta-analysis," *PLoS One*, vol. 8, no. 8, p. e71731, 2013.

[17] F. Kuhn and G. Gini, "Complete and early vitrectomy for endophthalmitis (CEVE) as today's alternative to the endophthalmitis vitrectomy study," in *Vitreo-retinal Surgery*, pp. 53–68, Springer, Berlin, Heidelberg, 2007.

[18] M. Nagpal, P. Jain, and K. Nagpal, "Pars plana vitrectomy with or without silicone oil endotamponade in surgical management of endophthalmitis," *Asia-Pacific Journal of Ophthalmology*, vol. 1, no. 4, pp. 216–221, 2012.

9

Giant Cell Reparative Granuloma of the Orbit: Clinicopathological Characteristics and Treatment

Álvaro Bengoa-González,[1] Enrique Mencía-Gutiérrez,[1] Beatriz Alonso-Martín,[1] Bianca-Maria Laslău,[1] Elena Salvador,[2] Ana-Belén Enguita-Valls,[3] and María-Dolores Lago-Llinás[1]

[1]*Ophthalmology Department, 12 de Octubre Hospital, Complutense University, 28041 Madrid, Spain*
[2]*Radiology Department, 12 de Octubre Hospital, Complutense University, 28041 Madrid, Spain*
[3]*Pathology Department, 12 de Octubre Hospital, Complutense University, 28041 Madrid, Spain*

Correspondence should be addressed to Enrique Mencía-Gutiérrez; emencia.hdoc@salud.madrid.org

Academic Editor: Kamal Kishore

Giant cell reparative granuloma (GCRG) is a rare fibroosseous lesion uncommonly seen in the orbital area. Although benign, it is known to be recurrent and locally destructive. We report two cases of GCRG of the orbit. In both cases, computed tomography revealed a heterogeneously growing well-defined mass, arising from the roof of the orbit, affecting the cortex, and invading the orbit. In the first case, the mass extended into the anterior cranial fossa. Magnetic resonance imaging with gadolinium showed, in both cases, a cystic character of the lesion with fluid levels. The surgical treatment was performed via an upper crease incision. An ultrasonic aspirator system was used to remove the tumor tissue and its extension into cranial fossa. Careful histopathologic analysis established the diagnosis of GCRG. Symptoms resolved completely with no evidence of recurrence after a follow-up of 18 and 14 months, respectively. We present the clinicopathological and radiological findings, and we describe the surgical approach. As a rare entity, GCRG of the orbit should be considered in differential diagnosis of fibroosseous orbital masses. Complete surgical excision carries a low risk of recurrence.

1. Introduction

Giant cell reparative granuloma (GCRG) is an uncommon osteolytic lesion that typically develops in the jawbone [1, 2], although it has also been described in other locations such as maxilla, sphenoid, ethmoid, and temporal bones and it also can be found occasionally in the small bones of the hands and feet [3].

It was Jaffe [4], who suggested this term in 1953 to describe lesions of the mandible and maxilla that were thought to occur as a nonneoplastic reaction secondary to an intraosseous hemorrhage. GCRG of the orbit is a very rare occurrence and was first reported by Sood et al. in 1967 [3–6].

It is included within a group of orbital fibroosseous lesions, among which are the osteoma, ossifying fibroma, fibrous dysplasia, osteoblastoma, osteoclastoma, brown tumor of hyperparathyroidism, and the aneurysmal bone cyst [1], with overlapping clinical and histopathologic features [7].

We have found 10 cases of GCRG with orbital involvement published in the medical literature [5], and only two of them had intracranial invasion [8, 9].

We present two cases of orbital GCRG, one of them with extension into the anterior cranial fossa. We describe the clinical, histological, and radiological characteristics and the surgical approach to removing them using an ultrasonic surgical aspirator device.

2. Case Presentation

2.1. Case 1. A 37-year-old male presented with proptosis, fullness of the right upper eyelid, and inferior displacement

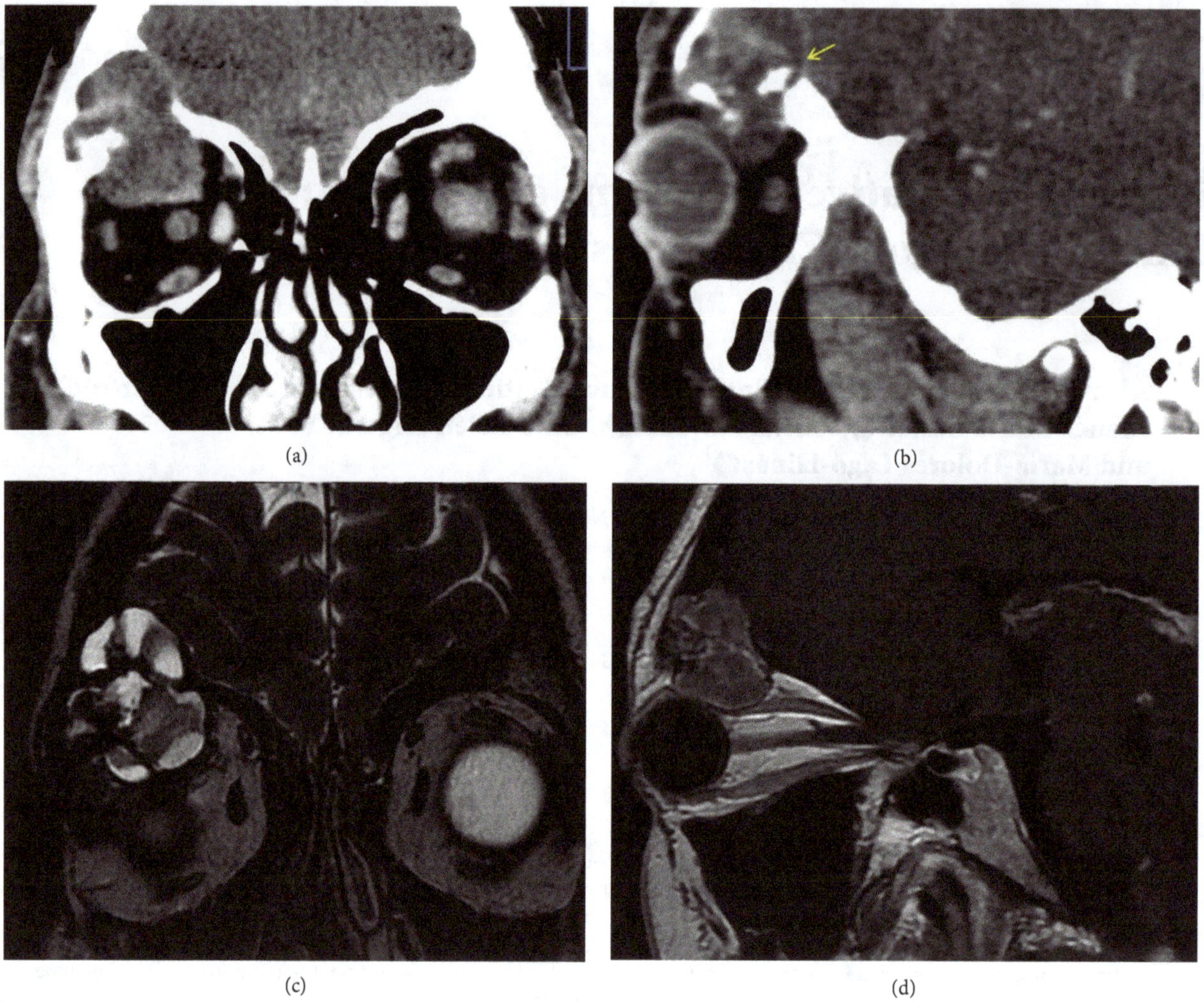

FIGURE 1: (a, b) Contrast-enhanced coronal and sagittal CT images, demonstrating an expansive lesion arising from the roof of the right orbit with a heterogeneous enhancement and soft tissue attenuation. Inside view of the lesion reveals several small foci of mineralization (arrow). The lesion shows the osseous expansive changes, with thinning of superior and inferior wall of the roof which leads to an invasion over the frontal sinus and into the orbit. (c) Coronal T2-weighted MRI shows a well-defined lesion with a low-signal-intensity margin representing either osseous sclerosis or a pseudocapsule. The lesion shows a multilobulated lytic pattern which reveals markedly increased signal intensity, reflecting the expansive cystic component, and low signal intensity in the small solid regions. (d) Sagittal postcontrast T1-weighted MR image shows a well-encapsulated mass with homogenous contrast enhancement.

of the right eye that had progressed gradually over several months. There was no history of pain, loss of visual acuity (VA), or diplopia. Ocular motility examination revealed a slight limitation of motion in supraduction. The patient reported no previous episodes of inflammation, sinus infection, or trauma. Fundus examination was normal. General physical examination and routine blood tests were within normal limits. Contrast-enhanced coronal and sagittal computed tomography (CT) images showed a lytic lesion arising from the roof of the right orbit, with heterogeneous captation, relatively hypocaptant with hypodense areas, and small foci of mineralization within the lesion. The mass had a thinning effect on the superior wall of the roof, without breaking it, and extended over the anterior cranial fossa. It also disrupted the inferior wall of the roof and invaded the orbit, displacing the superior rectus muscle and the globe inferiorly (Figures 1(a) and 1(b)). Magnetic resonance imaging (MRI) revealed a well-defined, heterogeneously enhancing mass, measuring 30 mm × 19 mm × 27 mm, hyperintense on T1-weighted images, and with lobulated, "pseudonodular" appearance on T2-weighted images, with markedly increased signal intensity, reflecting the expansible cystic component (Figures 1(c) and 1(d)). An orbitotomy was performed via an upper eyelid crease incision, and a red-yellowish friable mass, with evidence of dark coagulated blood, and fragments of bone tissue within the soft tissue was observed (Figure 2(a)). A tissue sample was taken for histopathological study, and then, an ultrasonic aspirator system (SONOPET®, Stryker, Kalamazoo, MI, USA) was used to remove the tumor. The handpiece of this device, with a soft tissue straight tip attached, was used to aspirate and separate the tumor from the surrounding heathy tissue, preventing damage to it. The handpiece is lightweight and ergonomic, allowing it to be inserted into narrow spaces with poor visibility,

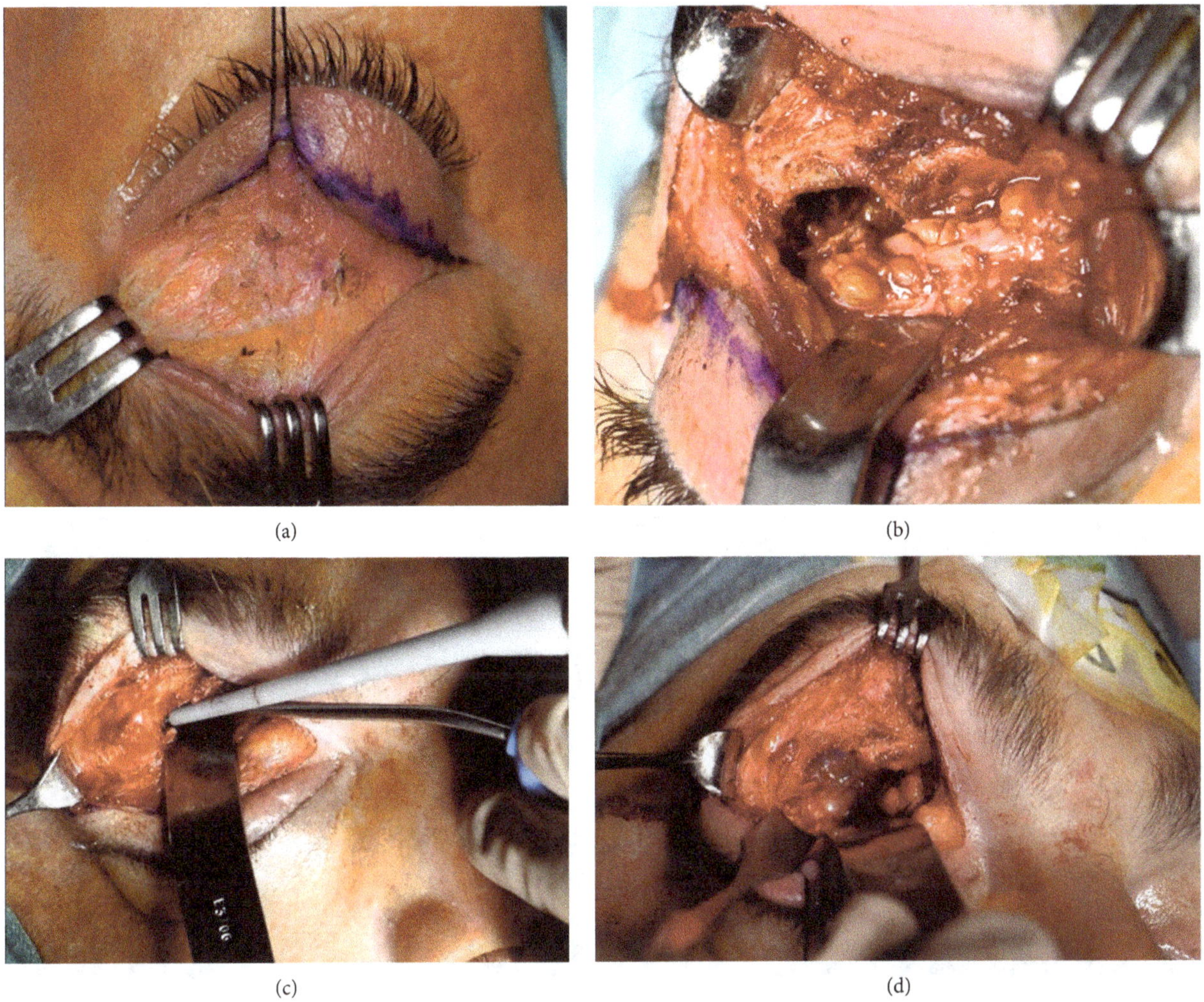

FIGURE 2: (a) Surgical approach through an upper eyelid crease incision to access the orbital roof. Intraoperative photograph showing bone destruction in the roof of the orbit and the presence of a red-yellowish mass, with evidence of dark coagulated blood and fragments of bone within the soft tissue. The tumor extends into the anterior cranial fossa. (b) The handpiece of SONOPET® ultrasonic aspirator used for aspiration and emulsification of the tumor tissue in the superior orbit and its extension into cranial cavity. (c) Resection of abnormal tissue from the upper orbit and its extension into anterior fossa.

thus making possible the approach to the cranial fossa through the orbital roof (Figure 2(b)). Moreover, with the Spetzler micro claw tip, the lateral edge of the orbital roof was sculpted to gain visibility and access to the cranial fossa. Once the tumor tissue was removed, we performed a curettage, removing the capsule and the tissue attached to the cortical surface of bone (Figures 2(c) and 2(d)). During these surgical maneuvers, a leak of cerebral spinal fluid, originating in the innermost part of the cavity, was noted and sealed with human fibrinogen/human thrombin, TachoSil®, Talceda Austria GmbH, Linz, Austria, efficiently. Oral treatment with antibiotics was prescribed for 1 week. Symptoms resolved and there was no evidence of recurrence after 18 months of follow-up.

2.2. Case 2. A 39-year-old male was referred to our oculoplastic service complaining of gradually progressive proptosis, and right upper eyelid swelling. The VA and ocular motility examination were normal. He had previous episodes of sinusitis and endoscopic surgical repair of the right frontal sinus. Orbital CT revealed a cystic mass measuring 30 mm × 15 mm × 20 mm that eroded the orbital roof, with thinning and pushing the cortex, but without invading the cranial cavity (Figures 3(a)–3(c)). MRI showed a well-defined mass, adjacent to the frontal sinus, of heterogeneous tissue. The majority of the tumor had high signal intensity on the T2-weighted image, with low signal areas which represented the solid component of the tumor (Figure 3(c)). Surgical treatment was performed via an upper eyelid crease incision. Gross examination of the specimen showed a soft, friable, red-bluish hemorrhagic tissue with small fragments of bone tissue within. A tissue sample was taken, followed by surgical excision using the ultrasonic aspirator system. The curettage was carried out eliminating the attachment to the orbital walls without incident. Symptoms resolved completely without recurrence after 14 months of follow-up. The histopathological study of both cases showed similar features. It consisted of a cellularity with a fibrohistiocytic appearance,

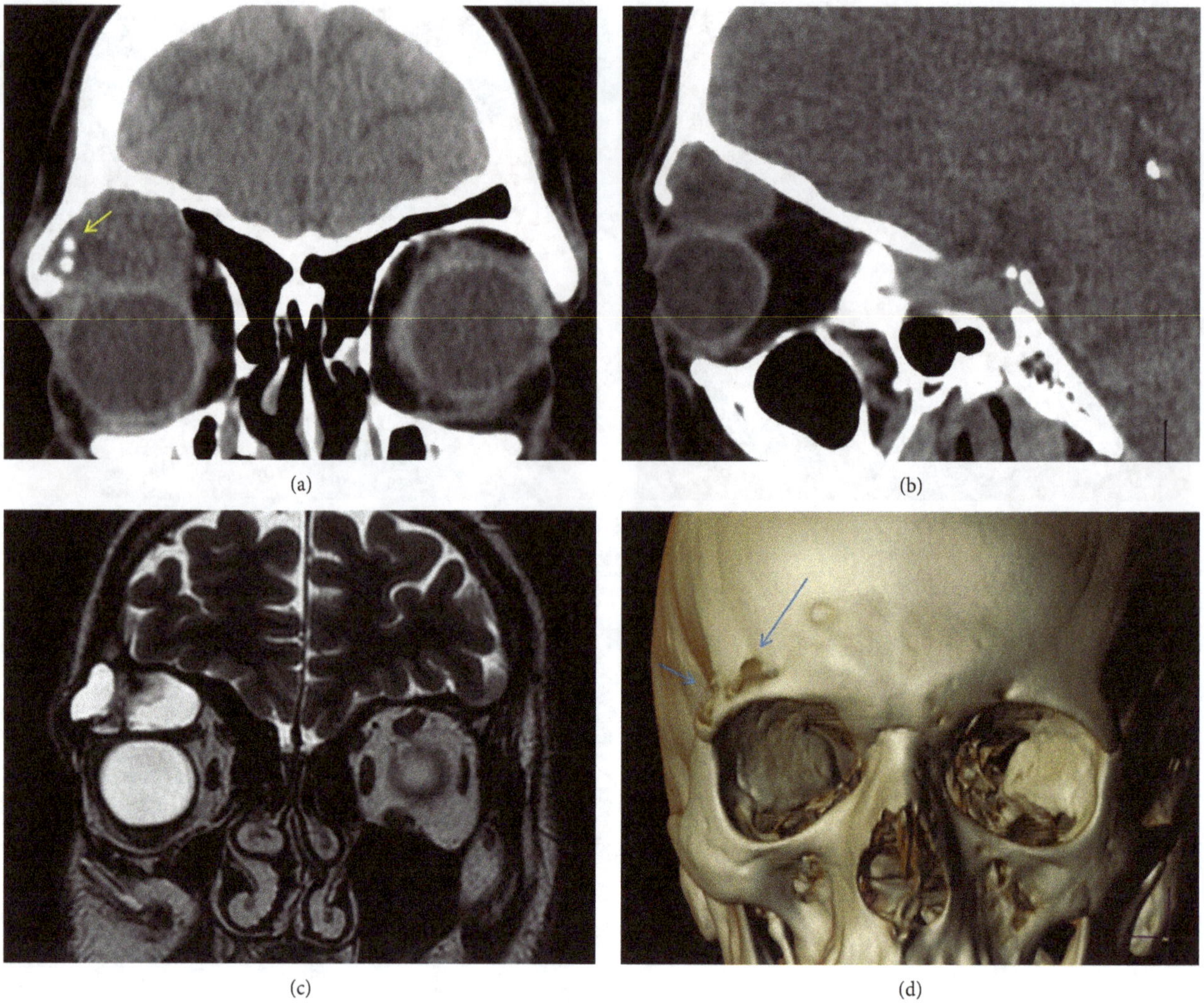

FIGURE 3: (a, b) Coronal and sagittal CT images, demonstrating an expansive lesion arising from the roof of the right orbit with soft tissue attenuation. Small foci of mineralization (arrow) into the lesion are presented. The lesion protrudes into the orbit. (c) Coronal T2-weighted MR image shows a well-defined lesion arising from the bone with an extraosseous component. The majority of the tumor has high signal intensity on the T2-weighted image, with low signal areas which represent the solid component of the tumor. (d) Volume-rendered 3D-CT reconstruction images show lytic areas with bone destruction in the roof of the orbit.

without atypia, with xanthomized cells as well as pigmented areas with hemosiderin deposits. In addition, there was a foreign body reaction and cholesterol crystals. Osteoid tissue was not identified. There were no areas of malignancy (Figures 4(a) and 4(b)). These findings led to the diagnosis of reparative giant cell granuloma in both cases. The biochemical study of the blood, including electrolytes, was within normal values.

3. Discussion

GCRG of the orbit is a benign fibrous lesion, although it can expand aggressively and can be locally destructive [1, 3], which happened in the cases which we present.

The etiology of this tumor remained unclear [8] but may be related to a reparative granulomatous response to an intraosseous hemorrhage [1, 5]. It is thought that chronic inflammation and trauma to the paranasal sinuses could produce intraosseous hemorrhage that initiates the reparative process [10], which might be the etiology of the second case we presented, although a history of trauma or chronic sinusitis has never been consistently demonstrated in all patients with GCRG [3, 10].

GCRG occurs more frequently in women and in the first two decades of life [11]. Almost all previously published orbital cases have been reported in patients under 40 years of age, like those presented in this study, but Pherwani et al. reported [3] a GCRG in an 85-year-old patient.

The clinical signs that our patients mainly manifested were proptosis, upper eyelid fullness, periorbital inflammation, lower displacement of the globe, and impaired extraocular movements; these signs and symptoms are in line with those described in the medical literature [1, 8, 9, 12]. Although not in our patients, other symptoms such as headache [13], decreased VA [9], orbital deformity [6, 9], and diplopia [14] have also been reported.

Most of the published cases of GCRG of the orbit affected the roof and/or the lateral orbital wall, as in our cases, but it

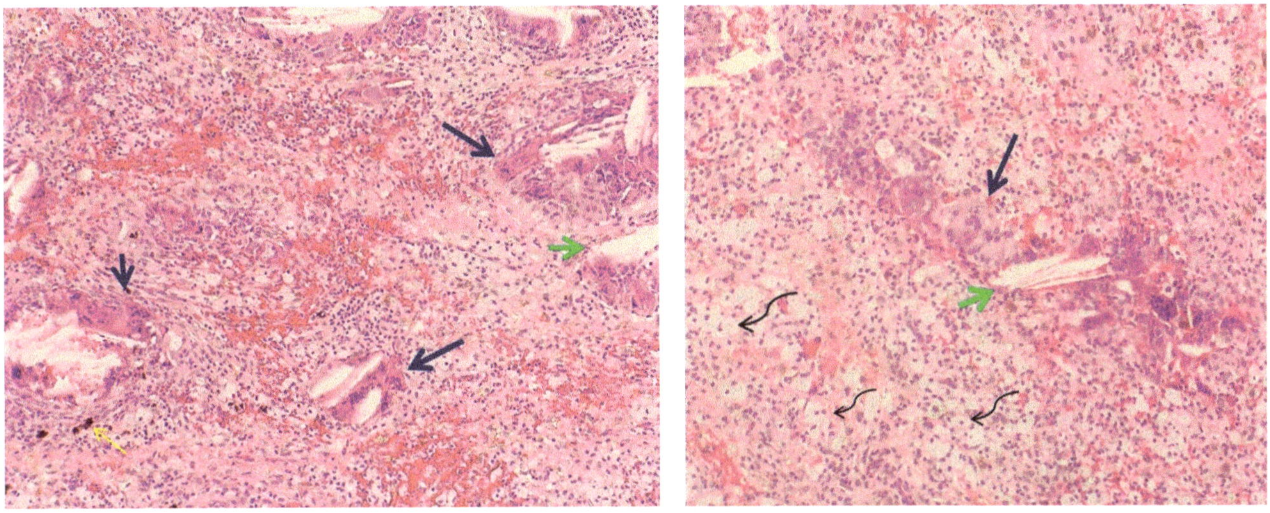

(a) (b)

FIGURE 4: (a, b) Histopathology (hematoxylin and eosin stain (40x) showing multinucleated foreign body giant cells (cholesterol crystals) with xanthomized cells, presence of hemosiderin deposition, and lymphocytic inflammatory infiltrate. Multinucleated giant cells (thick blue arrows), cholesterol crystals (short green arrows), xanthomized cells (wavy black arrows), and hemosiderin deposits (fine yellow arrow).

TABLE 1: Giant cell reparative granuloma cases involving the orbit.

Authors	Number cases	Side, location in the orbit
Bengoa-González A et al., current study	2	Right, superior, one extending anterior cranial fossa
2013, Chawla et al. [5]	1	Right, lateral
2005, Pherwani et al. [3]	1	Left, superomedial
2005, D'Ambrosio et al. [12]	1	Left, optic strut, and anterior clinoid process
2003, Font et al. [14]	1	Bilateral, lateral, and inferior
1999, Mercado et al. [1]	1	Left, lateral and posterior, and sphenoid bone
1988, Rootman et al. [15]	1	No data, superior extending anterior cranial fossa
1985, Sebag et al. [8]	1	Right, superolateral, and roof
1984, Scully et al. [13]	1	Right, posterior, lateral, and central
1981, Hoopes et al. [9]	1	Right, superior, lateral, and posterior
1967, Sood et al. [6]	1	Left, medial, and ethmoid sinus

can also affect the inferior, central, and medial portion of the orbit (Table 1) [1, 3, 5, 6, 8, 9, 12–15].

Treatment of GCRG is surgical excision, which is usually done with total resection or local curettage [1, 16], although complete surgical resection could not be done safely in some cases, due to tumor location and proximity to delicate structures [17].

Imaging findings of GCRG are not specific, thus making it very difficult to distinguish from other osteolytic bone lesions [18]. In both of our cases, the CT scan showed a heterogeneously growing [1] well-defined mass arising from the roof of the orbit, affecting the cortex and invading the orbital space. In the first case, cortical thinning and bulging were observed, as noted by Sebag et al. [8], who describe a cavity that invades the cranial fossa. Although in the first case the CT scan did not show a cortical tear, and a connection to the extradural space was ruled out, when detaching the mass tissue from the thin layer of the cortical bone, we observed a CSF leak which was sealed with TachoSil® (human fibrinogen/human trombin) efficiently.

Given the location and extent of the mass, an upper eyelid crease approach was used to access the superior orbital space, the orbital roof, and cranial fossa extension. Intraoperatively, bone destruction of the orbital walls was noted, and detached bone fragments were observed among soft tissues.

On gross inspection, the tumor may appear as a friable red-bluish mass [1], although it may also be cystic, bluish, fluctuating, and multiloculated, containing dark coagulated blood [1, 5, 8]. Histologically, GCGR is characterized by the presence of multinucleated giant cells, with or without new bone formation, intermingled with inflammatory cells, and focal areas of hemorrhage [18].

The GCGR of the orbit is very similar to the brown tumor of hyperparathyroidism, although in the latter the serum levels of calcium are usually high and those of phosphorus are low [1, 3]; its levels were normal in our cases.

It is important to distinguish GCRG from other tumors, such as osteoclastoma, also known as giant cell tumor, for management and prognosis. Osteoclastoma is a giant cell tumor within the bone [1] that mostly involves the epiphysis of long bones [9, 10]. It usually appears in the third to fourth decade of life, being very rare in those under 18 years of age. This tumor is composed of multinucleated giant cells distributed diffusely and evenly, whereas in GCGR the multinucleated giant cells are smaller, irregular, and clustered around hemorrhagic foci [1, 5]. New bone foci can also be observed in GCGR, but not in osteoclastoma [9, 10, 19].

Eosinophilic granuloma is the bone variant of histiocytosis X or Langerhans cell histiocytosis and generally occurs in the first decade of life [20]. In the cases presented, the histological image and the immunohistochemical profile ruled out that these were cases of an eosinophilic granuloma nor were cystic images observed that would have led to the diagnosis of an aneurysmal bone cyst; in addition, this bone cyst more frequently is located in vertebrae and metaphysis of long bones [12].

In both cases, an ultrasonic aspirator system was used to remove the tumor. The SONOPET® ultrasonic aspirator is a handheld surgical tool that allows access to small operative fields, such as the orbit [21]. The design of the handpiece and its weight allowed us to maneuver it for the extraction of tumors that are difficult to reach, as was the situation in the cases we present. In our first case, the mass expanded into the cranial fossa and was removed using an orbital approach, thus avoiding a craniotomy, as performed by other authors [8, 22, 23].

This ultrasonic system allowed us to sculpt the bone precisely, when an improvement of visibility was needed, as in the first case presented, and to remove the abnormal tissue, regardless of its consistency, with no traction nor sharp excision. It enables work near areas such as the dura mater without damaging the adjacent tissues.

We think, as do other authors [24, 25], that this device is particularly helpful in removing and sculpting, in a simple, secure, and precise way, infiltrative orbital masses with difficult anatomical access, as was the situation in our cases [26].

The recurrence rate of these tumors can be between 10 and 15% of the cases that have been incompletely removed, as has been seen in other published cases [6, 9]. The mean interval from the initial treatment to recurrence has been described around 19 months [27]; therefore, our patients need continuous follow-up on a regular basis due to the relatively short follow-up time of our two cases. Although spontaneous resolution has been documented [10], recurrences might be treated with reoperation or radiotherapy, options that can help in achieving complete remission [4, 12]. However, radiotherapy is generally not advisable due to the risk of carcinomatous or sarcomatous transformation and should be reserved for patients who are not surgical candidates [9].

4. Conclusions

In conclusion, the orbital GCGR, although rare, should be included in the differential diagnosis of fibroosseous lesions or other orbital masses. Although it is more frequent in young or middle-aged patients it must be considered in older patients too. The surgical resection of this lesion is usually possible and can be curative, relieving ocular symptoms.

Consent

Informed consent was obtained from all individual participants included in the study.

References

[1] G. V. Mercado, C. L. Shields, K. Gunduz, J. A. Shields, and R. C. Eagle Jr., "Giant cell reparative granuloma of the orbit," *American Journal of Ophthalmology*, vol. 127, no. 4, pp. 485–487, 1999.

[2] J.-L. Yu, L. M. Qu, J. Wang, and H. Y. Huang, "Giant cell reparative granuloma in the temporal bone of the skull base: report of two cases," *Skull Base*, vol. 20, no. 6, pp. 443–448, 2010.

[3] A. A. Pherwani, D. Brooker, and B. Lacey, "Giant cell reparative granuloma of the orbit," *Ophthalmic Plastic and Reconstructive Surgery*, vol. 21, no. 6, pp. 463–465, 2005.

[4] H. L. Jaffe, "Giant-cell reparative granuloma, traumatic bone cyst, and fibrous (fibro- osseous) dysplasia of the jawbones," *Oral Surgery, Oral Medicine, and Oral Pathology*, vol. 6, no. 1, pp. 159–175, 1953.

[5] B. Chawla, S. Khurana, and S. Kashyap, "Giant cell reparative granuloma of the orbit," *Ophthalmic Plastic and Reconstructive Surgery*, vol. 29, no. 4, pp. e94–e95, 2013.

[6] G. C. Sood, S. R. K. Malik, D. K. Gupta, and P. K. Kakar, "Reparative Granuloma of the Orbit: Causing Unilateral Proptosis," *American Journal of Ophthalmology*, vol. 63, no. 3, pp. 524–527, 1967.

[7] J. A. Shields, *Orbital Osseous, Fibro-Osseous, and Cartilaginous Tumors, Diagnosis and Management of Orbital Tumors*, WB Saunders, Philadelphia, 1989.

[8] J. Sebag, P. Chapman, J. Truman, and R. R. Riemersma, "Giant cell granuloma of the orbit with intracranial extension," *Neurosurgery*, vol. 16, no. 1, pp. 75–78, 1985.

[9] P. C. Hoopes, R. L. Anderson, and F. C. Blodi, "Giant cell (reparative) granuloma of the orbit," *Ophthalmology*, vol. 88, no. 12, pp. 1361–1366, 1981.

[10] S. Hirschl and A. Katz, "Giant cell reparative granuloma outside the jaw bone: diagnostic criteria and review of the literature with the first case described in the temporal bone," *Human Pathology*, vol. 5, no. 2, pp. 171–181, 1974.

[11] C. Reis, J. M. Lopes, E. Carneiro et al., "Temporal giant cell reparative granuloma: a reappraisal of pathology and imaging features," *AJNR American Journal of Neuroradiology*, vol. 27, no. 8, pp. 1660–1662, 2006.

[12] A. L. D'Ambrosio, S. C. Williams, A. Lignelli et al., "Clinicopathological review: giant cell reparative granuloma of the orbit," *Neurosurgery*, vol. 57, no. 4, pp. 773–778, 2005.

[13] L. F. Sinks and D. L. Gang, "Case records of the Massachusetts General Hospital. Weekly clinicopathological exercises. Case 10-1984. Proptosis of the eye of an eight-year-old boy," *New England Journal of Medicine*, vol. 310, no. 10, pp. 642–648, 1984.

[14] R. L. Font, G. Blanco, C. N. Soparkar, J. R. Patrinely, and M. L. Ostrowski, "Giant cell reparative granuloma of the orbit associated with cherubism," *Ophthalmology*, vol. 110, no. 9, pp. 1846–1849, 2003.

[15] J. Rootman and D. Selva, *Primary Bone Tumors of the Orbit. Diseases of the Orbit*, Lippincott Williams & Wilkins, Philadelphia, 1988.

[16] G. A. Smith and P. H. Ward, "Giant-cell lesions of the facial skeleton," *Archives of Otolaryngology*, vol. 104, no. 4, pp. 186–190, 1978.

[17] F. Ung, K. K. Li, D. A. Keith, and M. J. McKenna, "Giant cell reparative granuloma of the temporal bone: case report and review of the literature," *Otolaryngology–Head and Neck Surgery*, vol. 118, no. 4, pp. 525–529, 1998.

[18] X. Hu, T. Yuan, L. Lou, Y. Wang, Y. Liu, and G. Quan, "Cervical-thoracic epidural giant cell reparative granuloma: case report and review of the literature," *World Neurosurgery*, vol. 136, pp. 66–69, 2020.

[19] E. M. Tallan, K. D. Olsen, T. V. McCaffrey, K. K. Unni, and B. A. Lund, "Advanced giant cell granuloma: a twenty-year study," *Otolaryngology–Head and Neck Surgery*, vol. 110, no. 4, pp. 413–418, 1994.

[20] J. A. Shields and C. L. Shields, *Osseous, fibroosseous, and cartilaginous tumors. Atlas of Orbital Tumors*, Lippincott Williams & Wilkins, Philadelphia, 2nd edition, 1999.

[21] K. Kim, T. Isu, R. Matsumoto, M. Isobe, and K. Kogure, "Surgical pitfalls of an ultrasonic bone curette (SONOPET) in spinal surgery," *Neurosurgery*, vol. 59, 4 Supplement 2, pp. ONS390–ONS393, 2006.

[22] I. Vrcek, V. Starks, R. Mancini, and G. Gilliland, "Use of an ultrasonic bone curette (Sonopet) in orbital and oculoplastic surgery," *Proceedings (Baylor University Medical Center)*, vol. 28, no. 1, pp. 91–93, 2015.

[23] J. A. Sivak-Callcott, J. V. Linberg, and S. Patel, "Ultrasonic bone removal with the Sonopet Omni: a new instrument for orbital and lacrimal surgery," *Archives of Ophthalmology*, vol. 123, no. 11, pp. 1595–1597, 2005.

[24] S. Y. Sun, K. Stewart, S. Lyford-Pike, J. A. Garrity, A. R. Harrison, and A. Mokhtarzadeh, "Ultrasonic aspiration for debulking infiltrative masses of the orbit," *Ophthalmic Plastic and Reconstructive Surgery*, vol. 36, no. 2, pp. 198–201, 2020.

[25] E. J. Wladis and T. J. Kenning, "Cavitron ultrasonic surgical aspirator-assisted resection of combined orbital and intracranial tumors," *Orbit*, vol. 33, no. 3, pp. 234-235, 2014.

[26] Á. Bengoa-González, M. D. Lago-Llinás, E. Mencía-Gutiérrez, A. Martín-Clavijo, E. Salvador, and M. Gimeno-Carrero, "Surgical removal of orbital tumors by orbital approach using ultrasonic surgical system SONOPET®," *Orbit*, pp. 1–10, 2021.

[27] B. R. Chrcanovic, C. C. Gomes, and R. S. Gomez, "Peripheral giant cell granuloma: an updated analysis of 2824 cases reported in the literature," *Journal of Oral Pathology & Medicine*, vol. 47, no. 5, pp. 454–459, 2018.

10

Gas Expansion Three Days after Pars Plana Vitrectomy with Sulfur Hexafluoride 20% Tamponade following Carbon Monoxide Toxicity and Oxygen Therapy

Mojtaba Abrishami, Mehrdad Motamed Shariati, Ali Bolouki, and Ghodsieh Zamani

Eye Research Center, Mashhad University of Medical Sciences, Mashhad, Iran

Correspondence should be addressed to Mehrdad Motamed Shariati; mehrdad_shariati2005@yahoo.com

Academic Editor: Stephen G. Schwartz

Purpose. To report an unusual case of gas expansion following oxygen therapy in a patient with sulfur hexafluoride (SF_6) 20% tamponade after pars plana vitrectomy. *Case Report.* A 40-year-old man came to the clinic with severe ocular pain and redness and also vision decrease in his left eye three days after uncomplicated 23-gauge pars plana vitrectomy, internal limiting membrane peeling combined with phacoemulsification, and using 20% SF_6 injection as a tamponade agent due to significant cataract and a full-thickness macular hole. In ophthalmic examinations of his left eye, high intraocular pressure (approximately 70 mmHg), a flat anterior chamber, and a gas-filled vitreous cavity were found. The patient had been hospitalized the day before due to carbon monoxide poisoning and had undergone oxygen therapy with a pure 100% mask for three hours. *Conclusion.* It seems that oxygen therapy or carbon monoxide poisoning increases the volume of gas in the patient's vitreous cavity and the nonexpansile percentage of SF_6 expands.

1. Introduction

Pars plana vitrectomy normally ends with an empty vitreous cavity which usually needs tamponade. The physical properties of the gases (air, sulfur hexafluoride (SF_6), perfluoroethane (C_2F_6), and perfluoropropane (C_3F_8)) include interfacial surface tension and buoyancy, which have led to their use as tamponing agents in vitreoretinal surgeries for many years [1]. Because of the lower density, gas bubbles float on the surface of liquids. A small bubble of gas can cover a large area of the retina following the surgery [2]. The use of gases in vitreoretinal surgeries has known side effects such as raised intraocular pressure (IOP), gas migration, and cataract formation [3, 4]. Increased IOP is a vision-threatening complication following gas injection which mainly occurs due to gas expansion. The lower water solubility of pure gases (SF_6, C_2F_6, and C_3F_8) than nitrogen leads to dissolving nitrogen in gas and increasing its volume. This is especially exacerbated when the patient is anesthetized with nitrous oxide (N_2O) gas [2]. To prevent gas expansion, the surgeon dilutes the gas with air before injection [5]. The highest concentration of gas in the vitreous space that does not expand is called the isovolumic concentration. Studies have shown that this concentration is 20-25%, 16%, and 14-18% for SF_6, C_2F_6, and C_3F_8, respectively [3, 5].

In this report, we are going to introduce an unusual case of gas expansion following oxygen therapy for carbon monoxide (CO) poisoning three days after pars plana vitrectomy with a nonexpansile percentage of diluted SF_6 (20%) injection as a tamponade.

2. Case Presentation

A 40-year-old man came to the clinic because of decreased vision in his left eye. He underwent phacoemulsification with posterior chamber intraocular lens combined with 23-gauge pars plana vitrectomy, internal limiting membrane peeling, and 20% SF_6 injection as a tamponading agent due to significant cataract and a full-thickness macular hole. The surgery was done under general anesthesia, and it was uncomplicated. The N_2O gas was not used during the operation. After the fluid-air exchange, the surgeon used the following technique for gas-air exchange to ensure the accuracy of the injected gas concentration. Ten milliliters (ml) of pure SF_6 (Alcon, Inc., Fort Worth, TX) was drawn up in a 50 ml syringe and diluted with room air through a Millipore filter. One of the sclerotomies was sutured with coated Vicryl (polyglactin 910) 7-0 suture (Ethicon, Johnson & Johnson, Raritan, NJ), and then, the 50 ml isovolumic concentration of SF_6 (20% SF_6) was flushed into the vitreous cavity through the other two sclerotomies. Finally, all sclerotomies were sutured while the intraocular pressure (IOP) seems normal. The morning after surgery, the patient was examined. Besides mild corneal edema, the rest of the examinations were unremarkable. The anterior chamber was deep and formed, and the vitreous cavity was filled with gas. The IOP was 12 mmHg. After 3 days, he referred with pain and redness in his left eye. The best-corrected visual acuity was hand motion (HM) detection. In ophthalmic examinations of his left eye, we found high IOP (approximately 70 mmHg with Goldmann applanation tonometer), diffuse corneal microcystic edema, and forward dislocation of the IOL and iris diaphragm with the flat anterior chamber, and a gas-filled vitreous cavity (Figure 1). The patient had been hospitalized the day before due to carbon monoxide poisoning and had undergone oxygen therapy with a pure 100% mask for three hours. We prepared the patient to be transferred to the operating room for gas adjustment surgery. Under sterile conditions and local anesthesia, 0.4 milliliters of gas was aspirated from the vitreous cavity with a 27-gauge needle in the operating room. Two hours after the surgery, the IOP reached 10 mmHg with no IOP lowering medications. In the next 2 weeks of follow-up examinations, there was no IOP rise and the patient needs no antihypertensive medications.

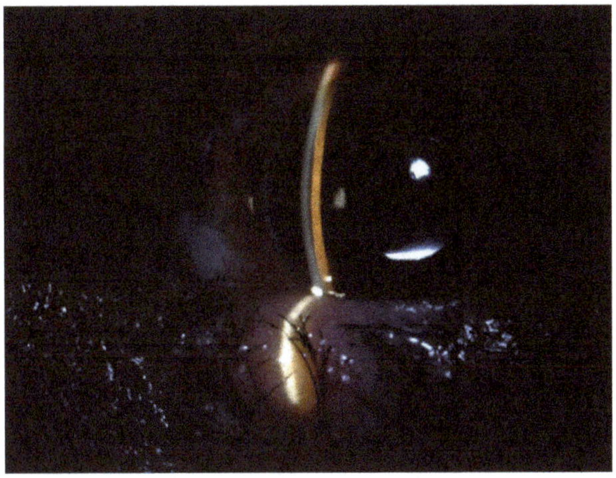

FIGURE 1: Forward dislocation of posterior chamber intraocular lens and iris with shallow anterior chamber.

3. Discussion

Sulfur hexafluoride is a nontoxic, inert, and insoluble gas in aqueous humor. When pure SF_6 is injected into the eye, it will expand because the rate at which nitrogen dissolves in gas is greater than the gas absorption into the surrounding tissue fluid compartment. This increase in volume stops when the concentration of nitrogen in the gas and blood reaches equilibrium. The absorption of the gas approximated a first-order kinetic equation concerning bubble volume [2].

During the expansion phase, intraocular pressure will rise and it will be sight threatening [6]. Using an isovolumic concentration of SF_6 (20%) makes this complication the minimum. Even when the isovolumic concentration of gas is injected into the vitreous cavity, it is recommended not to use N_2O for anesthesia [5]. In this case, due to not using N_2O gas throughout the surgery, an increase in gas volume following the dissolution of nitrogen seems unlikely.

One of the most common post pars plana vitrectomy complications in gas-filled eyes is IOP rise [6–8]. Different mechanisms have been reported including open-angle due to gas expansion and angle-closure as a result of anterior displacement of the lens-iris diaphragm and iridocorneal apposition. Among the risk factors for increasing IOP are the patient's older age, the surgeon's mistake in estimating the gas concentration, and previous scleral buckle surgery [9–11]. This IOP increment can be extremely harmful to patients with impaired optic nerve head circulation. In our case, the surgeon used the most accurate method available to inject the gas at the desired concentration. As described earlier, in this method, first, the pure gas is diluted to the desired concentration and then lavaged inside the vitreous space. This technique is safer than injecting a small volume of pure gas into an air-filled eye to achieve a diluted gas mixture because the volume of the air in the vitreous cavity cannot be determined with sufficient accuracy. Furthermore, the patient's IOP was within the normal range on the first day after the surgery, while in the case of injection of higher concentrations of gas, we should have seen an increase in IOP during this period [11]. It can be concluded that the hypothesis of increasing the gas volume due to injection of incorrect concentration seems unlikely.

Although we do not know the exact amount and duration of the patient's treatment with oxygen, it seems that oxygen therapy following carbon monoxide poisoning increases the volume of gas in the patient's eye three days after the surgery. Oxygen (O_2) therapy in patients with CO poisoning separates CO molecules from hemoglobin (Hb) by competition mechanism. This process occurs in the respiratory system. Besides, the binding of the CO molecules to Hb is much stronger than that of O_2 to Hb [12]. According to this knowledge, the rate of release of CO molecules from Hb in peripheral tissues is low and the possibility of gas expansion due to the dissolution of CO molecules seems illogical. Following O_2 therapy, a higher percentage of Hb is saturated with oxygen, and it is possible that an increase in gas volume occurred following the dissolution of the released oxygen in the vitreous cavity.

Given that increased IOP following gas dilation can be potentially blinding, it is best to warn patients and other clinical staff to consult with an ophthalmologist for a vitrectomized and gas-filled patient who needs oxygen therapy.

Consent

Consent was obtained from the patient to publish examinations and imaging.

References

[1] B. Gupta, J. E. Neffendorf, and T. H. Williamson, "Trends and emerging patterns of practice in vitreoretinal surgery," *Acta ophthalmologica*, vol. 96, no. 7, pp. e889–e890, 2018.

[2] J. T. Thompson, "Kinetics of intraocular gases: disappearance of air, sulfur hexafluoride, and perfluoropropane after pars plana vitrectomy," *Archives of Ophthalmology*, vol. 107, no. 5, pp. 687–691, 1989.

[3] E. J. Sigler, J. C. Randolph, S. Charles, and J. I. Calzada, "Intravitreal fluorinated gas preference and occurrence of rare ischemic postoperative complications after pars plana vitrectomy: a survey of the American Society of Retina Specialists," *Journal of Ophthalmology*, vol. 2012, 5 pages, 2012.

[4] P. Kanclerz and A. Grzybowski, "Complications associated with the use of expandable gases in vitrectomy," *Journal of ophthalmology*, vol. 2018, 7 pages, 2018.

[5] M. Shunmugam, S. Shunmugam, T. H. Williamson, and D. A. Laidlaw, "Air-gas exchange reevaluated: clinically important results of a computer simulation," *Investigative Ophthalmology & Visual Science*, vol. 52, no. 11, pp. 8262–8265, 2011.

[6] L. T. Lim, E. Y. Ah-Kee, B. P. House, and J. D. Walker, "The management of gas-filled eyes in the emergency department," *Case Reports in Emergency Medicine*, vol. 2014, Article ID 347868, 3 pages, 2014.

[7] M. G. Krzystolik and D. J. D'Amico, "Complications of intraocular tamponade: silicone oil versus intraocular gas," *International ophthalmology clinics*, vol. 40, no. 1, pp. 187–200, 2000.

[8] D. M. Rooney, M. H. Oltmanns, M. R. Sapp, and R. E. Morris, "Necrosis of the retina and uveal tract secondary to expanding gas tamponade," *Retinal Cases and Brief Reports*, vol. 15, no. 5, pp. 523–526, 2021.

[9] D. P. Han, H. Lewis, F. H. Lambrou Jr., W. F. Mieler, and A. Hartz, "Mechanisms of intraocuular pressure elevation after pars plana vitrectomy," *Ophthalmology*, vol. 96, no. 9, pp. 1357–1362, 1989.

[10] S. Chang, H. A. Lincoff, D. J. Coleman, W. Fuchs, and M. E. Farber, "Perfluorocarbon gases in vitreous surgery," *Ophthalmology*, vol. 92, no. 5, pp. 651–656, 1985.

[11] C. J. Chen, "Glaucoma after macular hole surgery," *Ophthalmology*, vol. 105, no. 1, pp. 94–100, 1998.

[12] S. R. Thorn and L. W. Keim, "Carbon monoxide poisoning: a review epidemiology, pathophysiology, clinical findings, and treatment options including hyperbaric oxygen therapy," *Journal of Toxicology: Clinical Toxicology*, vol. 27, no. 3, pp. 141–156, 1989.

11

Ophthalmic Surgery in Patients with Left Ventricular Assist Devices

George A. Dumas, Ayesha S. Bryant, and Gwendolyn L. Boyd

University of Alabama at Birmingham, Department of Anesthesiology and Perioperative Medicine, Birmingham, Alabama, USA

Correspondence should be addressed to George A. Dumas; gadumas@uabmc.edu

Academic Editor: Nicola Rosa

The newer generation of left ventricular assist devices (LVADs) are commonly used as destination therapy; these devices have demonstrated improved outcomes and increased survival. Given the longer lifespan, it is not surprising that patients with LVADS are increasingly presenting with noncardiac, chronic diseases and interventions for their treatment. This includes ophthalmic procedures in patients with LVAD. There is a paucity of literature about the experiences and outcomes in this cohort of patients presenting for ophthalmologic surgery. Here we present a case series consisting of 7 patients with LVAD that underwent 10 ophthalmic surgeries. No adverse events including intraoperative hemodynamic instability or respiratory compromise occurred. All patients had an on-time discharge with no 30-day recidivism. Most patients underwent a phacoemulsification with intraocular lens implantation and received a topical with intracameral anesthetic. We attribute these successful outcomes to a standardized clinical workflow consisting of careful preoperative screening, communication and presence of VAD coordinator, continuation of antithrombotics, monitoring based on presence of pulsatile flow, and a plan for rapid transfer if needed.

1. Introduction

Left ventricular assist devices (LVADs) are being encountered more frequently in patients undergoing ophthalmic procedures but there is little information or experience with this patient population in the outpatient setting. LVADs provide mechanical circulatory support for patients with advanced heart failure. In the 1990s, LVADs were initially developed as a bridge to cardiac transplantation in patients with advanced cardiac failure [1]. As these devices have evolved over time, LVADs have been increasingly used as destination therapy [2]. Newer second generation devices, including the Heartmate II, use axial continuous flow for circulatory support [1]. Third generation devices, including HeartWare and DuraHeart, use centrifugal continuous flow [1]. Outcomes have been improved with the newer continuous flow LVADs [1]. The number of patients using these devices has increased accordingly and lifespans of these patients have also been increased [3]. Often, patients survive several years on these devices and develop noncardiac chronic diseases [4]. As overall quality of life improves for these patients, vision related quality of life should be addressed as well. Since quality of life is enhanced with improved vision, we present a case series of ophthalmic procedures performed on this challenging patient population.

2. Case Presentation

The University of Alabama's Institutional Review Board approved conduct of this study. Findings from the medical records of seven patients with LVADs undergoing 10 ophthalmic surgery procedures are summarized in Table 1. The median patient age was 72 years (range, 40-78). LVAD type was the Heartmate II (Thoratec, Pleasanton, CA). All patients were continued on their antithrombotic medications perioperatively. Cataract surgery performed under topical with intracameral anesthesia, without any sedation, was the most common scenario (8 cases). The longest case (59 min), phaco/IOL/vitrectomy/ERM peel, was performed with retrobulbar block on a patient taking uninterrupted Coumadin 2 mg qod and 3 mg qod with INR 1.8. One corneal case involving EDTA chelation, keratectomy, and amniotic membrane placement was performed under sub-Tenon's block on a

TABLE 1: Patient characteristics and intraoperative data of patients with Left Ventricular Assist Device (LVAD) that underwent ophthalmic surgery.

Case	Age/gender	LVAD type	Procedure	Anesthesia	Sedation	Surgical time (mins)	OR time (mins)
1	72 /M	Heartmate II	Phaco/Iol	Topical+ intracameral	none	10	57
2	72 /M	Heartmate II	Phaco/Iol	Topical+ intracameral	none	16	53
3	73 /M	Heartmate II	Phaco/Iol	Topical+ intracameral	none	6	32
4	72 /M	Heartmate II	Phaco/Iol	Topical+ intracameral	none	17	32
5	59 /F	Heartmate II	Phaco/Iol	Topical+ intracameral	none	10	34
6	59 /F	Heartmate II	Phaco/Iol	Topical+ intracameral	none	6	30
7	40 /F	Heartmate II	EDTA scrub/keratectomy/AMT	Sub-Tenon's block	none	22	48
8	78 /M	Heartmate II	Phaco/Iol/vitrectomy/IVA/ERM peel	Retrobulbar block	none	59	82
9	78 /M	Heartmate II	Phaco/Iol	Topical+ intracameral	none	8	29
10	52M	Heartmate II	Phaco/Iol	Topical+ intracameral	none	15	37

LVAD: left ventricular assist device, M: male, F: female, Phaco/lol: phacoemulsification with intraocular lens implantation, EDTA: ethylenediamine-tetraacetic acid, AMT: amniotic membrane transplantation, IVA: intravitreal avastin, and ERM: epiretinal membrane.

patient taking uninterrupted Coumadin 3 mg qd, aspirin 325 mg qd, and plavix 75 mg qd with INR 1.5. Median surgical and operating room times were 12.5 mins (range, 6-59) and 35.5 mins (range, 29-82), respectively. Supplemental oxygen was administered to all patients. Noninvasive blood pressure (NIBP) monitoring was utilized without Doppler assistance in all patients. Pulse oximetry was utilized in all cases with a monitored waveform and oxygen saturation recorded. No cases of respiratory or hemodynamic compromise were noted and blood loss was negligible in all cases. No complications were noted during the perioperative time through same day discharge. All patients had an on-time discharge with no 30-day recidivism.

3. Clinical Workflow

The surgical procedures were coordinated through the University of Alabama's Heart Failure Program (HFP). A ventricular assist device (VAD) coordinator from the HFP familiar with the patient and their LVAD accompanied the patient to the ambulatory surgery unit and remained with the patient through discharge. The coordinator monitored flow, rpm, pulsatility index, and mean pressure on the flow console which they brought with them. The Heartmate II's have long lasting batteries and are smaller than previous generation LVADs which enhanced mobility. Our anticoagulation protocol for patients that received blocks (retrobulbar and sub-Tenon's) was to continue these medications as prescribed by cardiology throughout the perioperative period. We routinely block anticoagulated patients in our facility provided their therapies are not supratherapeutic. While the ambulatory facility did not house their own intensive care unit, X-ray capability, blood bank, or extensive lab capabilities, there was a process for rapid direct transfer to the University's Heart Failure Unit if needed. The patients were uniformly pleased to have their ophthalmic procedures performed and reported minimal discomfort.

Our series included seven LVAD patients who underwent 10 ophthalmic surgeries. Other reports in the literature cite the management of up to three LVAD patients having four cataract surgeries [5, 6]. In our experience, these procedures can be safely performed in a resource limited ambulatory facility, such as an ambulatory surgery center, provided a close working relationship with the VAD center is in place. The advantages of working with the VAD center include in-depth knowledge of the patients and their devices as well as a plan in place to facilitate rapid transfer to a higher acuity setting if needed. An advantage of utilizing an ambulatory center, provided this is where the clinician performs the vast majority of their cases, includes familiarity with staff, equipment, and supplies. The patients in this series all had enough pulsatile flow to allow use of NIBP monitors and pulse oximetry. In patients without pulsatile flow, other monitoring options exist. Options for blood pressure monitoring in patients without pulsatile flow include use of Doppler ultrasound while slowly deflating the blood pressure cuff, placement of an arterial catheter under ultrasound guidance, and intermittently turning down the flow on continuous flow devices to allow pressure measurement via oscillometry. For periodic oxygenation monitoring in patients without pulsatile flow, options include intermittently turning down the flow on continuous flow devices for pulse oximetry and arterial blood gas sampling from an arterial line. For continuous oxygenation monitoring in patients without pulsatile flow, options include use of cerebral oximetry, which does not require pulsatile flow, and continuous central venous saturation catheters. A monitoring plan should be in place for patients without pulsatile flow, particularly if surgery will take place at an ambulatory surgery center. While sedation may be helpful in some cases, it was not necessary in these highly motivated patients.

In summary, during the preoperative period, it is necessary to know the type of LVAD, to continue antithrombotics, and have the VAD coordinator on site. Intraoperatively, usual monitors may be used with pulsatile flow but Doppler ultrasound, arterial catheterization, cerebral oximetry, and intermittently decreasing device flow may be required in patients without pulsatile flow. Sedation is not always required. Postoperatively, patients are expected to go home, but a transfer plan to a higher acuity facility should be in place.

Authors' Contributions

All authors (George A. Dumas MD, Ayesha S. Bryant MSPH, MD, Gwendolyn L. Boyd MD) have made substantial contributions to this case series report (acquisition of data and interpretation of findings), participated in the writing of the manuscript and/or critical review of the report, provided final approval of this version for publication, and agree to be accountable for all aspects of the work including its accuracy and integrity.

References

[1] S. Kadakia, R. Moore, V. Ambur, and Y. Toyoda, "Current status of the implantable LVAD," *General Thoracic and Cardiovascular Surgery*, vol. 64, no. 9, pp. 501–508, 2016.

[2] P. Sutcliffe, M. Connock, R. Pulikottil-Jacob et al., "Clinical effectiveness and cost-effectiveness of second- and third-generation left ventricular assist devices as either bridge to transplant or alternative to transplant for adults eligible for heart transplantation: Systematic review and cost-effectiveness model," *Health Technology Assessment*, vol. 17, no. 53, pp. 171–499, 2013.

[3] M. Stone, J. Hinchey, C. Sattler, and A. Evans, "Trends in the management of patients with left ventricular assist devices presenting for noncardiac surgery: A 10-year institutional experience," *Seminars in Cardiothoracic and Vascular Anesthesia*, vol. 20, no. 3, pp. 197–204, 2016.

[4] S. H. McKellar, D. S. Morris, W. J. Mauermann, S. J. Park, and S. P. Zietlow, "Evolution of general surgical problems in patients with left ventricular assist devices," *Surgery*, vol. 152, no. 5, pp. 896–902, 2012.

[5] A. O. Eghrari, R. J. Rivers, M. Alkharashi, F. Rajaii, D. Nyhan, and S. Sikder, "Cataract surgery in patients with left ventricular assist device support," *Journal of Cataract & Refractive Surgery*, vol. 40, no. 4, pp. 675–678, 2014.

[6] A. Yang and J. Liu, "Sequential cataract surgeries in a patient with a left ventricular assist device (LVAD)," *BMJ Case Reports*, Article ID 162018, 2018.

12

Argon Laser Synechiolysis for Irido-Corneal Adhesion

Saeed Shokoohi-Rad, Samaneh Gholamhoseinpour-Omran, Hamed Hosseinikhah-Manshadi, and Mohammad Baghi Yazdi

Eye Research Center, Mashhad University of Medical Sciences, Mashhad, Iran

Correspondence should be addressed to Saeed Shokoohi-Rad; shokoohirads@gmail.com

Academic Editor: Kamal Kishore

Purpose. To introduce a new method for treating irido-corneal adhesion (ICA) by using argon laser. *Case Presentation.* A 60-year-old woman with advanced glaucoma who is undergoing trabeculectomy. In follow-up visits, choroidal effusion and iridocorneal adhesion were seen in the examination. The massive choroidal effusion was treated with medical therapy. In further follow-up examination, ICA was repaired with argon laser. *Result.* Early laser treatment prior to surgical management is suggested in postoperative synechia. *Conclusion.* Early argon laser synechiolysis is a less-invasive procedure which prevents probable surgical complications such as local detachment of Descemet's membrane or bleeding in surgical synechiolysis.

1. Introduction

There has been great progress in uses of lasers for many forms of procedures to treating glaucoma. Some of the procedures include argon laser trabeculoplasty, selective laser trabeculoplasty, endoscopic cyclophotocoagulation, and laser-assisted deep sclerotomy. Other applications of laser procedures such as suture lysis, bleb reopening, and iris adhesion lysis for posterior and anterior synechiae exist in this treatment field [1].

In this study, we introduce one of the laser technique applications for irido-corneal adhesion (ICA) which is formed sometimes after trabeculectomy in patients with advanced glaucoma. In this case, we reported a patient with early successful treatment of irido-corneal adhesion with argon laser synechiolysis.

2. Case Presentation

A 60-year-old woman was referred to and eye hospital for continuing glaucoma management. The patient had history of angle closure glaucoma and cataract surgery of the right eye last year. In the initial evaluation, best corrected vision for both the right and left eyes was 6/10; relative afferent pupillary defect (RAPD) was 2+ for the right eye. The right eye was pseudophakic. Intraocular pressure (IOP) was 25 mmHg while using brimonidine tartrate 0.2%, dorzolamide 2%, timolol 0.5%, and latanoprost. IOP for the left eye was 10 mmHg without medication. The cup-to-disc ratio was recorded 100% for the right and 80% for the left eye. Both eyes had 270 degrees of peripheral anterior synechiae in gonioscopy.

The patient was a candidate for right eye trabeculectomy. Surgery was concluded by an experienced surgeon in glaucoma without complications during the operation. At follow-up visits, days 1 and 3 and a week after surgery, the eye was moderately injected, IOP was 12,9,11, respectively, and funduscopy was normal.

Two weeks after surgery, the patient returned again to the glaucoma clinic with complaints of decreased visual acuity. The intraocular pressure (IOP) was 17 for the right eye, and anterior chamber was flat symmetrically at peripheral and central, grade 2, and the bleb was low lying and focal (not diffuse). The diagnosis was malignant glaucoma, and soon, IZHV (irido zonular hyaloid vitrectomy) was done for patient. According to the probable mechanism of malignant glaucoma, most of aqueous misdirection fluids are accumulated and lobulated around the equator of lens;

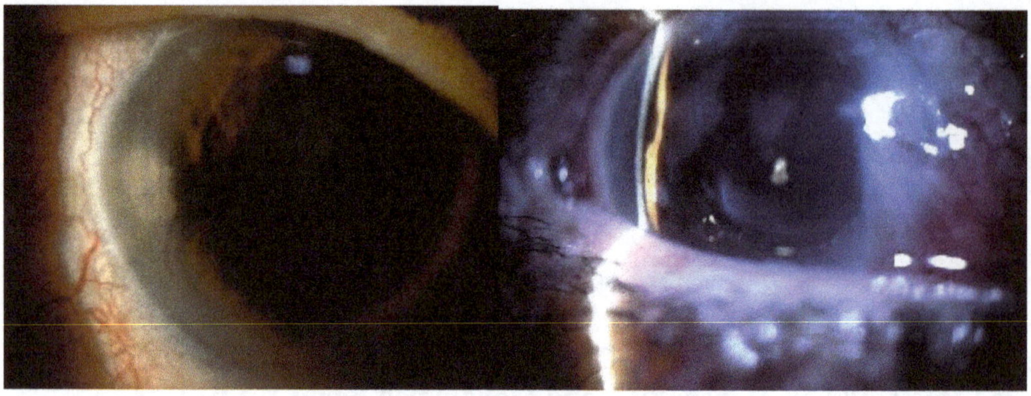

FIGURE 1: Slit lamp photograph of the right eye shows focal irido-corneal adhesion before argon laser synechiolysis.

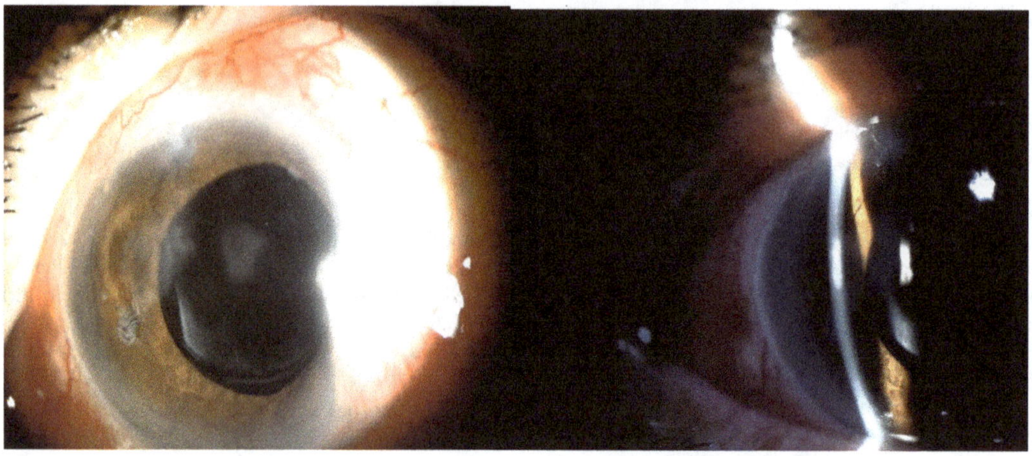

FIGURE 2: Slit lamp photograph of the same eye after argon laser synechiolysis showing symmetric deep anterior chamber.

hence, the preferred intervention for this kind of patient is IZHV [2, 3]. Based on a review by Debrouwere et al., IZHV was a treatment of choice in management of malignant glaucoma in comparison with posterior YAG capsulotomy [4].

In the next follow-up, nearly 10 days after IZHV, IOP was 7 mmHg, and on B-scan examination, nonmassive choroidal effusion was seen, since there was no indication of surgery for the patient; the patient was treated with tablet prednisolone 50 mg daily and followed closely. ICA (about one clock hour) was observed after healing of the choroidal effusion (Figure 1).

Then, the patient undergone argon laser synechiolysis with spot size 100 micron, 0.1 second, and power 400 mW near the adhesion site. The anterior chamber was immediately deepened and formed in 360 degrees after argon laser synechiolysis. In subsequent follow-ups, the IOP was 11 mmHg, and anterior chamber was deep and formed, and there was no choroidal effusion (Figure 2).

Due to successful experience of this case, since ICA is a common complication in anterior segment surgeries (including DSAEK, PK, and Phaco) in the future, argon laser can be used as a supporting treatment for this complications.

3. Discussion

Laser treatment in glaucoma continues to evolve with attitude towards primary and earlier intervention. Initial usage of argon laser trabeculoplasty was demonstrated by Wise and Witter which was effective for lowering intraocular pressure (IOP) [5, 6].

Development of new laser techniques results to be an essential role for glaucoma treatment. Laser technique is a safe and effective therapeutic approach for posttrabeculectomy suture lysis, closing cyclodialysis cleft, enlarging miotic pupil, and removing peripheral anterior synechiae from the angle of cornea [7].

Peripheral anterior synechiae in early stage is removed by setting (400–800 mW, 0.1–0.2 second, 50–100 μm spot size) as same as iridoplasty. It is essential to break down irido-corneal adhesin after trabeculectomy or penetrating keratoplasty in early stage. In our case, this procedure fourteen days after adhesion formation was successful, hence seems argon laser is not effective for chronic form of synechiae due to firmly adherent of iris to cornea [8].

Laser technique can reduce some surgical complication, for example, anterior synechiae removal by surgical dissection may have risks of local detachment of Descemet's membrane or bleeding. In this case, we support argon laser for lysis irido-corneal adhesion with nearly half of the mentioned power and spot size in early stage.

Consent

Consent for publication was acquired from the patient.

Authors' Contributions

All the authors contributed significantly to this report, and all authors agree to be accountable for all aspects of the work. All authors read and approved the final manuscript.

References

[1] F. Ekici, M. Waisbourd, and L. J. Katz, "Current and future of laser therapy in the management of glaucoma," *The Open Ophthalmology Journal*, vol. 10, no. 1, pp. 56–67, 2016.

[2] S. T. Ruben, J. Tsai, and R. A. Hitchings, "Malignant glaucoma and its management," *British Journal of Ophthalmology*, vol. 81, no. 2, pp. 163–167, 1997.

[3] H. Shahid and J. F. Salmon, "Malignant glaucoma: a review of the modern literature," *Journal of Ophthalmology*, vol. 2012, 6 pages, 2012.

[4] V. Debrouwere, P. Stalmans, J. Van Calster, W. Spileers, T. Zeyen, and I. Stalmans, "Outcomes of different management options for malignant glaucoma: a retrospective study," *Clinical and Experimental Ophthalmology*, vol. 250, no. 1, pp. 131–141, 2012.

[5] J. B. Wise and S. L. Witter, "Argon laser therapy for open-angle glaucoma," *Archives of Ophthalmology*, vol. 97, no. 2, pp. 319–322, 1979.

[6] J. B. Wise, "Long-term control of adult open angle glaucoma by argon laser treatment," *Ophthalmology*, vol. 88, no. 3, pp. 197–202, 1981.

[7] J. J. Meyer and S. D. Lawrence, "What's new in laser treatment for glaucoma," *Current Opinion in Ophthalmology*, vol. 23, no. 2, pp. 111–117, 2012.

[8] Y. El-Shabrawi, "Management of posterior synechiae, peripheral anterior synechiae, iridocorneal adhesions, and iridectomy," in *Surgical Management of Inflammatory Eye Disease*, Springer, Berlin, Heidelberg, 2008.

13

Orbital Cavernous Hemangioma Presenting with a Dome-Shaped Maculopathy-Like Appearance on Swept-Source Optical Tomography Imaging

Şükran Bekdemir,[1] **Ahmet Kaan Gündüz**,[2] **and Cevriye Cansız Ersöz**[3]

[1]*Ophthalmology Clinic, Polatlı Duatepe State Hospital, Ankara, Turkey*
[2]*Department of Ophthalmology, Ankara University Faculty of Medicine, Ankara, Turkey*
[3]*Department of Pathology, Ankara University Faculty of Medicine, Ankara, Turkey*

Correspondence should be addressed to Ahmet Kaan Gündüz; drkaangunduz@gmail.com

Academic Editor: Kevin J. Blinder

A 43-year-old patient presented with painless proptosis, limited upgaze, and vision loss in the right eye. Funduscopic examination revealed right optic disc edema and subtle macular compression. Swept-source optical coherence tomography (SS-OCT) revealed a smooth contoured elevation of the posterior pole without any distortion of retinal structures, an appearance closely simulating dome-shaped maculopathy. Swept-source optical coherence tomography angiography (SS-OCTA) revealed normal retinal and choroidal vasculature. Orbital magnetic resonance imaging demonstrated a well-circumscribed intraconal mass compressing the globe and optic nerve in the right orbit. An anterior orbitotomy was performed, whereby the tumor was totally excised and diagnosed histopathologically as cavernous hemangioma. This case represents an orbital cavernous hemangioma touching the eyeball and producing compression of the posterior pole presenting with a dome-shaped maculopathy-like appearance on SS-OCT. SS-OCT and SS-OCTA are important noninvasive tools for evaluating the retinal and choroidal effects in orbital tumors.

1. Introduction

Orbital cavernous hemangioma or orbital venous malformation by the newer nomenclature is the most common benign orbital tumor in adults. It typically presents with unilateral progressive painless proptosis in middle-aged females. Other presenting features include vision loss, restricted eye movements, diplopia, choroidal folds, and optic disc edema [1, 2]. Orbital imaging with computed tomography and magnetic resonance imaging (MRI) usually demonstrates a round- or oval-shaped well-circumscribed orbital tumor and may identify features such as optic nerve or globe compression. In recent years, optical coherence tomography (OCT) and optical coherence tomography angiography (OCTA) have become important diagnostic tools in evalauating retinal and choroidal diseases.

We herein report an interesting case of orbital cavernous hemangioma touching the eyeball and producing compression of the posterior pole simulating the appearance of dome-shaped maculopathy (DSM) on swept-source optical coherence tomography (SS-OCT).

2. Case Presentation

A 43-year-old male presented with vision loss in the right eye of 2-month duration. No history of systemic or ocular disease and trauma was present. Thyroid function tests were within normal limits. There was no edema or ecchymosis on either side. Visual acuity was 20/400 OD and 20/20 OS. There was no myopia or hypermetropia in either eye. Intraocular pressures were 17 mmHg OU. There was no relative afferent pupil defect bilaterally. Eye motility was normal in both eyes with the exception of limited upgaze in the right eye. There was 7 mm proptosis on the right side (Figure 1(a)). Fundus examination revealed prominent optic

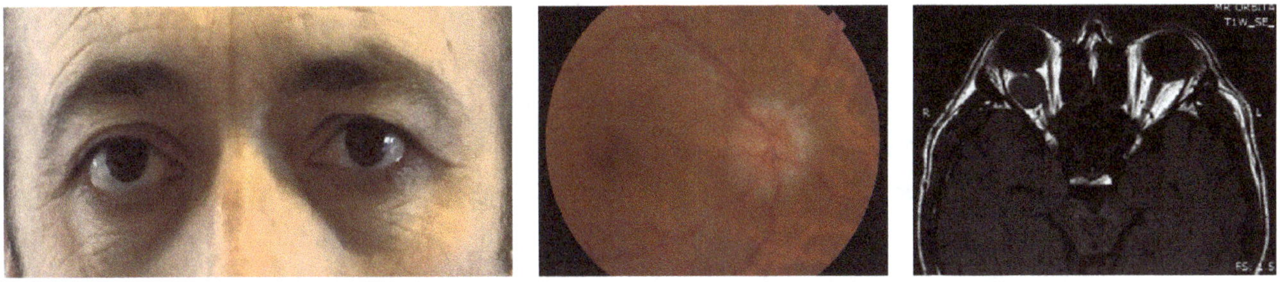

(a) (b) (c)

FIGURE 1: (a) Facial appearance of the patient at presentation. (b) Color fundus photograph of the right eye shows prominent optic disc edema and subtle macular compression. (c) Orbital T1-weighted axial magnetic resonance imaging shows an intraconal tumor isointense to the extraocular muscles producing compression of the globe and indenting the optic nerve.

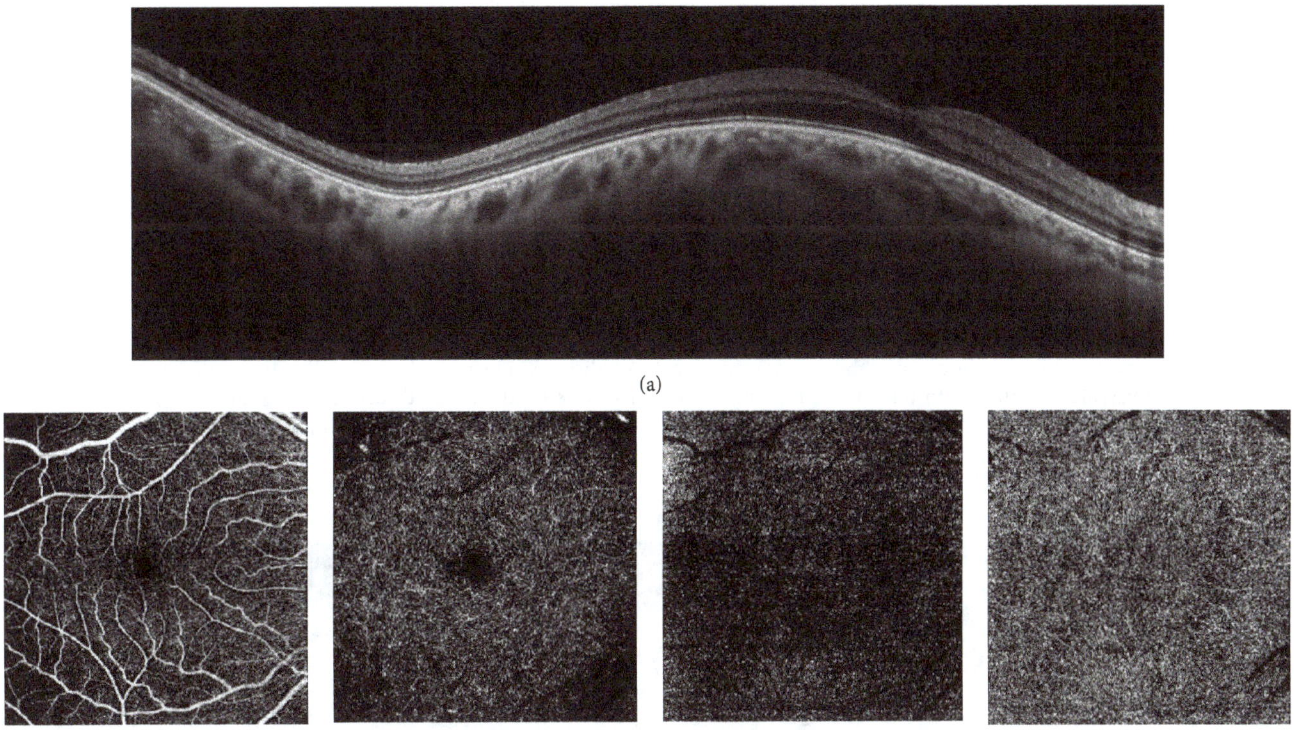

(a)

(b) (c) (d) (e)

FIGURE 2: (a) Swept-source optical coherence tomography through the fovea reveals a smooth contoured elevation of the posterior pole without any distortion of retinal structures, giving a dome-shaped maculopathy-like appearance. (b-e) Swept-source optical coherence tomography angiography images of superficial retinal plexus (b), deep retinal plexus (c), outer retina (d), and choriocapillaris (e) show normal retinal and choroidal vasculature patterns.

disc edema, subtle macular compression, and normal retinal vessels. Choroidal folds were not present (Figure 1(b)). Anterior segment and fundus examination in the left eye were normal. The patient underwent orbital MRI, which revealed an intraconal ovoid tumor compressing the globe posteriorly. The tumor displaced the lateral rectus laterally and optic nerve superomedially. The mass was isointense with respect to the extraocular muscles on T1-weighted images, hyperintense on T2-weighted images, and demonstrated contrast enhancement (Figure 1(c)).

SS-OCT (DRI OCT Triton plus, Topcon, Tokyo, Japan) operating at a speed of 100.000 A-scans/second revealed a smooth contoured elevation of the posterior pole without any distortion of retinal structures, an appearance closely simulating DSM (Figures 2(a)). There was no retinal traction or choroidal folds. Subfoveal choroidal thickness as measured by the automated choroidal scleral interface segmentation was 284 μm. Scleral thickness could not be measured. Swept-source optical coherence tomography angiography (SS-OCTA) revealed normal vascularisation in superficial and deep retinal plexi, outer retina, and choriocapillaris (Figure 2(b)–2(e)). An anterior orbitotomy was performed via the inferotemporal skin incision, and the tumor was totally removed with the help of a cryoprobe. The base

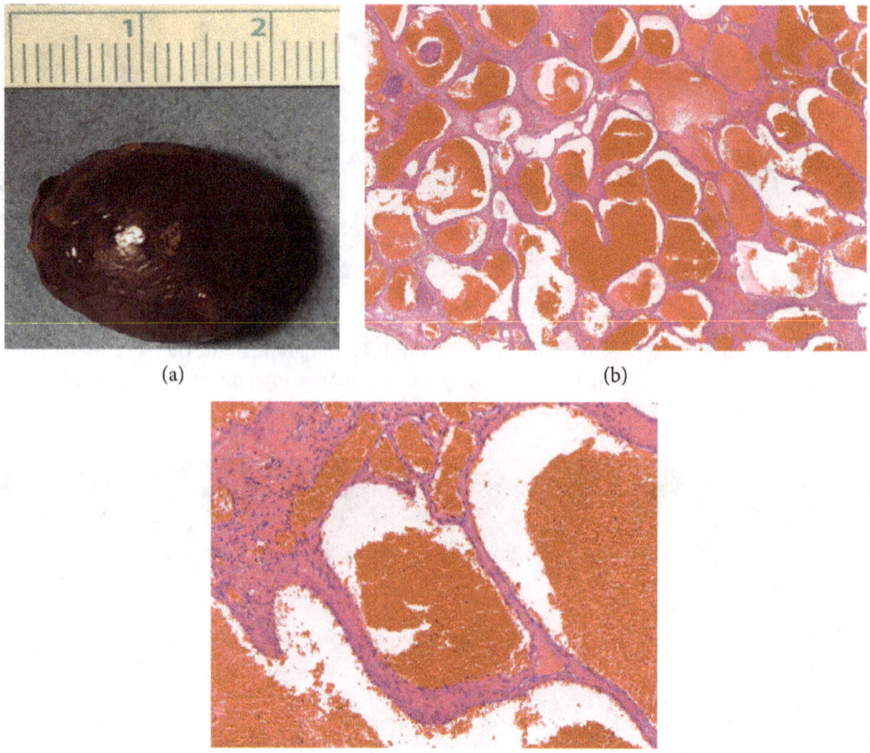

(a) (b) (c)

Figure 3: (a) Gross appearance of the excised orbital tumor showing the reddish well-circumscribed mass. (b) Histopathological examination reveals enlarged vascular channels with thick walls, the lumens of which were filled with erythrocytes, consistent with orbital cavernous hemangioma (H.E. × 20). (c) Higher magnification view of vascular structures lined by endothelium and filled with erythrocytes (H.E. × 100).

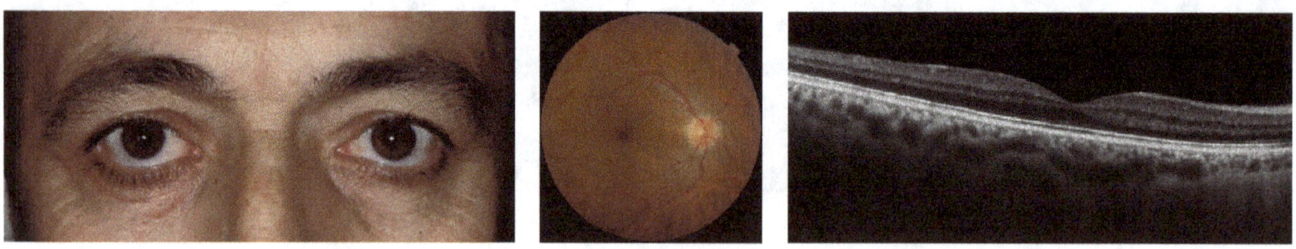

(a) (b) (c)

Figure 4: (a) Clinical appearance of the patient one month after orbitotomy showing that the right inferotemporal orbitotomy skin incision has nicely healed. (b) Fundus photograph shows significant resolution of optic disc edema and no macular compression. (c) Swept-source optical coherence tomography shows complete resolution of dome-shaped maculopathy-like appearance.

diameters of the excised reddish, smooth edged, capsulated mass measured approximately 2.5 × 1.5 cm (Figure 3(a)). Histopathological examination revealed enlarged vascular channels with thick walls, the lumens of which were filled with erythrocytes. The histopathological diagnosis was rendered as orbital cavernous hemangioma (Figures 3(b) and 3(c)). Ophthalmological examination 1 month after the surgery showed that the right orbitotomy skin incision had nicely healed (Figure 4(a)). Visual acuity improved to 20/20, and optic disc edema resolved significantly in the right eye (Figure 4(b)). SS-OCT showed complete resolution of the DSM-like appearance at the posterior pole (Figure 4(c)).

3. Discussion

Optical coherence tomography is a method that provides high-resolution cross-sectional imaging in biological tissues. In ophthalmology, it is widely used for noninvasive imaging of the posterior pole including the optic disc, macula, and choroid, in addition to anterior segment structures [3]. In our case, there was elevation in the macular area due to the orbital mass which compressed the globe from the posterior aspect. SS-OCT revealed the presence of a smooth contoured elevation of the posterior pole, an appearance closely simulating DSM. There was no distortion of retinal structures on SS-OCT and no retinal and choroidal vasculature changes were noted on SS-OCTA.

Dome-shaped maculopathy was first described as anterior protrusion of macula in the posterior staphyloma area of highly myopic patients. Subsequent studies indicated that DSM may also be present without posterior staphyloma [4, 5]. Although the pathophysiology is not clear, mechanisms such as localized thickening of the choroid, vitreoretinal traction, and posterior eye-wall collapse have been suggested as responsible factors. Subsequently, focal thickening of the subfoveal sclera has been proposed as a more likely mechanism, though the reason for the thickening is unknown [6]. Dome-shaped maculopathy is associated with high myopia (>6 diopters and axial length >26.5 mm) and its presence is positively correlated with the severity of myopic maculopathy. The prevalence of DSM in the general population is unknown. However, unilateral or bilateral DSM occurs in 10-20% of highly myopic patients [7–10]. Dome-shaped maculopathy was subsequently reported to occur in hereditary retinal dystrophies, central serous chorioretinopathy, and also in hypermetropic and emmetropic patients [5]. Dome-shaped maculopathy can be complicated by serous retinal detachment, choroidal neovascularization, and macular retinal pigment epithelial atrophy [8]. Our case was not myopic or hypermetropic in either eye. In addition, there were no evidence of other retinal problems alluded to in previous studies as possible etiologic factors for DSM. Choroidal thickness measurement was normal.

This case presents an interesting example of a DSM-like appearance on SS-OCT diagnosed in a patient with globe compression by an orbital cavernous hemangioma. Indirect ophthalmoscopy, fluorescein angiography, B mode ultrasonography, and MRI may be helpful in identifying globe compression caused by orbital tumors. Optical coherence tomography and OCTA, as noninvasive diagnostic tools, may reveal the retinal and choroidal changes better in such circumstances and without injection of dye.

Acknowledgments

The study was conducted according to the ethical tenets outlined in the Declaration of Helsinki as amended in 2013.

References

[1] J. Yan and Z. Wu, "Cavernous hemangioma of the orbit: analysis of 214 cases," *Orbit*, vol. 23, no. 1, pp. 33–40, 2004.

[2] J. A. Shields, C. L. Shields, and R. C. Eagle, "Cavernous hemangioma of the orbit," *Archives of Ophthalmology*, vol. 105, no. 6, p. 853, 1987.

[3] M. L. Gabriele, G. Wollstein, H. Ishikawa et al., "Optical coherence tomography: history, current status, and laboratory work," *Investigative Ophthalmology & Visual Science*, vol. 52, no. 5, pp. 2425–2436, 2011.

[4] D. Gaucher, A. Erginay, A. Lecleire-Collet et al., "Dome-shaped macula in eyes with myopic posterior staphyloma," *American Journal of Ophthalmology*, vol. 145, no. 5, pp. 909–914.e1, 2008.

[5] M. H. Errera, M. Michaelides, P. A. Keane et al., "The extended clinical phenotype of dome-shaped macula," *Graefe's Archive for Clinical and Experimental Ophthalmology*, vol. 252, no. 3, pp. 499–508, 2014.

[6] Y. Imamura, T. Iida, I. Maruko, S. A. Zweifel, and R. F. Spaide, "Enhanced depth imaging optical coherence tomography of the sclera in dome-shaped macula," *American Journal of Ophthalmology*, vol. 151, no. 2, pp. 297–302, 2011.

[7] A. Chebil, B. Ben Achour, N. Chaker, L. Jedidi, F. Mghaieth, and L. el Matri, "Choroidal thickness assessment with SD-OCT in high myopia with dome-shaped macula," *Journal Français d'Ophtalmologie*, vol. 37, no. 3, pp. 237–241, 2014.

[8] H. Ohsugi, Y. Ikuno, K. Oshima, T. Yamauchi, and H. Tabuchi, "Morphologic characteristics of macular complications of a dome-shaped macula determined by swept-source optical coherence tomography," *American Journal of Ophthalmology*, vol. 158, no. 1, pp. 162–170.e1, 2014.

[9] I. C. Liang, N. Shimada, Y. Tanaka et al., "Comparison of clinical features in highly myopic eyes with and without a dome-shaped macula," *Ophthalmology*, vol. 122, no. 8, pp. 1591–1600, 2015.

[10] X. Zhao, X. Ding, C. Lyu et al., "Observational study of clinical characteristics of dome-shaped macula in Chinese Han with high myopia at Zhongshan Ophthalmic Centre," *BMJ Open*, vol. 8, no. 12, 2018.

14

Huge Lateral Rectus Solitary Plasmacytoma Causing Shunt Extrusion

Nikoo Hamzeh,[1] **Mona Safizadeh**,[2] **Zohreh Nozarian**,[3] **Hiva Saffar**,[4] **and Seyed Mohsen Rafizadeh**[1]

[1]*Orbital and Oculoplastics Service, Farabi Eye Hospital, Tehran University of Medical Sciences, Tehran, Iran*
[2]*Glaucoma Service, Farabi Eye Hospital, Tehran University of Medical Sciences, Tehran, Iran*
[3]*Pathology Department, Farabi Eye Hospital, Tehran University of Medical Sciences, Tehran, Iran*
[4]*Pathology Department, Shariati Hospital, Tehran University of Medical Sciences, Tehran, Iran*

Correspondence should be addressed to Seyed Mohsen Rafizadeh; mohsen_raf1354@yahoo.com

Academic Editor: Stephen G. Schwartz

A 54-year-old man with a history of radiotherapy for right maxillary sinus plasmacytoma 3 years previously was referred to an orbital clinic with progressive proptosis in his right eye. His vision had deteriorated after an initial improvement after phacoemulsification 2 years before. He had undergone shunt implantation and later shunt removal following plate extrusion with the diagnosis of neovascular glaucoma following CRVO. His vision remained at no light perception afterwards, despite a controlled IOP with topical medications. In his CT scan, a large orbital mass was seen with lateral rectus involvement. He underwent deep orbitotomy for tumor resection following worsening of symptoms, and his symptoms were improved afterwards. Pathology report was consistent with plasmacytoma with anaplastic features. After tumor resection, he underwent another course of radiotherapy with complete remission of symptoms afterwards.

1. Introduction

Plasmacytoma is a rare tumor of small round cell or plasmacyte origin which can occur in the setting of systemic multiple myeloma or as a solitary tumor [1]. Orbital and ocular plasmacytomas are extremely rare. They may originate from the bone when involving the orbit [2] and can mimic other ocular neoplasms such as lymphoma, metastases, chondrosarcoma, or giant cell tumors [3]. Plasmacytomas of the orbit can present with diplopia, proptosis [4], and symptoms of orbital cellulitis as well. They may show unspecific imaging characteristics and may not be distinguished from other ocular tumors which would make their diagnosis more difficult [3]. Extramedullary plasmacytomas have been reported in 3% of multiple myeloma patients [2], and different treatment approaches such as excision, radiotherapy, or higher radiation doses that may damage ocular structures have been proposed [5].

2. Case Presentation

A 54-year-old man with a history of radiotherapy for right maxillary sinus plasmacytoma 3 years ago was referred to an orbital clinic with progressive proptosis in his right eye. His left eye had a vision of 5/10 (Snellen acuity chart), and except for a cataract, his examination was unremarkable. He had undergone uncomplicated phacoemulsification 2 years ago in his right eye with a best corrected visual acuity (BCVA) of 1/10, after which he had reported vision improvement; however, his vision had started to deteriorate at 4 months postoperatively. Initial examinations at that time did not find a specific cause for the patient's

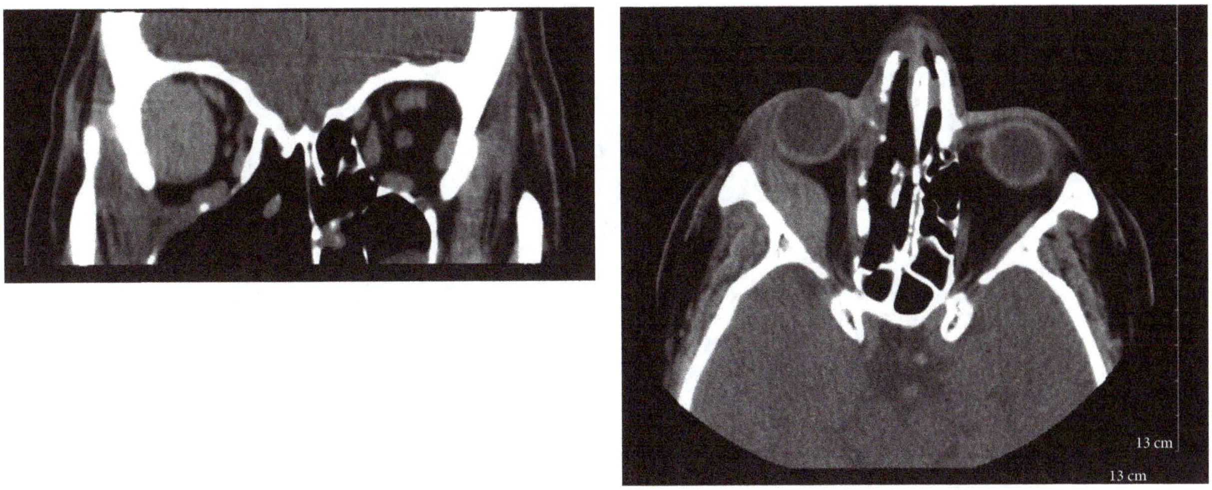

(a) (b)

Figure 1: Coronal (a) and axial (b) CT scans showing large orbital mass with lateral rectus involvement.

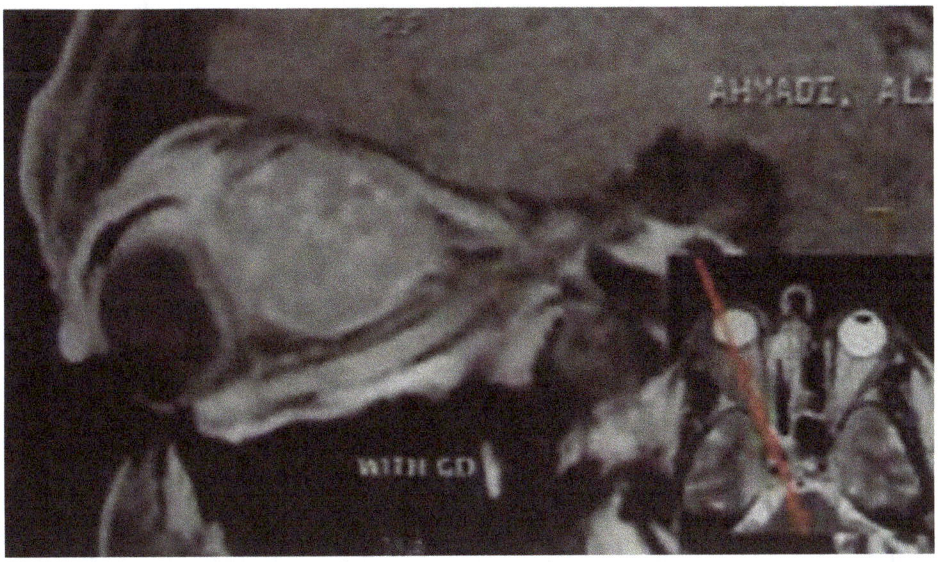

Figure 2: Sagittal MRI scan showing orbital mass with lateral rectus involvement.

vision loss. He had failed to follow up for subsequent examinations for 1.5 years afterwards.

He was referred to a glaucoma clinic with diagnosis of uncontrolled neovascular glaucoma (NVG) secondary to central retinal vein occlusion (CRVO) about 22 months after phacoemulsification. His vision was hand motion (HM) at that time, and he had mild proptosis in his right eye. Then, he underwent Ahmed glaucoma valve (AGV) implantation with intravitreal bevacizumab (IVB) injection. Panretinal photocoagulation was done after AGV implantation. However, AGV was removed 2 weeks later due to severe proptosis and plate extrusion. He was then referred to an orbital clinic with progressive proptosis and limitation of eye movement in all gazes. He had a vision of no light perception (NLP) at the time of examination with a pale optic disc and cup to disc ratio of 10/10. His intraocular pressure (IOP) was 18 mmHg with dorzolamide, timolol, brimonidine, and latanoprost. In his CT scan, a large orbital mass was seen with lateral rectus involvement (Figures 1 and 2) and he received intravenous Solumedrol. However, he became a candidate for deep orbitotomy following worsening of symptoms and the tumor was resected and sent for pathology. After that, his symptoms were improved. The specimen processed and stained by H/E stain and showed infiltration of almost monomorphic cells with plasmacytoid features and infiltration of soft tissue and striated muscle. Immunohistochemistry examination (IHC) was done for definite diagnosis. Tumor was diffuse and strongly positive for CD138, CD56, and lambda light chain and diffuse dot-like pattern for CD99 (Figure 3). Also, the tumor was negative for LCA, CD20, CD3, PAX5, TdT, S100, CD34, kappa, CK, chromogranin, and synaptophysin, which was consistent with plasmacytoma with anaplastic features. In general, this tumor seemed to be a recurrent lesion of a previous tumor in the right maxillary sinuses.

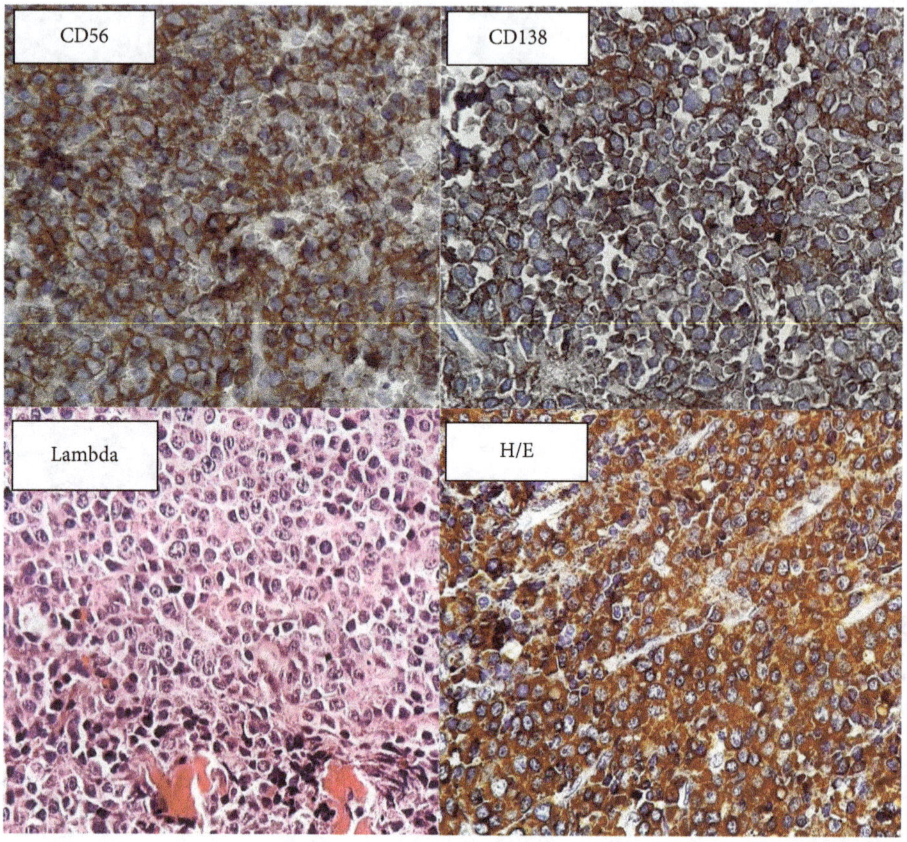

FIGURE 3: H/E-stained slide show plasmocytoid cells with infiltration of muscle fiber. (×400). Tumoral cells diffuse and strongly positive for CD138, CD56, and lambda light chain.

After tumor resection, he underwent another course of approximately 30 sessions of radiotherapy (overall dose of 60G) for complete remission of symptoms (Figure 4). Our patient underwent a systemic work up to exclude systemic multiple myeloma, and all results including protein electrophoresis and bone marrow biopsy and aspiration were negative for systemic involvement.

3. Discussion

Solitary plasmacytoma is a plasma cell tumor with no evidence of systemic involvement; however, when the disease has systemic manifestations, it is called multiple myeloma. Orbital plasmacytomas can originate from the bone (solitary plasmacytoma) or from soft tissue (extramedullary) or may be a manifestation of multiple myeloma at which the tumor can be significant and produce profound vision loss [6]. They can involve the orbit, conjunctiva [7], uvea, retina, lacrimal sac [8], and ciliary body. They present as an orbital mass, epibulbar mass [9], orbital abcess [6], chalazion [6], dacryocystitis [6], granulomatous uveitis or as an isolated mass in the rectus muscles [4, 10]. An increase in the IOP or neovascular glaucoma has also been reported in the iris and ciliary body plasmacytomas [11]. Most of the reported cases of ocular plasmacytomas have associations with systemic multiple myeloma, which makes our case unique that there was no systemic involvement of the disease in our patient.

Due to the diagnosis of the maxillary sinus plasmacytoma about 3 years ago, it seems that the orbital mass was caused by a recurrence of the maxillary sinus mass. In fact, it has been stated that for the complete treatment of this aggressive tumor, both surgical resection and adequate radiotherapy are required, and a shortcoming in either of these two modalities can lead to the recurrence of this tumor. However, it is possible that inadequate resection with surgery or inadequate radiotherapy in the treatment of a previous sinus plasmacytoma has led to recurrence of the tumor in orbit [12].

Any cause of reduced venous outflow and retinal ischemia can cause CRVO [13]. Retrobulbar masses can cause compression of the retinal artery and central retinal artery occlusion (CRAO) [14]. Any vascular damage such as tumor resection can release serotonin, and acting as a vasoconstrictor, it can cause transient arterial vasospasm and a subsequent CRAO which may be managed by immediate intervention [15]; however, those scenarios are unlikely in the setting of CRVO.

CRVO is caused by compression of venules while crossing arterioles causing thrombosis, stasis, turbulence, and a resultant venous outflow obstruction. Diabetes, hypertension, hyperlipidemia, open angle glaucoma, atherosclerosis, vasculitis, dysproteinemias such as Waldenstrom

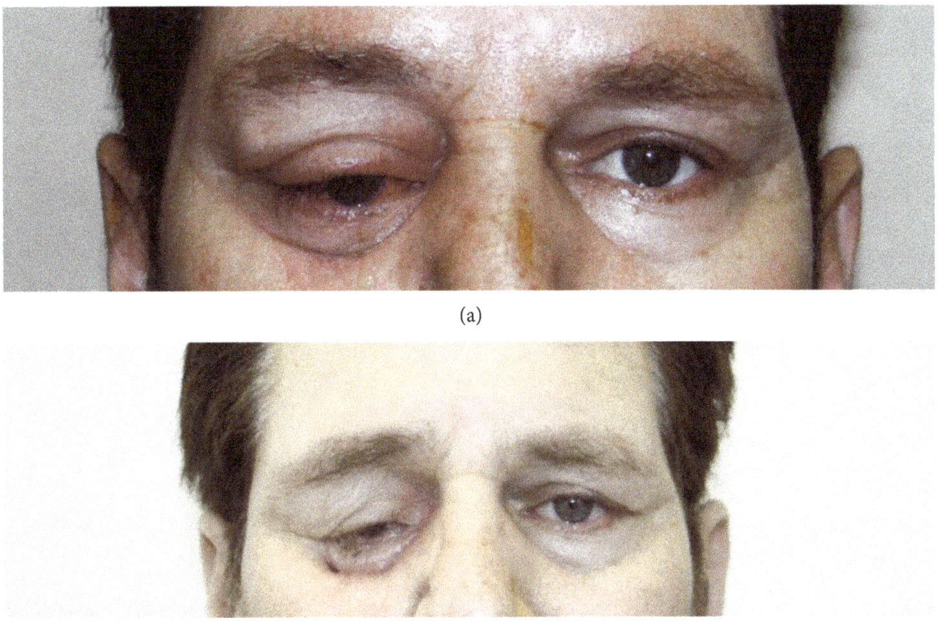

FIGURE 4: Preoperative (a) and postoperative (b) external pictures showing resolution of proptosis after orbitotomy.

macroglobulinemia and multiple myeloma, blood dyscrasias such as Polycythemia vera, and a hypercoagulable state are known risk factors for CRVO [16]. Any orbital lesion or process causing central retinal vein compression such as tumor or a carotid cavernous fistula can cause venous stasis and CRVO [13]. Retrobulbar external compression seen in thyroid eye disease or orbital masses can be accounted for CRVO as well.

In multiple myeloma, the viscosity of the venous blood flow increases due to hypercoagulopathy state, and as a result, the risk of vascular thromboembolic events, such as retinal venous occlusion, rises. Therefore, if a retinal venous occlusion occurs in the absence of common underlying diseases, one of the diseases that should probably be investigated is multiple myeloma. However, in plasmacytoma without systemic involvement, as in our case, there is no coagulation disorder and retinal vascular accident is unlikely. One possible explanation of retinal venous occlusion in this situation is the increase in intraorbital pressure as a result of the increase in the intraorbital volume due to a large tumor, which causes pressure on the central retinal vein, and consequently, venous turbulence and venous thrombosis may develop [13, 16].

Since our patient showed no evidence of systemic multiple myeloma and had none of the risk factors of CRVO, It is not clear whether his development of CRVO and subsequent NVG was due to ischemia because of previous radiotherapy or ischemic and compressive effects of the plasmacytoma; however, since he had an acceptable vision following radiotherapy for a few years and his vision improved after cataract surgery and only started to worsen few months later with the onset of proptosis, we can propose that the orbital lesion might have been a contributing factor to the development of CRVO.

Consent

Informed consent was obtained from the patient to report the case.

Authors' Contributions

All authors contributed to drafting or revising the article, gave final approval of the manuscript, and agree to be accountable for all aspects of the work.

References

[1] J. W. Adkins, J. A. Shields, C. L. Shields, R. C. Eagle, J. C. Flanagan, and P. C. Campanella, "Plasmacytoma of the eye and orbit," *International Ophthalmology*, vol. 20, pp. 339–343, 1997.

[2] C. N. Burkat, J. J. Van Buren, and M. J. Lucarelli, "Characteristics of orbital multiple myeloma: a case report and literature review," *Survey of Ophthalmology*, vol. 54, pp. 697–704, 2009.

[3] E. Wallace, Z. Stewart, D. Theriot et al., "Atypical presentation of extramedullary plasmacytoma," *Ochsner Journal*, vol. 18, pp. 101–103, 2018.

[4] N. Saffra, F. Gorgani, D. Panasci, and D. Kirsch, "Diplopia and proptosis due to isolated lateral rectus plasmacytoma in a patient with multiple myeloma," *BMJ Case Reports*, vol. 12, article e229178, 2019.

[5] S. S. Y. Wang, M. B. Lee, A. George et al., "Five cases of orbital extramedullary plasmacytoma: diagnosis and management of an aggressive malignancy," *Orbit*, vol. 38, pp. 218–225, 2019.

[6] D. J. Russell and S. R. Seiff, "Orbital plasmacytoma mimicking an orbital abscess," *Ophthalmic Plastic and Reconstructive Surgery*, vol. 33, pp. e32–e33, 2017.

[7] A. Bradley, A. Estes, L. Ulrich, D. Thomas, and D. Gay, "Epibulbar plasmacytoma masquerading as subconjunctival hemorrhage in a patient with multiple myeloma," *Cornea*, vol. 36, pp. 249–251, 2017.

[8] S. Pradhan and P. L. Custer, "Multiple myeloma presenting in the lacrimal sac," *American Journal of Ophthalmology*, vol. 141, pp. 563-564, 2006.

[9] K. J. Chin, S. Kempin, T. Milman, and P. T. Finger, "Ocular manifestations of multiple myeloma: three cases and a review of the literature," *Optometry - Journal of the American Optometric Association*, vol. 82, pp. 224–230, 2011.

[10] P. A. Tenzel, K. Mishra, A. Andron, R. C. Della Rocca, and H. S. Reddy, "Extramedullary plasmacytoma of the lateral rectus muscle," *Orbit*, vol. 36, pp. 78–80, 2017.

[11] H. Selvan, S. Kashyap, S. Sen, B. Chawla, N. Lomi, and V. Gupta, "Trabeculectomy in an unsuspected extramedullary iris–ciliary body plasmacytoma," *European Journal of Ophthalmology*, 2020.

[12] E. Cantone, A. M. Di Lullo, L. Marano et al., "Atrategy for the treatment and follow-up of sinonasal solitary extramedullary plasmacytoma: a case series," *Journal of Medical Case Reports*, vol. 11, p. 219, 2017.

[13] I. Kozak, S. M. Elkhamary, and T. M. Bosley, "Central retinal vein occlusion in a childhood optic nerve tumour," *Neuro-Ophthalmology*, vol. 40, pp. 35–39, 2016.

[14] U. Körner-Stiefbold, "Central retinal artery occlusion–etiology, clinical picture, therapeutic possibilities," *Therapeutische Umschau*, vol. 58, pp. 36–40, 2001.

[15] M. Naderan, M. T. Rajabi, S. Z. T. Mohammadi, and M. B. Rajabi, "Central retinal artery occlusion following orbital tumor resection: is rapid intervention effective?," *Indian Journal of Ophthalmology*, vol. 63, pp. 678–680, 2015.

[16] L. L. Lim, N. Cheung, J. J. Wang et al., "Prevalence and risk factors of retinal vein occlusion in an Asian population," *British Journal of Ophthalmology*, vol. 92, no. 10, pp. 1316–1319, 2008.

15

Postoperative Multimodal Analysis in Successful Gas Displacement of a Submacular Hemorrhage

Tatiana Urrea-Victoria, Emiliano Fulda-Graue, Miguel A. Quiroz-Reyes, Felipe Esparza-Correa, Alejandra Nieto-Jordan, Erick A. Quiroz-Gonzalez, and Federico Graue-Wiechers

Instituto de Oftalmología Fundacíon Conde de Valenciana (Non-profit Organization), Chimalpopoca 14, Colonia Obrera, Mexico City 06800, Mexico

Correspondence should be addressed to Miguel A. Quiroz-Reyes; drquiroz@prodigy.net.mx

Academic Editor: Takaaki Hayashi

In this report, we describe a case of timely gas vitrectomy to displace a moderate submacular hemorrhage from the submacular space without tPA, release vitreoretinal traction along the borders of a posterior retinal tear, and analyze postoperative multimodal imaging findings in a 34-year-old male patient whose right eye was injured by a stone. The patient underwent a successful nontissue plasminogen activator gas vitrectomy 3 days after the accident. A multimodal evaluation with spectral-domain optical coherence tomography (SD-OCT), 10-2 and 30-2 campimetry, microperimetry, multifocal electroretinography (mfERG), and visual evoked potentials was performed 6 months after the accident. The multimodal imaging tests yielded abnormal foveal SD-OCT patterns, with a fibrous sealed tear in the retinal pigment epithelium. Campimetry showed low levels of retinal sensitivity; microperimetry and mfERG revealed a subnormal retinal response and a reduction in the N1 and P1 wave amplitudes. The visual evoked potential responses were normal. Multidisciplinary examination at 6 months postoperatively revealed a structurally and functionally abnormal macula. The retina remained attached. Our functional findings indicate that submacular hemorrhage should be treated in a timely manner to minimize photoreceptor damage.

1. Introduction

Closed-globe blunt ocular trauma mechanisms can rupture the vascular choroid and result in central vision-threatening submacular hemorrhage (SMH) [1]. This condition is defined as the presence of a significant hemorrhage under the neurosensory macula [2], which is generally caused by the contusional breakdown of the blood–retina barrier [3]. Besides ocular trauma, the most common conditions that may cause an SMH are pathological myopia, pathological submacular choroidal neovascularization, polypoidal choroidal vasculopathy, arterial macroaneurysms, and presumed ocular histoplasmosis syndrome [2, 4]. Blunt ocular trauma with SMH is a major cause of severe vision loss [4], usually affecting young patients and causing several pathological conditions such as commotion retinae, choroidal rupture, macular hole, subretinal and macular hemorrhage, retinal vascular rupture, vitreous hemorrhage, retinal pigment epithelial edema and healed scarring, retinal dialysis, macular infarction, traumatic optic neuropathy, optic nerve avulsion [2], and even retinal tears. Clinical and histopathological studies have shown that prolonged contact of the blood catabolic products with photoreceptors in the subretinal space worsens the prognostic and visual outcomes [5].

Postcontusional choroidal rupture usually runs vertical and temporal to the optic nerve disc and sometimes runs through the foveal center, with different and significant amounts of secondary hemorrhagic macular detachment in 66% of cases, resulting in poor visual outcomes, particularly when the SMH persists for several days [2, 3].

Here, we describe the case of a patient with a trauma-related SMH complicated with a large tractional posterior

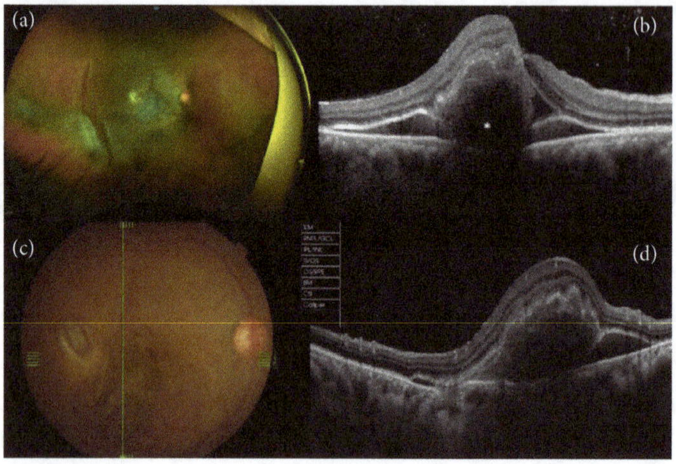

Figure 1: (a) A wide-field preoperative photograph shows limited moderate submacular hemorrhage associated with a parafoveal choroidal rupture and an irregular-shaped posterior retinal tear. (b) A swept-source cross-sectional optical coherence tomography (OCT) image in the horizontal plane shows a submacular hemorrhage that appears hyperreflective; it is hemoglobin-rich (*) and hyporeflective when the serous component is predominant. Due to the presence of blood, there is attenuation of the IS/OS (inner segment/outer segment) band and RPE (retinal pigment epithelium) line. (c) Posterior pole preoperative clinical photography and (d) corresponding swept-source cross-sectional OCT image in the vertical plane depict an elevated preoperative central submacular hemorrhage and an RPE attenuation-like defect.

paramacular retinal tear; these two posttraumatic lesions were not connected or tunneled together at the level of the subretinal space since this would have facilitated its simultaneous surgical approach to treat this condition only with gas vitrectomy pneumatic displacement of the blood and release of the vitreoretinal traction complemented with laser retinopexy, without the use of tissue-plasminogen activator (tPA) to avoid additional potential retinal toxic damage. We would like to emphasize the efficacy of our simplified surgical approach and the importance of timing in surgical intervention to achieve adequate anatomical and functional recovery with minimal sequalae at the subclinical level as demonstrated by the multimodal imaging structural and functional evaluations.

2. Case Presentation

The Retina Department at the *Instituto de Oftalmologia* Hospital, Mexico City, Mexico, provided authorization and released the electronic clinical record pertaining to this case report. This study adhered to the tenets of the Declaration of Helsinki and received approval from the institutional ethics committee (no reference number is usually provided for a case report by this institution). Written informed consent was obtained from the patient in accordance with the institutional guidelines. Data are available from the imageology and psychophysics laboratory at the Retina Department of the Institution.

A 34-year-old man presented with reduced central vision in his right eye 3 days after experiencing blunt trauma due to being struck by a stone. The preoperative best-corrected visual acuity (BCVA) was 1/200 in the affected eye. The intraocular pressure was 10 mmHg, and there was a pupillary sphincter rupture. On biomicroscopy assessment, the vitreous cavity showed partial posterior detachment with vitreoretinal traction around the edges of an irregular posterior retinal tear, with a very shallow subretinal fluid-like appearance and neuroretinal whitening around the tear. The rest of the retina was completely attached, and no communication between the posterior retinal tear and the SMH was documented on optical coherence tomography (OCT). The macula was dome-shaped and elevated because of the presence of a moderately thick SMH (Figures 1(a)– 1(d)). Cross-sectional images (Figures 1(b) and 1(c)) were acquired along the horizontal and vertical planes through the foveal center using a Swept-Source DRI Optical Coherent Tomography Triton device (Topcon Medical Systems, Inc., Oakland, NJ). An SS-OCT image crossing the retinal tear was not obtained.

Although only injection of an expansible gas bubble was considered the finding of a large posterior tear in the relatively young man, with traction of a nonliquefied vitreous cortex around the edges of the tear, allowed us to decide on the use of surgery as treatment modality. It is important to emphasize that it was not possible to drain the submacular hemorrhage through the retinal tear by avoiding concomitant retinal detachment. This would have facilitated the total transoperative removal of the submacular blood on the third day, when surgery was performed. However, it was decided not to use tPA because of its potential retinal toxicity, leaving only gas followed by strict postoperative prone position to achieve the pneumatic displacement of the blood.

Under local anesthesia and sedation, the patient underwent a pneumatic submacular blood displacement procedure, which involved a gas pars plana vitrectomy and the release of vitreoretinal traction around the retinal tear. Subsequently, central vitrectomy was performed with removal of the cortical vitreous body from the retinal surface, using a silicone-tipped cannula and active suction. The surgeon was careful to obtain a free and mobile posterior hyaloid membrane. Laser retinopexy was performed around the retinal tear, and an air-fluid exchange was conducted at the end of the surgical procedure using a mixture of nonexpandable 10% perfluoropropane gas (C_3F_8). Postoperatively, the

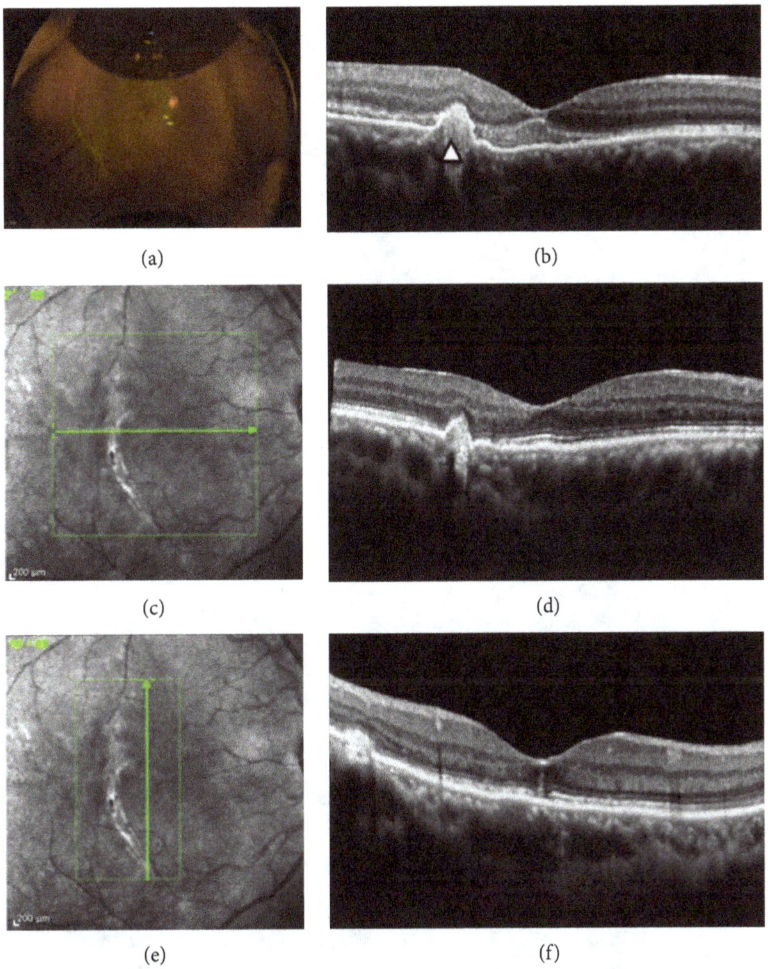

FIGURE 2: (a) Six weeks after surgery. The 20% remaining perfluoropropane (C_3F_8) bubble with a posterior temporal retinal tear treated with laser. (b) The 6-week spectral-domain optical coherence tomography (SD-OCT) corresponding to the submacular hemorrhage is almost completely reabsorbed. The IS/OS and external limiting membrane (ELM) lines show irregularity and are compacted against the protruded hyperreflective retinal pigment epithelium (arrowhead). The retinal pigment epithelium shows bulging without rupture but only mild disruption and fused IS/OS with the ELM (c, d). The 6-month postoperative cross-sectional horizontal and (e, f) vertical planes through the foveal center on SD-OCT.

patient was instructed to strictly remain in the prone position for 5 days and follow the protocol for recovery recommended for this type of blunt trauma treated with pneumatic submacular blood displacement. Local and systemic antibiotics were administered after the surgical procedure.

At the 6-week follow-up visit (Figures 2(a) and 2(b)), the blood had been inferiorly displaced, the BCVA was 20/140, eye pressure was normal, the retina was attached with some blood remnants inferiorly, and the macula had flattened, without underlying blood remnants. Figure 3 shows that the BCVA was 20/30, the medium was very clear, the retina was attached, and the posterior retinal tear had a tight seal with the retinal pigment epithelium (RPE). Postoperative multimodal imaging analysis was performed to obtain the structural and functional patterns such as BCVA, visual field testing evaluation, and multifocal electroretinography, and microperimetry evaluation. The postoperative spectral-domain optical coherence tomography (SD-OCT-Spectralis OCT, Heidelberg Engineering, Germany) pattern showed a resolved submacular hemorrhage, an ellipsoid (IS/OS) line, and external limiting membrane (ELM) SD-OCT biomarker lines preserved but distorted and fused with the protruding RPE line (Figure 4).

Figures 5(a) and 5(b) show the 10-2 and 30-2 automated central field testing (Visual Field Perimeter, Vision Monitor MonPackONE, MetroVision, France), which revealed mean deficits in the retinal sensitivity of 9.0 dB and 7.8 dB, respectively, at the central points of the stimuli. No other visual field changes were detected.

Figures 5(c) and 5(d) show that the N1 wave amplitude of the multifocal electroretinography (mfERG) (Electrophysiology Vision Monitor Analyzer MonPackONE, MetroVision, France). A 61-hexagon 30° test had decreased by 75.0%, 41.9%, 27.0%, 10.5%, and 6.15%, respectively, from the <2-degree to >15-degree central rings (normal range of the mean deficit allowed is 1-2%). The implicit time was shorter in the <2-degree central ring and slightly longer in the remaining central rings. The nV amplitude of the P1 waves significantly decreased with subnormal implicit times in all central rings studied in the affected eye, compared to the normal

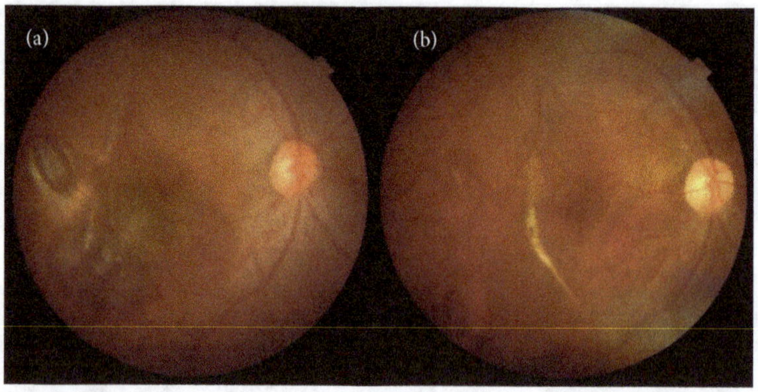

FIGURE 3: Preoperative and 6-month postoperative fundus color photographs. (a) Submacular hemorrhage associated with an adjacent parafoveal choroidal rupture. (b) Six months after surgery: a clinically normal foveal appearance and subretinal reparative scarring along the choroidal rupture temporal to the fovea.

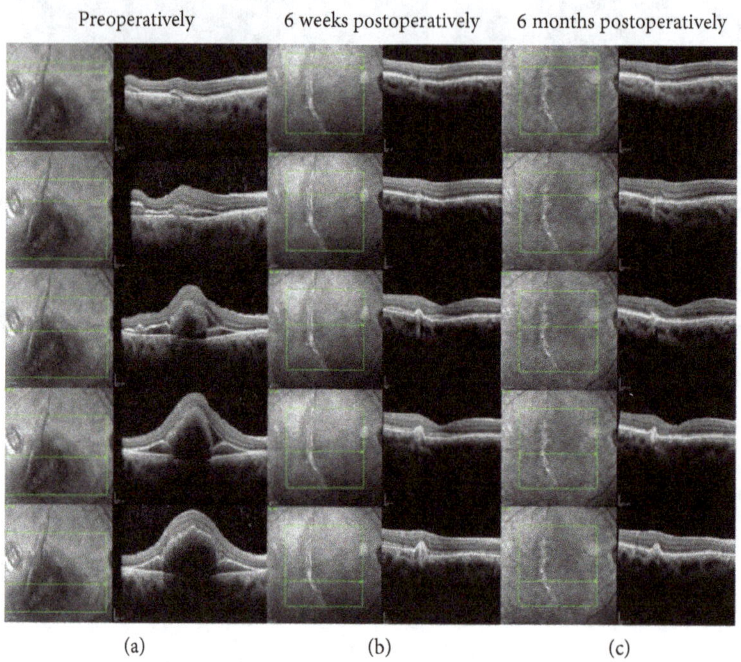

FIGURE 4: Preoperative spectral-domain optical coherence tomography (SD-OCT) of the corresponding macular locus images. Preoperative SD-OCT (left vertical column), 6-week postoperative SD-OCT (central vertical column), and 6-month postoperative comparative SD-OCT (right vertical column). (a–c) SD-OCT cross-sectional images acquired along the horizontal plane through the foveal center depict the involuted presence of blood and the sequential slow improvement of the retinal pigment epithelium, IS/OS, and external limiting membrane layers.

contralateral eye. Figure 5(d) shows the mfERG as a 3-D topographic field map of the macular function that shows subnormal foveal photoreceptor sensitivity with a normal spatial resolution due to stable fixation and location pattern.

On microperimetry (MP-3 MAIA Confocal Microperimetry, MetroVision, France), the fixation pattern was found to be stable, and the fixation location pattern was documented as foveocentral. The retinal sensitivity analysis map showed abnormal macular integrity with reduced sensitivity, mainly in the center of the fovea, as well as reduced sensitivity over the choroidal rupture. There was no correlation between the reduced retinal sensitivity locus and the corresponding retinal thickness on OCT (Figure 6). The visual evoked potentials (RETeval, LKC Technologies; Gaithersburg, MD) were measured with a midoccipital active scalp electrode placed (Oz) in the midline 3-4 cm above the inion, a reference electrode on the forehead, and the ground electrode placed on the earlobe where normal (Figure 7).

3. Discussion

Here, we have reported a case in which early treatment with gas vitrectomy yielded successful displacement of the submacular blood as well as release of vitreoretinal traction at the margins of the posterior tear. Moreover, a strict prone positioning regimen allowed the sealing of the tear, preservation

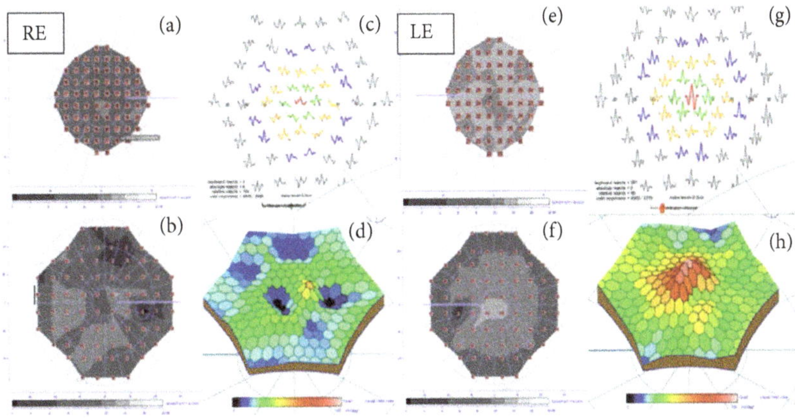

FIGURE 5: Comparative campimetric and multifocal electroretinography (mfERG). Right eye (a) 10-2 and (b) 30-2 visual field view testing show deficits in retinal sensitivity to the central points of the stimuli. The mean deficits are 9.0 and 7.8 dB, respectively, compared with the contralateral normal eye (normal mean deficit: 0.5-2.0 dB). (c) Subnormal retinal response and reduction of the N1 and P1 wave amplitudes. The 61-hexagon 30° test had decreased by 75.0%, 41.9%, 27.0%, 10.5%, and 6.15%, respectively, from the <2-degree to >15-degree central rings compared to the normal control parameters (normal range of the mean deficit permitted is 1-3%). (d) mfERG as a 3-D topographic field map of the macular function shows subnormal foveal photoreceptor sensitivity with a normal spatial resolution, due to stable fixation and location pattern. Left eyes comparative normal figures of the left eye show (e) 10-2, (f) 30-2, and (g, h) mfERG within the normal range.

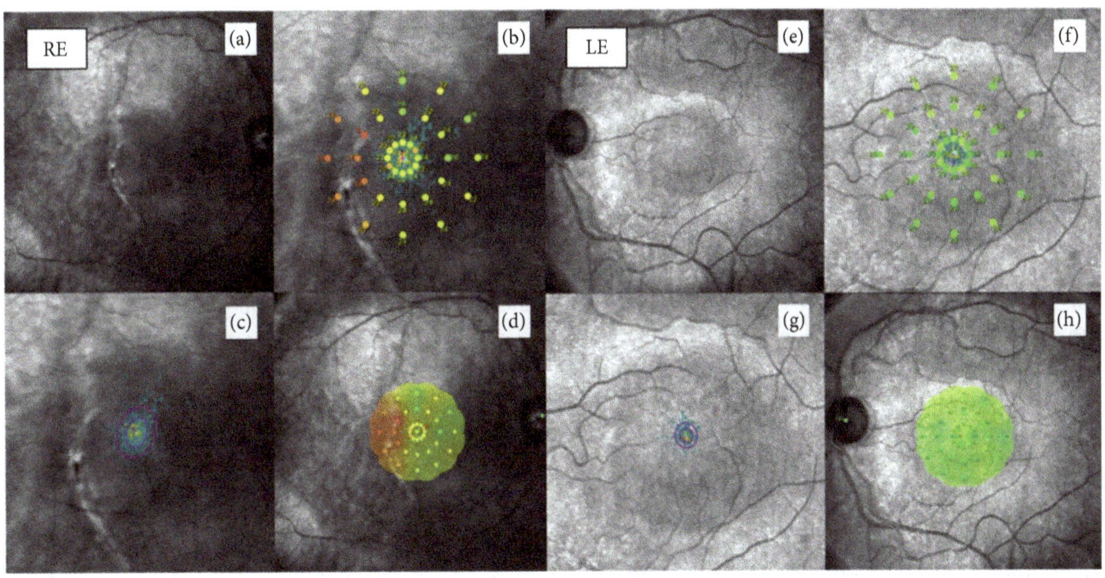

FIGURE 6: Comparative 6-month microperimetry. (a) The clinical aspect depicts a normal central fovea with a juxtafoveal choroidal rupture. (b) Retinal sensitivity measured with a microperimetry device (MAIA) shows a very diminished retinal sensitivity temporal to the fovea and an abnormal response 6 months following the surgery. The red figures and numbers indicate abnormally low retinal sensitivities (dB). (c) Stable foveal fixation pattern of the affected eye. (d) Corresponding foveal plotting with low retinal sensitivity on the temporal side of the fovea. (e–h) Correspond to normal left eye microperimetry.

of the retinal anatomical structure, and displacement of the submacular blood outside the central area of the macula; all the previous facts have also been demonstrated in other studies [1, 3, 4, 6]. The use of postoperative multimodal imaging analysis with serial SS-OCT, SD-OCT, mfERG, and microperimetry in this case highlights a possible clinical and functional contribution to the study and knowledge of this vision-threatening traumatic condition. Our analysis illustrated a point-to-point correlation between the disruption of the external layers of the retina (RPE, IS/OS band, and ELM line) and the reduced retinal sensitivity in the microperimetry and mfERG, as well as a good correlation between the SD-OCT microabnormalities in retinal thickness and the same retinal locus of reduced retinal sensitivity on microperimetry.

The main aspect to consider when managing this condition is rapid blood displacement [2]. The patient in our case only underwent gas vitrectomy with nonexpanding 10% C_3F_8 and received no tPA, which has been used previously [1, 6].

This patient showed choroidal rupture temporal to the fovea, similar to what was described in others studies [2],

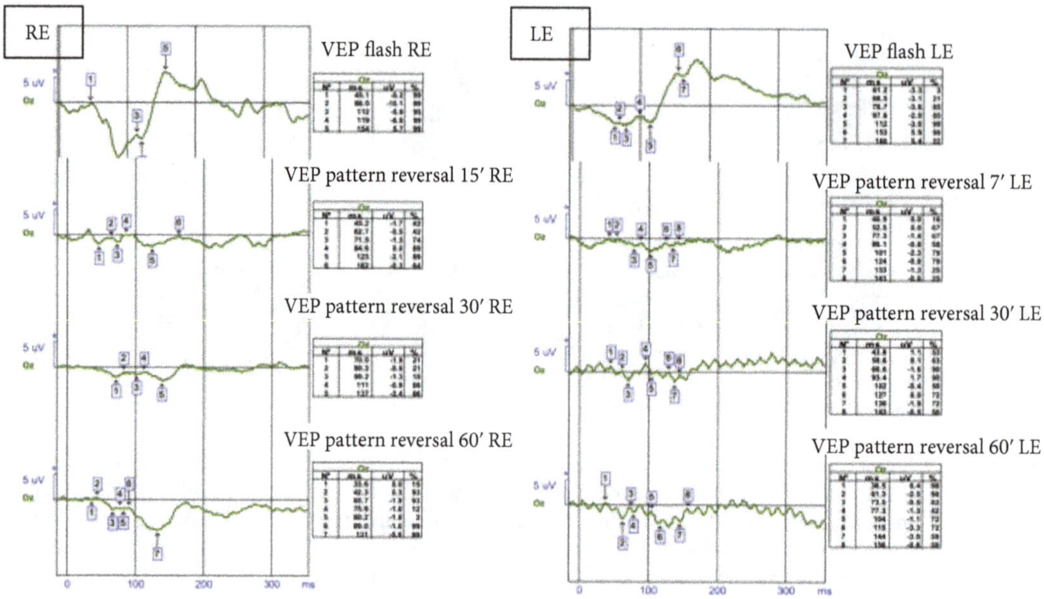

Figure 7: Visual evoked potentials. Comparative visual evoked potentials of the affected eye. N75-74.115 ms, P100-100.225 ms, and P135 were not recorded. Normal left eye VEP functional traces were considered between the normal ranges.

and did not show evidence of complications, such as choroidal neovascularization or subfoveal scarring (Figures 2(c)–2(f) and Figure 4(c)).

The natural course of SMH varies according to the etiology, duration, diameter, and thickness of the hemorrhage [7]. It has been reported that an SMH is a devastating complication of various pathological entities, and in the case of a large or massive SMH secondary to blunt trauma, the prognosis for visual recovery is usually poor, with the final BCVA ranging from 20/200 to light perception [8].

Numerous approaches have been described for the displacement of SMH, including vitrectomy with the use of intravitreal or subretinal recombinant tPA (r-tPA), intravitreal gas tamponade, postoperative positioning [4], and pneumatic displacement with or without tPAs [6]. Ultimately, the preferred technique is defined by the duration and the extent of the SMH in addition to the surgeon's skill and preference [9].

In 1991, Peyman et al. [10] first reported the visual outcomes of r-tPA-assisted SMH removal. In their study, 60% of patients demonstrated an improvement in BCVA by two or more lines. A less invasive procedure is described by Chen et al. [11] which comprised of an intravitreal injection of r-tPA and gas tamponade to facilitate lysis of the SMH. This procedure allows clinicians to avoid surgical intervention for draining an SMH [6]. Early studies used subretinal tPA and perfluorocarbon liquid to facilitate aspiration through a small retinotomy [6]. However, this technique has become less common because it is associated with poor postoperative visual acuity and a high rate of retinal detachment [6]. Balughatta et al. [5] recently reported a case series of C_3F_8 pneumatic displacement of limited traumatic SMH with excellent anatomical results and final visual acuities attributed only to gas injection and patient positioning, without surgery or the use of tPA.

In cases complicated by posterior retinal tears, we consider that the release of vitreoretinal traction is of paramount importance and the pneumatic displacement without tPA injection followed by a strict prone position, in cases complicated by posterior retinal tears such as the one reported here, is less invasive and potentially less toxic than the tPA-assisted surgical drainage of the SMH. The mechanism involves moving the blood away from the subfoveal space by using the long-acting gas buoyancy effect to displace the blood from the submacular foveocentral photoreceptors [1, 2, 4, 7, 11].

In this report, photoreceptor dysfunction was considered to be the result of blood pooling under the macula and contact with the central photoreceptors, although pneumatic displacement occurred within the first 3 days. We considered that the OCT changes in this case (Figures 1, 2, and 4(a)–4(c)) were consistent with disruption of the photoreceptors and demonstrated by the loss of regularity and compacting of the IS/OS and ELM SD-OCT biomarkers with some degree of irregular fibrous RPE changes. Furthermore, the quantification of the differential threshold of retinal sensitivity or visual field testing performed under different stimuli conditions (both background and stimuli) allowed us to detect subtle abnormalities with 10-2 and 30-2 visual field examinations (Figures 5(a) and 5(b)). The mfERG showed outer retinal and photoreceptor abnormalities, but to optimize its value, it is important to compare the mfERG results with those of concurrent automated visual fields. The visual evoked potentials elicited were in the normal range, excluding traumatic optic neuropathy. The microperimetry findings showed a satisfactory correlation between the microstructural SD-OCT macular pathology and the corresponding functional abnormality determined by microperimetry, visual field testing, and mfERG. However, there was no correlation between the localized locus of reduced macular sensitivity and the corresponding retinal thickness on

OCT (Figure 6). In this case, there were consistent changes in the microperimetry findings and deep abnormalities in the N1 wave assessed by the mfERG, which were indicative of localized outer retina and photoreceptor dysfunction, as previously noted.

We acknowledge the several inherent limitations and shortcomings of this case report. However, based on the analysis of our results as well as other findings reported on the literature, we can confirm that early non-tPA pneumatic displacement could be achieved without severe visual damage. Prospective and multicenter protocols are needed to improve the approach in severe or complicated cases of SMH, similar to the one reported here.

In summary, this report confirms that early removal of blood from beneath the macula within the first few days is important in cases of SMH. This case was complicated by the presence of a large posterior retinal tear and vitreoretinal traction, but vitreoretinal release and gas vitrectomy were sufficient to displace the submacular blood and maintain the retinal attachment with good anatomical and functional results. A few subclinical and consequently not significant abnormalities since they do not affect the quality of binocular vision were detected at the 6-month multimodal functional evaluation only with sophisticated diagnostic tools.

Our findings suggest that SMH should be treated as soon as possible to minimize photoreceptor damage. With early displacement of the hemorrhage, only subclinical damage ensues. We emphasize that if the blood stays in contact with the photoreceptors for a long time, the damage will be greater, with loss of vision and clinical sequelae. This report suggests retina surgeons to perform timely surgical techniques to allow displacement of blood from the submacular space and, thereby, open an innovative path to developing new drugs that could reduce the toxic effects of blood catabolism seen with the drugs currently in use.

Acknowledgments

We are deeply appreciative of Editage author services for their excellent assistance in the editing and formatting of this manuscript.

References

[1] S. Doi, S. Kimura, Y. Morizane et al., "Successful displacement of a traumatic submacular hemorrhage in a 13-year-old boy treated by vitrectomy, subretinal injection of tissue plasminogen activator and intravitreal air tamponade: a case report," *BMC Ophthalmology*, vol. 15, no. 1, pp. 1–4, 2015.

[2] G. Casini, P. Loiudice, M. Menchini et al., "Traumatic submacular hemorrhage: available treatment options and synthesis of the literature," *International journal of retina and vitreous*, vol. 5, no. 1, pp. 1–9, 2019.

[3] F. F. Malik and V. Poulaki, "Management of submacular hemorrhage," *International Ophthalmology Clinics*, vol. 54, no. 2, pp. 51–59, 2014.

[4] G. S. Gujral, M. Agarwal, R. Mayor, D. Shroff, J. Chhablani, and M. P. Shanmugam, "Clinical profile and management outcomes of traumatic submacular hemorrhage," *Journal of current ophthalmology*, vol. 31, no. 4, pp. 411–415, 2019.

[5] P. Balughatta, V. Kadri, S. Braganza et al., "Pneumatic displacement of limited traumatic submacular hemorrhage without tissue plasminogen activator: a case series," *Retinal Cases and Brief Reports*, vol. 13, no. 1, pp. 34–38, 2019.

[6] S. Sharma, J. B. Kumar, J. E. Kim et al., "Pneumatic displacement of submacular hemorrhage with subretinal air and tissue plasminogen activator: initial United States experience," *Ophthalmology Retina*, vol. 2, no. 3, pp. 180–186, 2018.

[7] K. Bae, G. E. Cho, J. M. Yoon, and S. W. Kang, "Optical coherence tomographic features and prognosis of pneumatic displacement for submacular hemorrhage," *PLoS One*, vol. 11, no. 12, article e0168474, 2016.

[8] V. R. Juncal, M. Hanout, F. Altomare et al., "Surgical management of submacular hemorrhage: experience at an academic Canadian centre," *Canadian Journal of Ophthalmology*, vol. 53, no. 4, pp. 408–414, 2018.

[9] G. Yiu and T. H. Mahmoud, "Subretinal hemorrhage," *Microincision Vitrectomy Surgery*, vol. 54, pp. 213–222, 2014.

[10] G. A. Peyman, N. C. Nelson, W. Alturki et al., "Tissue plasminogen activating factor assisted removal of subretinal hemorrhage," *Ophthalmic Surgery, Lasers and Imaging Retina*, vol. 22, no. 10, pp. 575–582, 1991.

[11] C. Y. Chen, C. Hooper, D. Chiu, M. Chamberlain, N. Karia, and W. J. Heriot, "Management of submacular hemorrhage with intravitreal injection of tissue plasminogen activator and expansile gas," *Retina*, vol. 27, no. 3, pp. 321–328, 2007.

16

Temporal Approach, Digitally Assisted Phacovitrectomy in a Patient with Severe Kyphosis due to Axial Spondyloarthritis

J. Rios-Nequis Geovanni, J. Abel Ramírez-Estudillo, L. Daniel Gutiérrez-García, Martin Jiménez-Rodríguez, and Arthur Levine-Berevichez

Fundación Hospital Nuestra Señora de la Luz IAP, Mexico

Correspondence should be addressed to J. Rios-Nequis Geovanni; nequismd@gmail.com

Academic Editor: Stephen G. Schwartz

Purpose. To describe a temporal approach, digitally assisted phacovitrectomy in a patient with severe kyphosis due to axial spondyloarthritis. *Case Report.* A 70-year-old male patient with proliferative diabetic retinopathy with vitreous hemorrhage and cataract and ankylosing spondylitis with severe kyphosis. A temporal approach, digitally assisted 25 G phacovitrectomy was performed with a Constellation platform and the NGENUITY visualization system. The Trendelenburg position was utilized. *Conclusion.* A temporal approach, digitally assisted phacovitrectomy may be used in select cases of severe kyphosis with positive outcomes.

1. Introduction

Ankylosing spondylitis is part of a spectrum of axial spondyloarthritis with HLA-B27-associated autoimmune inflammatory disease that classically causes spinal involvement. As the disease progresses, there is a decrease in the mobility of the spine and thorax [1]. These patients may pose a challenge for the ocular surgical approach. Techniques that use the Trendelenburg position have been described for retinal detachment surgery with scleral buckling [2]. The positioning of the patient and the stretcher is essential to perform the procedure. Advanced cases may require up to 90° of inclination [3]. Previous reports of temporal approach cataract surgery and the Trendelenburg position have also been reported [4].

In 2010, the first 3D visualization device for retina surgery known as the Digital Assisted Vitreoretinal Surgery (DAVS) was introduced; these systems are composed of 2 cameras linked to the surgical microscope, an image processor, and a high-resolution screen. They offer the advantage of improving the ergonomics of the surgeon, increasing the depth of field, and improving the magnification [5]. We present a case report of a patient with severe kyphosis who underwent temporal approach, digitally assisted phacovitrectomy using the Trendelenburg position.

2. Case Report

A 70-year-old male patient with a medical history of type 2 diabetes mellitus, ankylosing spondylitis, and severe kyphosis was referred to our institution due to visual loss of 4 months of evolution in the right eye secondary to proliferative diabetic retinopathy (PDR), vitreous hemorrhage (VH), and cataract. The patient underwent phacovitrectomy on a modular surgical table (Operon D860, Stryker, USA); a support pad was used on the head and neck (Figure 1). The patient was positioned in the Trendelenburg position, and a temporal approach was utilized. A 25 G valved system and Constellation platform (Alcon, Fort Worth, USA) with DAVS NGENUITY visualization system (Alcon, Fort Worth, USA) were used. The OPMI Lumera 700 microscope (Zeiss, Germany) was used with the RESIGHT noncontact visualization system (Zeiss, Germany) tilted to 30° (Figure 2). The trocars were placed at M7, M9, and M11 with the phacoemulsification incision at M8 in the clear cornea. Phacoemulsification was performed through a clear

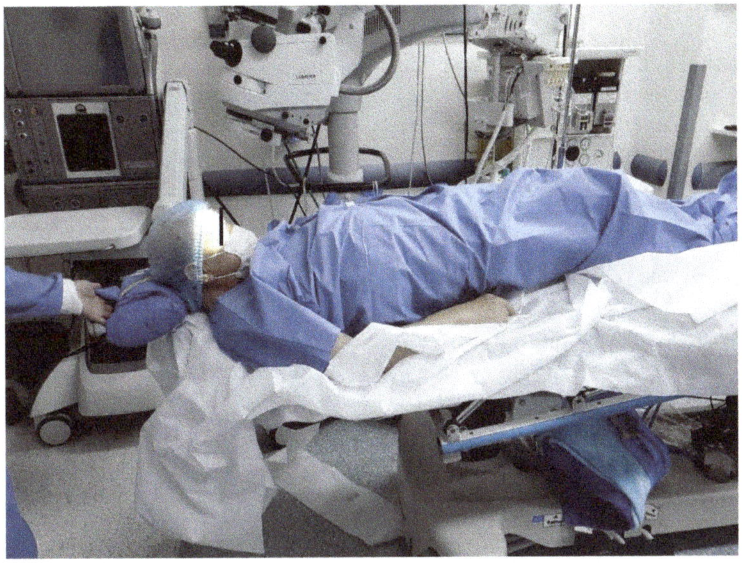

FIGURE 1: Patient in Trendelenburg position with a support pad on the head and neck in a modular surgical bed.

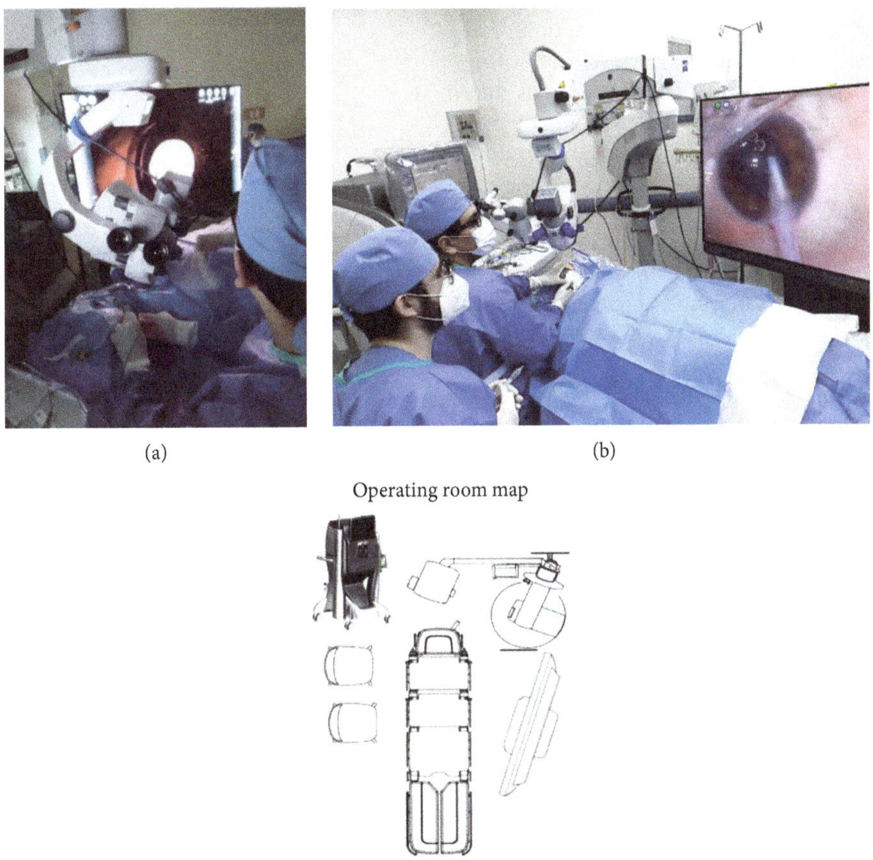

FIGURE 2: Operation room adaptation. (a) Surgical microscope OPMI Lumera 700 (Zeiss, Germany) with the RESIGHT noncontact visualization system (Zeiss, Germany) with an inclination of 30°. (b) Temporary phacovitrectomy approach with a high-resolution screen placed on one side of the surgical bed. (c) Representative map of the operating room.

corneal incision in the M8 meridian. A conventional 3-port vitrectomy was performed with previously described placement, applying panretinal photocoagulation and air tamponade without complications. The duration of the procedure was 40 minutes. The postsurgical best-corrected visual acuity was 20/40 after 12 months.

3. Discussion

To our knowledge, this is the first report of a temporal approach, digitally assisted phacovitrectomy using DAVS in the Trendelenburg position in a patient with severe kyphosis due to ankylosing spondylitis.

Skinner et al. reported the utility of DAVS in severe kyphosis with a superior approach. The severe kyphosis of our patient prevented us from performing a superior approach, for which we suggested doing it temporarily [6]. The DAVS system allows the high-resolution screen to be positioned at the surgeon's discretion, improving ergonomics and allowing the microscope to be adapted to inconvenient positions that could not previously be achieved with conventional microscopes. You et al. published the case of a patient with severe kyphosis with a curvature greater than 90° with rhegmatogenous retinal detachment operated with a conventional microscope; in this case, they required an extreme nonphysiological Trendelenburg position.

The Trendelenburg position allowed us a better exposure of the globe for intervention, without the negative physiological changes in cardiopulmonary function that may develop in the extreme position [7]. Close monitoring of the ventilatory and oximetric capacity is essential during the procedure. During the procedure, our patient presented adequate saturation, without presenting respiratory distress.

In conclusion, DAVS in conjunction with the Trendelenburg position may allow better patient and surgeon comfort in cases of severe kyphosis. This may allow retinal surgery to be performed more safely and efficiently in select patients.

References

[1] D. Yu, A. van Tubergen, J. Sieper, and P. Romain, "Clinical manifestations of axial spondyloarthritis (ankylosing spondylitis and nonradiographic axial spondyloarthritis) in adults," 2020, February 2021.

[2] D. S. Iaboni, M. E. Seamone, M. S. Stairs, D. M. O'Brien, M. S. Bisson, and R. R. Gupta, "Novel patient positioning apparatus for retinal surgery in a case of severe kyphosis," *Retinal Cases and Brief Reports*, vol. 13, no. 4, pp. 385–387, 2019.

[3] T. You, C. X. Huang, S. Chen et al., "Case report: extreme patient positioning for retinal surgery in advanced kyphosis," *Retinal Cases and Brief Reports*, vol. 9, no. 3, pp. 218-219, 2015.

[4] S. Prasad, G. G. Kamath, and R. P. Phillips, "Phacoemulsification in a patient with marked cervical kyphosis," *Journal of Cataract and Refractive Surgery*, vol. 26, no. 8, pp. 1258–1260, 2000.

[5] J. S. Agranat, J. B. Miller, V. P. Douglas et al., "The scope of three-dimensional digital visualization systems in vitreoretinal surgery," *Clin Ophthalmol*, vol. Volume 13, pp. 2093–2096, 2019.

[6] C. Skinner and C. Riemann, ""Heads up" digitally assisted surgical viewing for retinal detachment repair in a patient with severe kyphosis," *Retinal Cases & Brief Reports*, vol. 12, no. 3, pp. 257–259, 2018.

[7] C. Hewer, "The physiology and complications of the Trendelenburg position," *Canadian Medical Association Journal*, vol. 74, no. 4, pp. 285–288, 1956.

17

Challenges of Pediatric Cataract Surgery in a Case of Seasonal Hyperacute Panuveitis (SHAPU)

Pratap Karki,[1] Ranju Kharel Sitaula,[2] Anadi Khatri,[3] Sagun Narayan Joshi,[4] Haramaya Gurung,[5] Indraman Maharjan,[5] Ananda Kumar Sharma,[6] and Madan Prasad Upadhaya[7]

[1]*Department of Ophthalmology, Maharajgunj Medical Campus Tribhuvan University, Institute of Medicine, B. P. Koirala Lions Centre for Ophthalmic Studies, Maharajgunj, Kathmandu, Nepal*
[2]*Department of Ophthalmology, Maharajgunj Medical Campus, Institute of Medicine, Tribhuvan University, B. P. Koirala Lions Centre for Ophthalmic Studies, Maharajgunj, Kathmandu, Nepal*
[3]*Birat Medical College and Teaching Hospital Biratnagar, Nepal*
[4]*Dept of Ophthalmology, Maharajgunj Medical Campus, Tribhuvan University, Institute of Medicine, B.P. Koirala Lions Centre for Ophthalmic Studies, Maharajgunj, Kathmandu, Nepal*
[5]*Himalaya Eye Hospital, Pokhara, Nepal*
[6]*Department of Ophthalmology, Maharajgunj Medical Campus, Institute of Medicine, B.P. Koirala Lions Center for Ophthalmic Studies, Nepal*
[7]*Ophthalmology, Tribhuvan University, Chair Emeritus B.P Eye Foundation, Children Hospital for Eye, ENT and Rehabilitation (CHEERS), Bhaktapur, Nepal*

Correspondence should be addressed to Pratap Karki; karkipratap@gmail.com

Academic Editor: Huban Atilla

A four-year-old female child diagnosed as a case of severe Seasonal Hyperacute Panuveitis (SHAPU) underwent lens-sparing core vitrectomy in her left eye with intravitreal antibiotic and steroid. Patient responded well to treatment and intraocular inflammation subsided. However, three months later, she developed vision impairing dense cataract which also made posterior segment assessment difficult. Lens aspiration with primary posterior capsulotomy and anterior vitrectomy with intraocular lens (IOL) implantation was performed. However, four weeks later, the patient developed occlusio pupillae with iris bombe. She did not respond to medical management so synechiolysis with surgical iridectomy was performed after which a normal depth anterior chamber was attained. Synechia and iris bombe were also relieved, and vision was regained.

1. Introduction

Seasonal Hyperacute Panuveitis (SHAPU) is rare but devastating panuveitis reported from Nepal since last 46 years in autumn of every odd year. Most cases have been reported from hilly regions in and around Kaski district of Nepal. Association has been seen with direct physical exposure or vicinity to the white moths [1]. History of physical contact with moth was seen in 48.6% of SHAPU cases and 11.4% of control in a case control study [1]. It causes uniocular blindness and is the commonest cause of panuveitis among the Nepalese children [1–3]. In a previous study, 71.4% cases were children [1]. The role of white moths in SHAPU causation is still unclear, and studies are being conducted to evaluate, whether the SHAPU is due to the auto-immune response to the moth toxins or due to pathogens delivered by the moths over the ocular surface. Similarly, why it primarily affects children is still not understood.

Sudden onset of red eye with severe intraocular reactions, leukocoria, and hypotony are the characteristic features of

SHAPU. No standard treatment protocol for SHAPU has been developed over the past 46 years. So, for the wider coverage of both microbial and immunological aspects, a blanket therapy with antibiotics and steroid is used. The periocular injections and ocular surgery are carried depending upon the grading of SHAPU [4]. As an ocular emergency, severe SHAPU needs urgent intravitreal injections and vitrectomy with or without lensectomy. Visual rehabilitation after lensectomy in any SHAPU child remains a challenge. Herein, we report a SHAPU case which received immediate management with core vitrectomy but developed cataract for which she underwent intraocular lens (IOL) implantation. Soon she developed unexpected complications in the form of occlusio pupillae and iris bombe and presented as secondary angle closure with ocular hypertension. This is the first report of its kind related to SHAPU. The written consent from the legal parents has been obtained for the publication.

2. Case Report

A 4-year-female child from Kaski district, Pokhara, presented with sudden onset of redness, diminution of vision, and watering in her left eye for 2 days (Figure 1) on 10th September 2019. Pokhara is the same region which is known to have many reported cases of SHAPU in every SHAPU epidemic. On specific inquiry, there was history of sudden increase in white moth population in their area. However, there was no history of direct exposure of the child to the moths. The child had no complaints of pain and was cooperative during assessment. Visual acuity (VA) in her right eye was 6/6, N6. In the left eye, VA was hand movement close to the face with inaccurate projections of rays. Examination of the affected eye revealed circumcorneal congestion and clear cornea with dense anterior chamber reaction. There was a clump of thick exudates floating in the middle of anterior chamber along with 1 mm cream colored settled hypopyon (Figure 2). Leukocoria was present, and the fundal glow and fundus details were not visible. Ultrasound brightness (B) scan revealed dense vitreous hyperechoic opacities in the mid and postvitreous with thickened choroid. Echogenic impression revealed an attached retina (Figure 3). Intraocular pressure (IOP) was 8 mmHg with air puff tonometry. Her right eye was found to be normal in all aspects; routine blood investigations were normal.

With the diagnosis of left eye severe SHAPU, the child immediately underwent lens-sparing core vitrectomy under general anesthesia. Three sclerotomies were made 4 mm from the limbus, and the 20 gauge vitrectomy was performed at 1500 cuts/minute with vacuum at 350 mmHg. After removing core vitreous, the posterior hyaloid was left intact. Intraoperatively, no retinal necrosis was seen. Fluid air exchange was done at the end of procedure, and the sclerotomy sites were closed under air tamponade at 30 mmHg. Prior to the vitrectomy, diagnostic aqueous tap with 26 G needle and vitreous tap with 3 ml syringe was done (Figure 4). And at the end of vitrectomy, intravitreal antibiotics (vancomycin 1 mg/0.1 ml + ceftazidime 2.25 mg/0.1 ml) and intravitreal steroid dexamethasone (0.4 mg/0.1 ml) were given. The retina appeared intact so only air tamponade was used. After vitrectomy, the child was under moxifloxacin eyedrop and prednisolone acetate eye drop hourly and atropine thrice daily. Systemic antibiotic injection (ceftriaxone 250 mg × BD × 7 days) and oral steroid (1 mg/kg body weight) were administered on tapering dose. Diagnostic aqueous and vitreous tap did not reveal any microbial organisms on Gram, Giemsa, and KOH stain. The ocular fluid samples and blood samples, none grew any organism in Blood agar, Brain Heart Infusion broth, and Sabouraud dextrose agar.

By seventh postoperative day, her vision improved to 5/60 N10, the circumcorneal and conjunctival congestion reduced, hypopyon and exudates disappeared, and cellular reactions in anterior chamber decreased. Fundal glow was visible, but details could not be appreciated due to vitritis and onset of cataract.

On subsequent regular follow-up, her intraocular inflammation resolved, and her eye became quiet after 3 months, but her cataract gradually became dense in the left eye; fundus was not visible, but vitreous was clear with attached retina on USG B Scan. Her vision deteriorated to 2/60 N10; however, posterior segment appeared normal in repeat B scan.

After next 8 weeks quiescence of intraocular inflammation, she underwent lens aspiration with 3 mm primary posterior capsulotomy followed by anterior vitrectomy and primary intraocular lens implantation (PMMA-Fred Hollows Foundation Lens) in the bag without optic capture under general anesthesia. She was started on oral steroid at 0.5 mg/kg/body weight 7 days prior to surgery. Postoperatively, she had VA of 6/36 N10, and oral steroid was tapered over 3 weeks.

But one month after the cataract surgery, she presented with painful red eye, and examination revealed occlusio pupillae with iris bombe and shallow anterior chamber in the operated eye (Figure 5). The IOP was 22 mmHg with Goldmann applanation tonometer. She was kept under hourly prednisolone acetate 1% eyedrop, atropine thrice daily, and beta blockers twice a day. Subconjunctival injection of mydricaine was given in four quadrants. But no sign of relief of iris bombe noted. Next day, again under repeat general anesthesia, she underwent 360° synechiolysis with peripheral iridectomy (PI) at 2 o'clock with vitrectomy cutter (Figure 6). Intraocular lens was in situ at bag and was not removed during surgery. On 1st postoperative day, the child was comfortable with quiet eye, vision was 5/60 N10, anterior chamber was normal, PI was patent, intraocular lens was in position, and the fundus was normal. Her IOP was 12 and 13 mmHg without any antiglaucoma drugs. Her best corrected visual acuity in 6 months follow-up was 6/60 N10 and is under amblyopia therapy for visual rehabilitation.

3. Discussion

SHAPU causes severe intraocular inflammation which if not treated and controlled in time leads to permanent visual loss and hypotony. Mild to moderate cases respond well to timely intravitreal injection of antibiotics and steroid [4]. However, severe cases require core vitrectomy in combination with intravitreal injections.

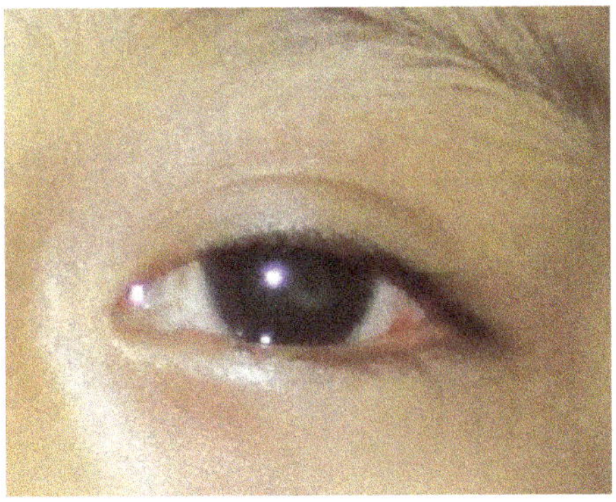

FIGURE 1: Presence of congestion and leukocoria in the left eye.

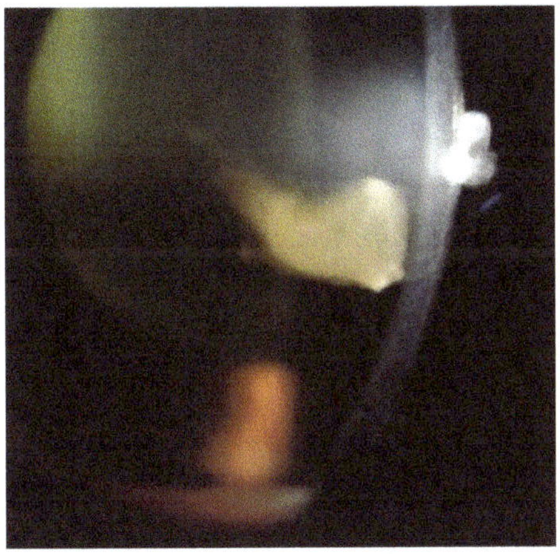

FIGURE 2: Slit view of the left eye showing an exudative clump in the middle of anterior chamber along with 1 mm cream colored settled hypopyon.

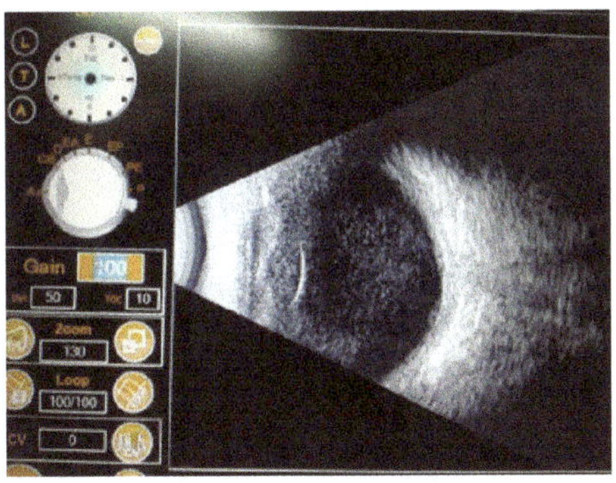

FIGURE 3: USG (B) scan showing multiple hyperechoic opacities in the mid and postvitreous with an attached retina.

Use of steroids and vitrectomy may predispose these cases to develop complicated cataract. Inadvertent lens touch can also cause cataract, although no so such event was noted in our case. Early cataract may sometimes be managed conservatively, and surgery can be delayed. Dense cataract however warrants early surgery not only for routine evaluation of the posterior segment but also to prevent amblyopia as SHAPU happens mostly in young children.

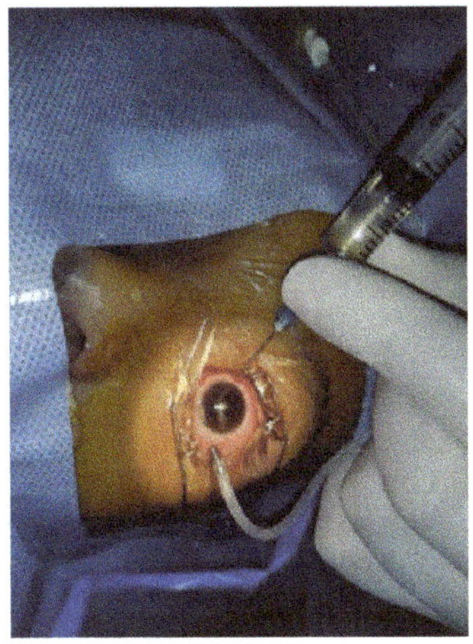

FIGURE 4: Diagnostic vitreous tap of the left eye showing light yellow aspirate in the syringe.

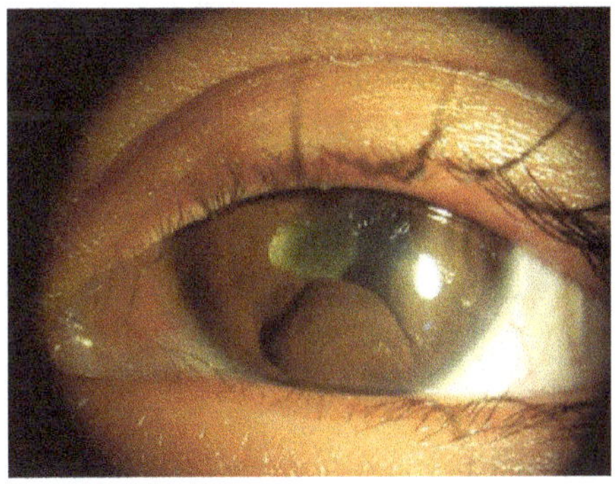

FIGURE 5: Occlusio pupillae with iris bombes at multiple areas in the left eye.

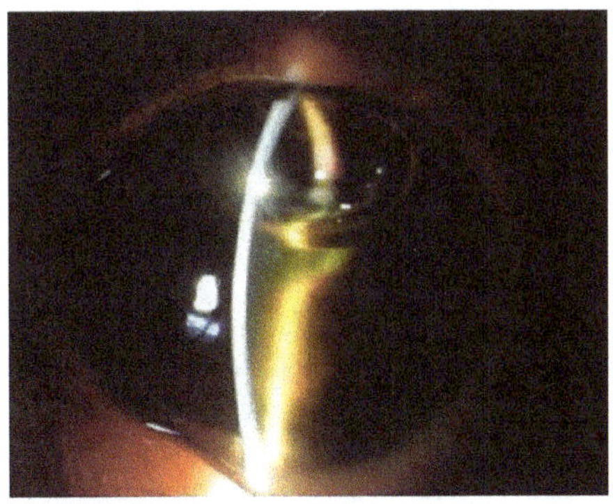

FIGURE 6: Slit lamp view of the left eye showing relieve of iris bombe after synechiolysis but presence of postoperative inflammatory reactions in the anterior chamber.

Decision for complete vitrectomy with primary lensectomy in a child with SHAPU has to be done judiciously. Entire removal of the vitreous with lensectomy may be fruitful to prevent subsequent recurrence and proliferative vitreoretinopathy. On the other hand, core vitrectomy without removal of cortical vitreous can be enough to remove the bulk of vitreous exudates without untoward damage to the fragile retina. Likewise, lensectomy at the same sitting can help to increase visibility during vitrectomy, but lens-sparing vitrectomy also proves worthy to prevent postoperative amblyopia in these young children [4].

Challenges of cataract surgery in patients with uveitis are well known. Good preoperative inflammation control is a prerequisite for surgery in these patients, and postoperative inflammation also needs to be controlled well [5]. However, in our case despite good preoperative inflammation control, patient developed postoperative complication resulting in synechia and iris bombe. This is a known postoperative complication of cataract surgery in patient with uveitis but had not been reported in any SHAPU cases earlier [6].

Severe inflammation associated with SHAPU especially in young children often predispose to severe postoperative inflammation and complications [7]. This poses a challenge when doing cataract surgery in these children with additional the threat of complications related to general anesthesia.

Primary vs. secondary intraocular lens implantation in pediatric uveitis cataract has been the topic of debate over decades. Doubtful outcome has been reported in uveitis cases with primary intraocular lens implantation [7]. We implanted the primary intraocular lens in this case for early visual rehabilitation and for prevention of amblyopia. But, our experience with this case has shown better to avoid primary intraocular lens to reduce further intraocular inflammation-related complications in a SHAPU case.

4. Conclusion

Cataract surgery can have severe postoperative inflammation in children with SHAPU despite good preoperative control. Our experience in this case suggests avoiding primary intraocular lens implantation while doing cataract surgery in these patients.

References

[1] M. P. Upadhyay, R. Kharel Sitaula, A. Manandhar et al., "The risk factors of Seasonal Hyperacute Panuveitis," *Ophthalmic Epidemiology*, vol. 28, no. 3, pp. 250–257, 2021.

[2] R. Kharel (Sitaula), A. Khatri, N. Sunam Gamal, A. Kumar Sharma, and D. Narayan Shah, "Patterns of uveitis among Nepalese population presenting at a tertiary referral eye care centre in Nepal," *New Frontiers in Ophthalmology*, vol. 5, no. 3, 2019.

[3] A. Manandhar, "Patterns of uveitis and scleritis in Nepal: a tertiary referral center study," *Ocular immunology and inflammation*, vol. 25, Supplement 1, pp. 54–62, 2017.

[4] R. Kharel Sitaula, A. Khatri, P. Karki et al., "Classification of Seasonal Hyperacute Panuveitis (SHAPU)," *Ocular Immunology and Inflammation*, pp. 1–5, 2021.

[5] C. J. Chu, A. D. Dick, R. L. Johnston, Y. C. Yang, and A. K. Denniston, "Cataract surgery in uveitis: a multicentre database study," *British Journal of Ophthalmology*, vol. 101, no. 8, pp. 1132–1137, 2017.

[6] A. Haripriya and A. Eliza, "Managing cataract surgery in uveitis," *Community Eye Health Journal*, vol. 31, no. 104, pp. 82-83, 2019.

[7] S. Yangzes, N. G. Seth, R. Singh et al., "Long-term outcomes of cataract surgery in children with uveitis," *Indian Journal of Ophthalmology*, vol. 67, no. 4, pp. 490–495, 2019.

18

Massive Orbital Myiasis Caused by *Sarcophaga argyrostoma* Complicating Eyelid Malignancy

Anfisa Ayalon,[1,2] Veronika Yehezkeli,[1,2] Yossi Paitan,[2,3] Krzysztof Szpila,[4] Kosta Y. Mumcuoglu,[5] and Elad Moisseiev[1,2]

[1]*Department of Ophthalmology, Meir Medical Center, Kfar Saba, Israel*
[2]*Sackler School of Medicine, Tel Aviv University, Tel Aviv, Israel*
[3]*Clinical Microbiology and Virology Laboratories, Meir Medical Center, Kfar Saba, Israel*
[4]*Department of Ecology and Biogeography, Faculty of Biology and Environmental Protection, Nicolaus Copernicus University, Toruń, Poland*
[5]*Parasitology Unit, Department of Microbiology and Molecular Genetics, The Hebrew University-Hadassah Medical School, Jerusalem, Israel*

Correspondence should be addressed to Anfisa Ayalon; doctor.anfi@gmail.com

Academic Editor: Cristiano Giusti

Purpose. To report a case of massive orbital myiasis caused by the larvae of *Sarcophaga argyrostoma*, complicating eyelid malignancy. *Observations.* A 98-year-old man first presented to our clinic noted to have a fast-growing lesion on his right upper and lower eyelids. Squamous cell carcinoma of the eyelids was highly suspected, and surgical excision was advised, but the patient refused any surgical or nonsurgical intervention. For the next eight months, the patient's family members continued to observe a high rate of tumor growth accompanied by deterioration of the general condition. During this whole period, the patient rejected admission to the hospital and was observed by nursing home staff. He was admitted to the emergency room in cachexic, unresponsive condition with fetid discharge and multiple live maggots crawling out from a large necrotic mass over the right orbit. On examination, no eyelids, eyeball, or other ocular tissue could be seen, while an extension of necrotic mass to forehead and midcheek was noted. Manual removal of larvae was performed. The patient passed away eight hours after his admission and larval removal. The maggots were identified as the third-instar larvae of *Sarcophaga argyrostoma. Conclusions and Importance.* This is the first reported case of home-acquired, massive orbital myiasis by *S. argyrostoma*. This case illustrates the crucial role of fly control as part of medical and home care in immobile patients. Moreover, it shows the importance of awareness by nursing home staff, paramedical, and medical personnel of possible myiasis, especially in bed-bound patients with skin malignancies and open wounds.

1. Introduction

Myiasis is a condition caused by the infestation of humans or animals by fly larvae of the order Diptera. According to the locality of the affected area, human myiasis is usually classified as cutaneous, oral, ocular, nasal, urogenital, and gastrointestinal. Facultative myiasis is caused by fly larvae which usually use decaying organic material such as feces and corpses as medium to develop and can rarely infest animals and humans, e.g., when they are affected by open infected wounds. Obligatory myiasis agents are able to penetrate also the intact skin and are always parasitic, e.g., the spotted flesh fly (*Wohlfahrtia magnifica*), which is common also in the Mediterranean countries [1]. *Sarcophaga argyrostoma* is a cosmopolitan and synanthropic species and is known to cause facultative myiasis in humans and animals [2]. Nosocomial myiasis is a very infrequent phenomenon but can have legal consequences and economic burden and cause

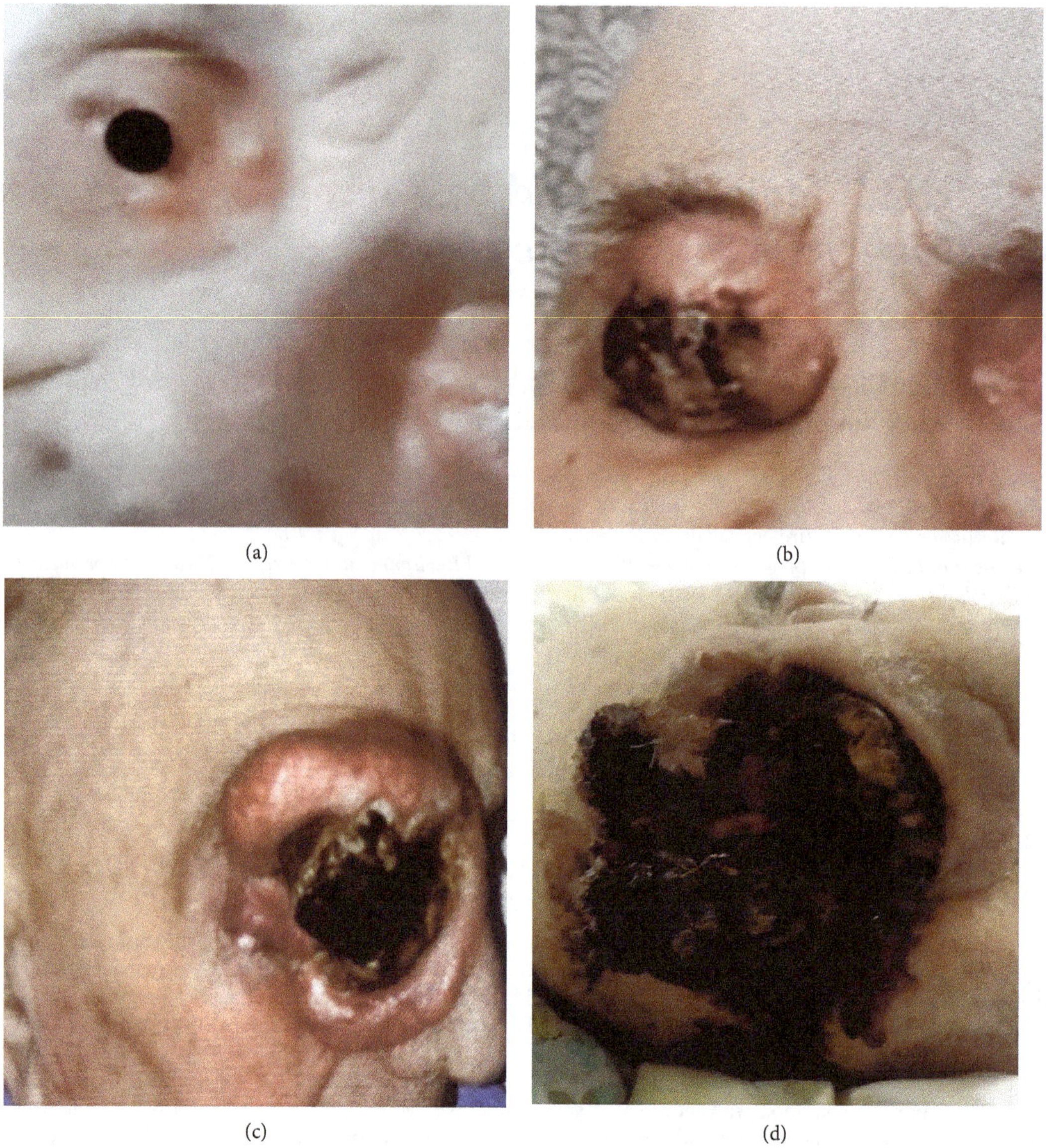

Figure 1: (a) Patient at the first presentation to the oculoplastic clinic. Note nodule-like lesions on the nasal part of his right upper and lower eyelids. (b, c) The high rate of tumor growth. Large, indurated tumor with ulcerated center can be seen. (d) Eight months after the first examination. Large ulcerated squamous cell carcinoma in the right orbital area, note the extension of necrotic mass to forehead and midcheek with multiple maggots.

prolonged hospitalization, disability, and even death [3–5]. Exposed skin malignancies and open wounds are risk factors of myiasis, especially in immobile patients [6].

We report a case of home-acquired orbital myiasis caused by larvae of *S. argyrostoma*, complicating course of eyelid malignancy.

2. Case Report

A 98-year-old man with a history of ischemic heart disease, dyslipidemia, and cerebral stroke was first referred to our oculoplastic clinic due to fast-growing lesions in both eyelids from the right side. Squamous cell carcinoma of the eyelids was highly suspected, but the patient refused any further diagnostic or treatment procedures, including biopsy or surgical removal of the lesions (Figure 1(a)). Over the next eight months, the patient refused admission to the hospital and was observed at his home by nursing home staff. The patient's family (members) continued to note a high rate of tumor growth accompanied by deterioration of the general condition (Figures 1(b) and 1(c)). During this period, the patient became unresponsive, cachexic, and had a large orbital tumor mass. When admitted to the emergency room, fetid discharge and multiple live maggots crawling out from a large necrotic over the right orbit could be seen, while he showed a markedly deteriorated general status. On examination, no eyelids, eyeball, or other ocular tissue could be seen on the right side of his face while the necrotic mass extended to forehead and midcheek (Figure 1(d)). Despite intensive treatment, the patient passed away eight hours later. Overall,

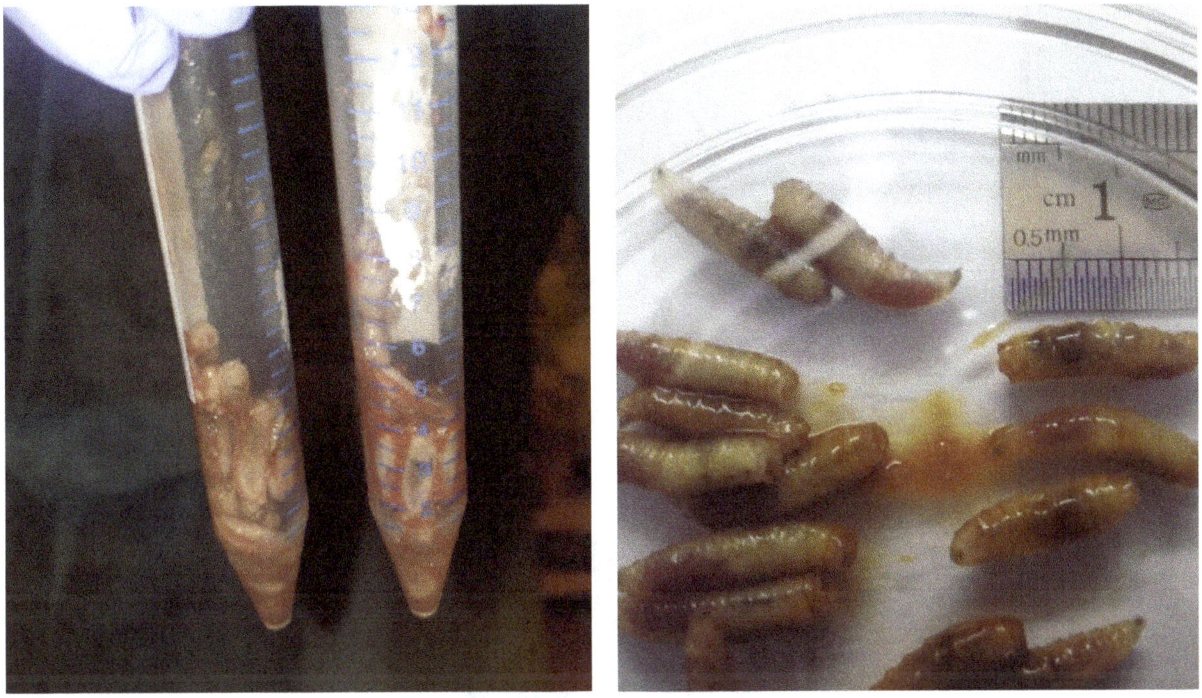

(a) (b)

FIGURE 2: (a, b) Maggots collected after removal from the patient.

32 larvae were removed from the patient and morphologically identified as the third larval instars of *S. argyrostoma* [7–9] (Figures 2 and 3).

3. Discussion

Squamous cell carcinoma (SCC) is reported as the second most common nonmelanoma skin cancer and the second most common eyelid malignancy [10, 11]. Advanced SCC is challenging to treat and is also a risk factor for unintended infestation with fly larvae. According to the literature, ophthalmomyiasis is a condition that can be seen in all age groups and, depending on the site of larval invasion, can be classified into external, internal, or orbital [6]. Orbital myiasis is a very rare form of this condition and occurs when large numbers of larvae invade the orbit and destroy its contents [12]. Due to medicolegal and sanitary issues, it is very important to record and correctly identify the species involved in myiasis, especially in cases of nosocomial acquired one. Hospital acquired ophthalmomyiasis by *S. argyrostoma* was reported only once in the literature [13]. There are previous reports of orbital myiasis, complication course of eyelid tumor [6, 14], but to the best of our knowledge, our report is the first one that describes a case of home-acquired orbital myiasis caused by *S. argyrostoma*. The main predisposing factors for the infestation in our patient included a very large area of necrotic tissue offered by the tumor, the patient's poor general condition with multiple medical comorbidities, advanced age, and lack of hygiene and fly control.

Due to lack of standard protocols, management of myiasis can be challenging and should be first focused on its prevention. Awareness by nursing home staff, paramedical, and medical personnel to possible myiasis in immobile patients with skin malignancies and open wounds is crucial. Screens on the windows could prevent flies from entering the rooms were immobilized patients and those with chronic wounds are living or hospitalized, while it is important to eliminate existing flies with insecticides. Proper wound care, hygiene, and adequate nutrition also play an important role in the recovery [14].

Treatment should aim to remove maggots completely, and the simplest measures are irrigation and mechanical removal [10]. Surgical debridement of local site with the use of topical agents, like turpentine oil, chloroform, ethyl chloride, phenol, and olive oil, and systemic treatment with ivermectin were described to be effective in the literature [15, 16]. Although topical and systemic treatments were shown to be effective in the management of myiasis, it should be kept in mind that such insecticides kill larvae in the deep layers of the wound and without removal of neutralized decomposing larvae body intoxication can be initiated. It should be also remembered that third-instar larvae usually stay for additional 1-3 days on the wound and leave the human body to pupate in a dry environment. In the literature, there are few reported cases of orbital myiasis and no previous reports of orbital myiasis caused by *S. argyrostoma*. Our patient had an unlikely course and outcome of the eyelid squamous cell carcinoma due to his refusal of any treatment and late presentation. The present case illustrates the importance of prevention and monitoring by medical personnel in immobile and debilitated patients.

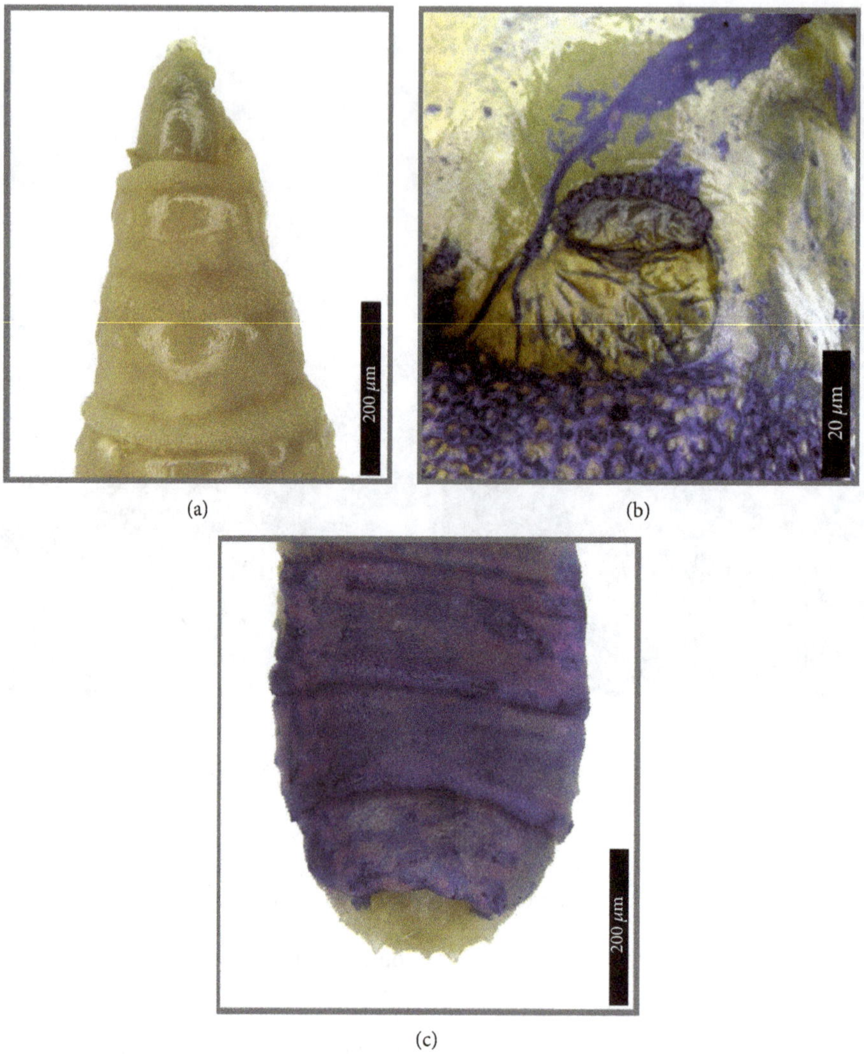

FIGURE 3: Third-instar larva of *Sarcophaga argyrostoma*. (a) Pseudocephalon and thoracic segments, dorsal view. (b) First thoracic segment, anterior spiracle, contrasted with ink marker. (c) Sixth and seventh abdominal segments and anal division, dorsal view, contrasted with ink marker.

4. Conclusion

Myiasis is a possible complication of untreated eyelid malignancies. To the best of our knowledge, we reported the first case of massive orbital myiasis caused by *S. argyrostoma*. There is a crucial role of fly control as part of medical and home care in immobile patients.

Moreover, our case shows the importance of awareness by nursing home staff, paramedical, and medical personnel of possible myiasis, especially in bad-bound patients with skin malignancies and open wounds.

Authors' Contributions

AA, VY, YP, KS, KYM, and EM were responsible for data collection, analysis, and writing/preparation of the manuscript. All authors attest that they meet the current ICMJE criteria for authorship.

Acknowledgments

KS was supported financially by the Polish National Science Centre (grant no. 2012/07/B/NZ8/00158).

References

[1] K. Y. Mumcuoglu, "Other ectoparasites: leeches, myiasis and sand flies," in *Manson's Tropical Diseases*, J. Farrar, P. J. Hotez, T. Junghanss, G. Kang, D. Lalloo, and N. J. White, Eds., pp. 843–847, Elsevier, 2014.

[2] F. Zumpt, "Myiasis in man and animals in the Old World," in *A textbook for physicians, veterinarians and zoologists*, Butterworth & Co. (Publishers) Ltd., London, 1965.

[3] M. Dutto, M. Pellegrino, and S. Vanin, "Nosocomial myiasis in a patient with diabetes," *The Journal of Hospital Infection*, vol. 83, no. 1, pp. 74–76, 2013.

[4] M. Dutto and M. Bertero, "Cutaneous superficial myiasis: report of a rare nosocomial parasitic disease caused by *Sarcophaga* spp. (Diptera, Sarcophagidae)," *Central European Journal of Public Health*, vol. 19, no. 4, pp. 232–234, 2011.

[5] A. Giangaspero, M. Marangi, A. Balotta, C. Venturelli, K. Szpila, and A. Di Palma, "Wound myiasis caused by *Sarcophaga (Liopygia) argyrostoma* (Robineau-Desvoidy) (Diptera: Sarcophagidae): additional evidences of the morphological identification dilemma and molecular investigation," *ScientificWorldJournal*, vol. 2017, article 9064531, 9 pages, 2017.

[6] J. C. Yeung, C. F. Chung, and J. S. Lai, "Orbital myiasis complicating squamous cell carcinoma of eyelid," *Hong Kong Medical Journal*, vol. 16, no. 1, pp. 63–65, 2010.

[7] J. Sanjean, "Taxonomic studies of *Sarcophaga* larvae of New York, with notes on the adults," *Memoirs of the Cornell University Agricultural Experimental Station*, vol. 349, pp. 1–115, 1957.

[8] K. Szpila, R. Richet, and T. Pape, "Third instar larvae of flesh flies (Diptera, Sarcophagidae) of forensic importance - critical review of characters and key for European species," *Parasitology Research*, vol. 114, no. 6, pp. 2279–2289, 2015.

[9] N. Ubero-Pascal, A. Paños, M.-D. García, J.-J. Presa, B. Torres, and M.-I. Arnaldos, "Micromorphology of immature stages of *Sarcophaga (Liopygia) cultellata* Pandellé, 1896 (Diptera: Sarcophagidae), a forensically important fly," *Microscopy Research and Technique*, vol. 78, no. 2, pp. 148–172, 2015.

[10] U. Wollina, "Myiasis on squamous cell carcinoma of skin," *Wiener Medizinische Wochenschrift*, vol. 165, no. 3-4, pp. 79–82, 2015.

[11] D. M. Reifler and A. Hornblass, "Squamous cell carcinoma of the eyelid," *Survey of Ophthalmology*, vol. 30, no. 6, pp. 349–365, 1986.

[12] M. S. Sachdev, H. Kumar, Roop, A. K. Jain, R. Arora, and V. K. Dada, "Destructive ocular myiasis in a noncompromised host," *Indian Journal of Ophthalmology*, vol. 38, no. 4, pp. 184–186, 1990.

[13] S. Graffi, A. Peretz, A. Wilamowski, H. Schnur, F. Akad, and M. Naftali, "External ophthalmomyiasis caused by a rare infesting larva, *Sarcophaga argyrostoma*," *Case Reports in Ophthalmological Medicine*, vol. 2013, Article ID 850865, 2 pages, 2013.

[14] S. J. Khardenavis, S. Kulkarni, V. Khardenavis, and A. Deshpande, "Ophthalmomyiasis in a case of basal cell carcinoma of eyelid," *BMJ Case Reports*, vol. 2018, 2018.

[15] L. K. S. Kumar, S. Manuel, T. V. John, and M. P. Sivan, "Extensive gingival myiasis - diagnosis, treatment, and prevention," *Journal of Oral and Maxillofacial Pathology*, vol. 15, no. 3, pp. 340–343, 2011.

[16] A. Jain, "Myiasis in patients with oral squamous cell carcinoma - a systematic review and protocol for management," *Oral and Maxillofacial Surgery*, vol. 23, no. 3, pp. 265–269, 2019.

19

Large Orbital Pediatric Intraosseous Hemangioma

Colin Bacorn and Lily Koo Lin

Department of Ophthalmology and Vision Science, University of California Davis Health, Sacramento, CA, USA

Correspondence should be addressed to Lily Koo Lin; lklin@ucdavis.edu

Academic Editor: Huban Atilla

A five-year-old male presenting with progressive right facial swelling underwent multiple biopsies before being diagnosed with a polyostotic frontal-zygomatic primary intraosseous hemangioma. Intraosseous hemangiomas are rare, more frequently afflict adult females, and very rarely involve the orbit. Our case with bony destruction and surrounding soft tissue mass measured 5.3 cm in a child mimicked a more ominous malignancy. This case is unique with its rapid progression and largest reported size, leading to additional challenges such as difficulty in achieving an adequate tissue sample and in the surgical management with respect to significant blood loss in a small child.

1. Introduction

Primary orbital intraosseous hemangiomas in children are exceedingly rare [1–5]. Intraosseous hemangiomas are more common in adult females and typically involve the vertebral body and calvarium with the frontal bone making up approximately 45% of reported calvarial cases [6]. Skull tumors may be more common in children while vertebral lesions are identified more frequently in middle aged adults [7]. Involvement of the facial bones is less common [8]. It is important to consider the possibility of this rare tumor preoperatively as life-threatening blood loss during surgical excision can be encountered [9–12].

2. Case Presentation

A five-year-old male with no medical or ophthalmologic history presented with one month of a progressively enlarging right facial mass. There was no prior trauma. This painless mass was firm to palpation and measured 3 cm in greatest dimension on initial presentation. Computed tomography (CT) of the orbits revealed a lytic osseous-based mass arising within the right zygoma (Figures 1(a) and 1(b)). The lesion exhibited a nonossified component within the orbit and exerted mass effect on the globe without evidence of scleral invasion. Based on these imaging characteristics, the primary differential diagnosis was Ewing's sarcoma but metastasis was also considered. Further systemic workup with CT of the chest, abdomen, and pelvis as well as a technetium bone scan failed to demonstrate other lesions or evidence of a primary malignancy. Fine-needle biopsy of the mass was inconclusive, showing only compact and woven bone, and the patient was referred for incisional biopsy. Approximately two months following symptom onset, the lesion had continued to enlarge and measured 5 cm in the largest dimension. An incisional biopsy was performed of just the soft tissue component and was again nondiagnostic and without malignant cells.

Based on these results, the patient was referred to our oculoplastic service for further management. Ophthalmic examination revealed best corrected visual acuity of 20/25 in the right eye and 20/20 in the left eye with normal stereopsis. The right bony orbital mass was noted (Figure 2) with relative proptosis of 2 mm of the right eye. There was no relative afferent pupillary defect or deficit of extraocular motility. The rest of his ophthalmic examination was normal. Magnetic resonance imaging (MRI) of the orbits was significant for a 5.3 cm mass with suggestion of intralesional vascular

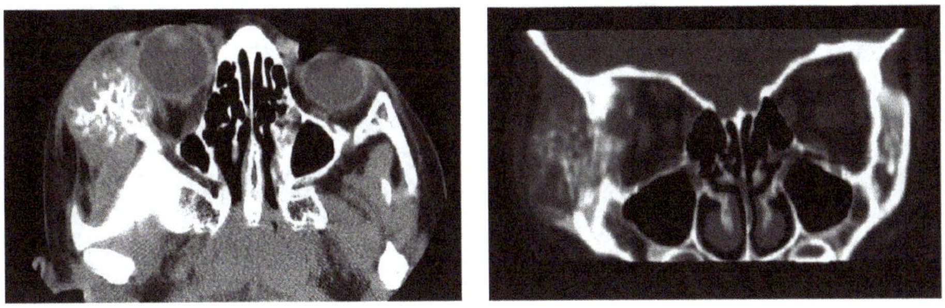

(a) (b)

Figure 1: (a) Axial and (b) coronal noncontrast computed tomography (CT) of the orbit of an osteolytic lesion with a large soft tissue component involving the right frontal and lateral orbit and zygomatic arch. A sunburst- or honeycomb-type pattern of new bone formation is seen.

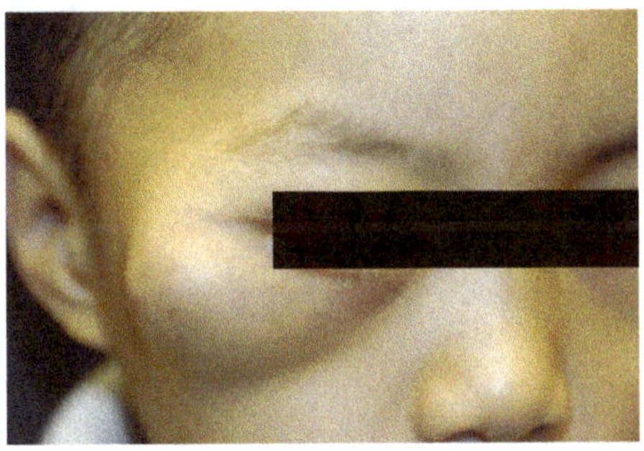

Figure 2: External photograph of patient's right facial mass involving the lateral orbit.

channels (Figures 3(a) and 3(b)). A third biopsy was performed via lateral orbitotomy with excision of a 5 cm × 6 cm bony mass. Intraoperatively, the mass was noted to be composed of numerous cystic spaces containing blood vessels and sanguineous material (Figure 4). Complete excision necessitated sacrifice of portions of the lateral and inferior orbital rims. The remaining intact bone was burred smooth, and a reconstructive implant was not necessary. Bone wax, diamond burr, cautery, and TISSEEL fibrin sealant (Baxter Healthcare Corporation, Westlake Village, CA, 91362 USA) were all employed to achieve hemostasis. The patient was typed and cross-matched due to approximately 150 milliliters of blood loss; however, given he remained hemodynamically stable both during and after surgery, ultimately no blood transfusion was administered. The final histopathology revealed reactive intratrabecular spaces containing numerous proliferated, small capillary-sized and dilated thin-walled blood vessels. The single layer of endothelial lining in the proliferating capillary vessels and blood-filled channels within bone confirmed a diagnosis of interosseous capillary hemangioma (Figure 5). Cytogenetic testing revealed normal karyotype supporting a diagnosis of intraosseous hemangioma. Postoperative examination demonstrated acceptable cosmesis (Figure 6). The patient has maintained best corrected visual acuity of 20/20 OD and 20/20 OS with full extraocular motility and without clinical evidence of recurrence eight years following excision.

3. Discussion

In children, a number of malignant orbital lesions can present with bone destruction such as Ewing's sarcoma, metastasis (osteosarcoma, neuroblastoma), Langerhans cell histiocytosis, leukemia, and rhabdomyosarcoma [1–5]. Although benign tumors such as fibrous dysplasia, juvenile ossifying fibromas, and intraosseous hemangiomas can demonstrate osteolytic activity, often, the initial goal is ruling out malignancy as was true in our case.

Primary orbital intraosseous hemangiomas in children are extremely rare. A recent case report and literature review identified 49 reported cases of zygomatic intraosseous hemangioma; only five of the patients were under the age of 18 at diagnosis and only seven were noted to have ocular findings [11]. None of these cases documented a lesion of our size (5 cm × 6 cm) in the zygomatic location. A separate study of 24 pediatric cases of cranial intraosseous hemangioma identified only four lesions with invasion into the orbit [13].

Clinically, these tumors often present as a subacute to chronic enlarging, firm, mass which may or may not be painful [14]. Occasionally, patients demonstrate multiple simultaneous lesions, although this is rare in the bones of the skull (10-15%) [15]. More rapid enlargement following trauma has also been reported. The diagnosis is often suggested by radiographic features including the classic description of a lytic lesion with "soap-bubble" or "sunburst" or "honeycomb" appearance; however, this pattern can be seen with other osteolytic etiologies as well [12]. MRI characteristics vary based on the tumor's fat composition and venous flow, but generally, these lesions exhibit either a high (high fat) or intermediate to low (low fat) T1-weighted signal and a heterogeneous, hyperintense T2-weighted signal and contrast enhancement [15–17].

Fine-needle aspiration is technically difficult in these bony tumors and may lack sufficient diagnostic accuracy as our case required excisional biopsy for diagnosis. Needle biopsy can disrupt the thin-walled blood vessels, so the specimen is nonspecific. Biopsy specimens without incorporating the bony component can also be nondiagnostic. Histologic subtypes have been classified as either cavernous, capillary, mixed, or scirrhous on the basis of the size of the vascular spaces and amount of connective tissue within the lesion

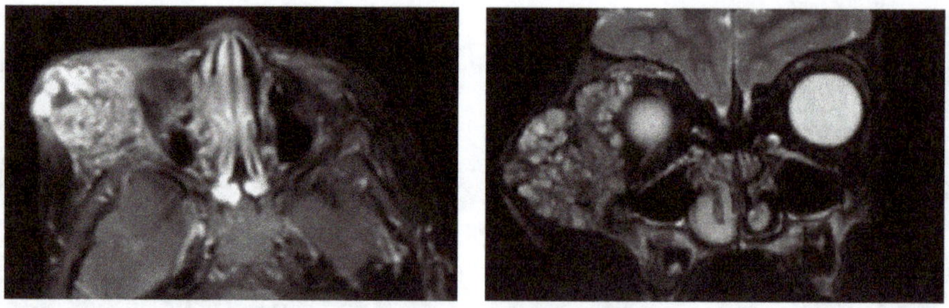

(a) (b)

Figure 3: (a) Axial T1-weighted postcontrast fat-saturated magnetic resonance (MR) image shows avid heterogenous enhancement of the soft tissue and intraosseous components. (b) Coronal T2-weighted fat-saturated noncontrast MR image shows the mass with multiple septations/cystic components.

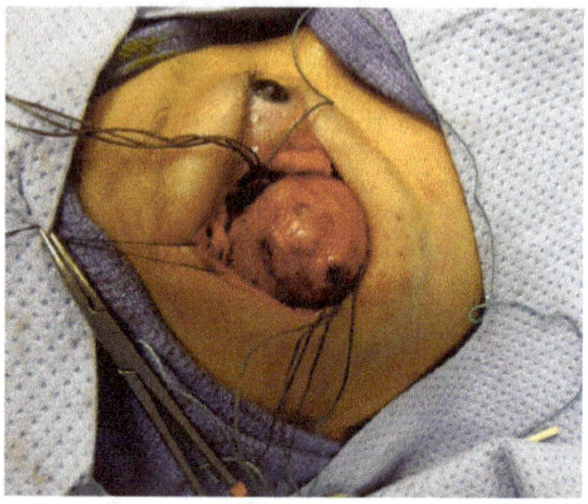

Figure 4: External photograph of the intraoperative gross appearance of the mass.

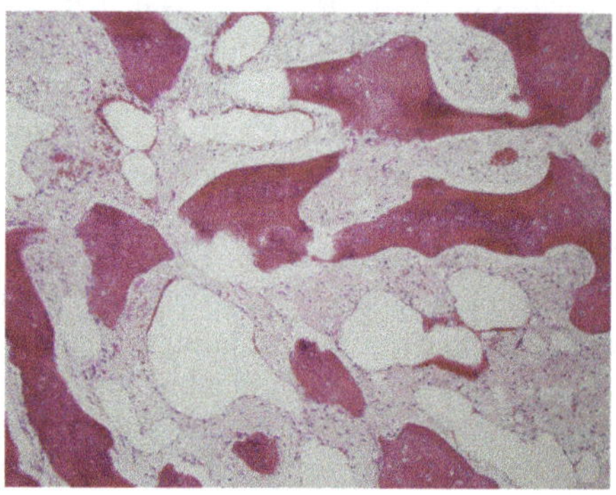

Figure 5: Low-power photomicrograph (original magnification, ×4; hematoxylin & eosin stain) shows dilated thin-walled vessels lined by flattened endothelial cells extending between scattered reactive bone trabeculae.

[11, 18]. While the diagnosis is often suspected on imaging features and gross examination intraoperatively or of the resected specimen, histopathologic examination is useful in differentiating these tumors from other vascular malformations and immunohistochemical analysis for Factor VIII, vimentin, CD31, and GLUT-1 may be appropriate in select cases [12, 19, 20].

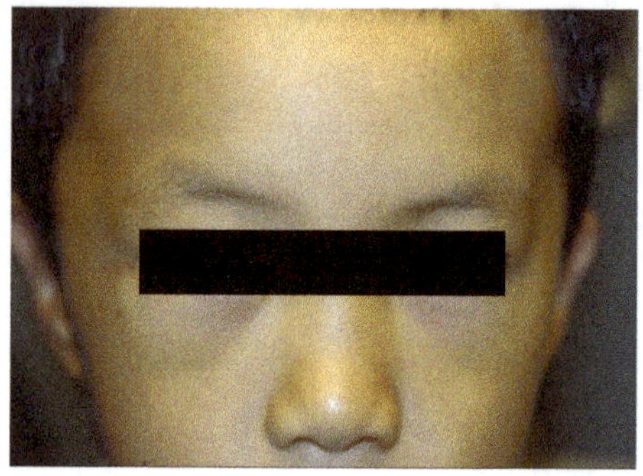

Figure 6: External photograph at the one-month postoperative visit, with resolution of the right orbital mass.

Treatment is typically total surgical excision with or without preoperative embolization [16, 21–25]. Given the age of our patient and both the invasiveness of angiography and the need for general anesthesia for the study, preoperative angiography was not pursued. Significant blood loss in the surgical resection of intraosseous hemangiomas has been well documented [9–12]. Our small patient's body weight was 19.3 kilograms at the time of his surgery, with an estimated blood volume (EBV) of 1351 milliliters (EBV = body weight (19.3 kg) × average blood volume of child (70 ml/kg)). Children may require red blood cell transfusion during or after surgery for an acute blood loss of greater than 10-15% EBV [26]. Our patient lost about 150 milliliters of blood intraoperatively, which placed him within this range. Given that he remained hemodynamically stable, and that transfusing red blood cells especially in children is not without risk, he did not ultimately receive a transfusion. However, this should be a consideration when surgically resecting intraosseous hemangiomas of this size in a small child. When lesions are inaccessible, or otherwise unresectable, radiotherapy has also been employed [27–29]. As in our case with 8-year follow-up, recurrence following complete excision is uncommon [29, 30]. Large pediatric intraosseous hemangiomas of the orbit are rare but should be remembered in the differential diagnosis of osteolytic lesions as surgical removal requires preoperative considerations such as the possibility of significant blood loss.

Acknowledgments

The authors thank Rebecca Sonu MD (El Dorado Pathology Medical Group, Placerville, CA) for her help with the histopathology image for this case.

References

[1] J. A. Shields, C. L. Shields, and R. Scartozzi, "Survey of 1264 patients with orbital tumors and simulating lesions: the 2002 Montgomery Lecture, part 1," *Ophthalmology*, vol. 111, no. 5, pp. 997–1008, 2004.

[2] G. Bonavolontà, D. Strianese, P. Grassi et al., "An analysis of 2,480 space-occupying lesions of the orbit from 1976 to 2011," *Ophthalmic Plastic and Reconstructive Surgery*, vol. 29, no. 2, pp. 79–86, 2013.

[3] B. V. Castillo and L. Kaufman, "Pediatric tumors of the eye and orbit," *Pediatric Clinics of North America*, vol. 50, no. 1, pp. 149–172, 2003.

[4] H. M. Alkatan, F. Al Marek, and S. Elkhamary, "Demographics of pediatric orbital lesions: a tertiary eye center experience in Saudi Arabia," *Journal of Epidemiology and Global Health*, vol. 9, no. 1, pp. 3–10, 2019.

[5] A. A. Rao, J. H. Naheedy, J. Y.-Y. Chen, S. L. Robbins, and H. L. Ramkumar, "A clinical update and radiologic review of pediatric orbital and ocular tumors," *Journal of Oncology*, vol. 2013, Article ID 975908, 22 pages, 2013.

[6] Y. Yang, J. Guan, W. Ma et al., "Primary intraosseous cavernous hemangioma in the skull," *Medicine*, vol. 95, no. 11, article e3069, 2016.

[7] C. Philpott, A. Wray, D. Mac Gregor, and L. Coleman, "Dural infantile hemangioma masquerading as a skull vault lesion," *American Journal of Neuroradiology*, vol. 33, no. 6, pp. E85–E87, 2012.

[8] S. Myadam, V. Kishan, A. Deepa, K. Shri Puja, and R. K. Divya, "Intraosseous hemangioma of the zygomatic bone: a rare site for hemangioma," *Medical Journal, Armed Forces India*, vol. 72, no. 1, pp. 85–87, 2016.

[9] L. Yu, L. Cai, G. R. Yu, Z. H. Zeng, and S. X. Tao, "Solitary giant hemangioma of the humerus," *Orthopedics*, vol. 32, no. 12, pp. 925–928, 2009.

[10] N. C. Charles and R. D. Lisman, "Intraosseous hemangioma of the orbit," *Ophthalmic Surgery and Lasers*, vol. 33, no. 4, pp. 326–328, 2002.

[11] D. B. Powers, E. Fisher, and D. Erdmann, "Zygomatic intraosseous hemangioma: case report and literature review," *Craniomaxillofacial Trauma and Reconstruction*, vol. 10, no. 01, pp. 1–10, 2017.

[12] S. Madge, S. Simon, Z. Abidin et al., "Primary orbital intraosseous hemangioma," *Ophthalmic Plastic and Reconstructive Surgery*, vol. 25, no. 1, pp. 37–41, 2009.

[13] G. L. Prasad and K. Pai, "Pediatric cranial intraosseous hemangiomas: a review," *Neurosurgical Review*, vol. 41, no. 1, pp. 109–117, 2018.

[14] A. M. Marcinow, M. J. Provenzano, R. K. Gurgel, and K. E. Chang, "Primary intraosseous cavernous hemangioma of the zygoma: a case report and literature review," *Ear, Nose, & Throat Journal*, vol. 91, no. 5, pp. 210–215, 2012.

[15] H. Kiratli and M. Orhan, "Multiple orbital intraosseous hemangiomas," *Ophthalmic Plastic and Reconstructive Surgery*, vol. 14, no. 5, pp. 345–348, 1998.

[16] Y. Suzuki, H. Ikeda, and K. Matsumoto, "Neuroradiological features of intraosseous cavernous hemangioma-case report," *Neurologia Medico-Chirurgica*, vol. 41, no. 5, pp. 279–282, 2001.

[17] A. Rigopoulou and A. Saifuddin, "Intraosseous hemangioma of the appendicular skeleton: imaging features of 15 cases, and a review of the literature," *Skeletal Radiology*, vol. 41, no. 12, pp. 1525–1536, 2012.

[18] C. A. Eliot and J. T. Castle, "Intraosseous hemangioma of the anterior mandible," *Head and Neck Pathology*, vol. 4, no. 2, pp. 123–125, 2010.

[19] N. Kadlub, L. Dainese, A. Coulomb-L'Hermine et al., "Intraosseous haemangioma: semantic and medical confusion," *International Journal of Oral and Maxillofacial Surgery*, vol. 44, no. 6, pp. 718–724, 2015.

[20] G. Yang, C. Li, X. Chen et al., "Large capillary hemangioma of the temporal bone with a dural tail sign: a case report," *Oncology Letters*, vol. 8, no. 1, pp. 183–186, 2014.

[21] J. S. Choi, Y. C. Bae, G. B. Kang, and K.-U. Choi, "Intraosseous hemangioma of the orbit," *Archives of Craniofacial Surgery*, vol. 19, no. 1, pp. 68–71, 2018.

[22] J. S. Brandner, Y. B. Rawal, L. J. Kim, and J. K. Dillon, "Intraosseous hemangioma of the frontal bone. Report of a case and review of the literature," *Journal of Oral and Maxillofacial Surgery*, vol. 76, no. 4, pp. 799–805, 2018.

[23] C.-Y. Wu, H.-M. Huang, D.-C. Chen, D.-Y. Cho, and S.-T. Wei, "Primary intraosseous hemangioma of the orbital roof: a pitfall of surgery," *The Journal of Craniofacial Surgery*, vol. 27, no. 6, pp. e580–e581, 2016.

[24] S. Koybasi, L. Saydam, and L. Kutluay, "Intraosseous hemangioma of the zygoma," *American Journal of Otolaryngology*, vol. 24, no. 3, pp. 194–197, 2003.

[25] B. H. Park, E. Hwang, and C. H. Kim, "Primary intraosseous hemangioma in the frontal bone," *Archives of Plastic Surgery*, vol. 40, no. 3, pp. 283–285, 2013.

[26] H. Rachel, "Transfusion principles in children," *Anaesthesia & Intensive Care Medicine*, vol. 10, no. 2, pp. 71–75, 2009.

[27] U. Singh, C. Kalavakonda, S. Venkitachalam, S. Patil, and R. Chinnusamy, "Intraosseous hemangioma of sella: case report and review of literature," *World Neurosurgery: X*, vol. 3, p. 100030, 2019.

[28] G. D. Rios Dias and A. A. Velasco Cruz, "Intraosseous hemangioma of the lateral orbital wall," *Ophthalmic Plastic and Reconstructive Surgery*, vol. 20, no. 1, pp. 27–30, 2004.

[29] M. Perugini, G. Renzi, G. Gasparini, G. Cerulli, and R. Becelli, "Intraosseous hemangioma of the maxillofacial district: clinical analysis and surgical treatment in 10 consecutive patients," *The Journal of Craniofacial Surgery*, vol. 15, no. 6, pp. 980–985, 2004.

[30] T. Gupta, G. E. Rose, M. Manisali, P. Minhas, J. M. Uddin, and D. H. Verity, "Cranio-orbital primary intraosseous haemangioma," *Eye*, vol. 27, no. 11, pp. 1320–1323, 2013.

20

Orbital Solitary Fibrous Tumor: Four Case Reports—Clinical and Histopathological Features

Carmen Navarro-Perea,[1] Cristina Calleja-García,[1] Álvaro Bengoa-González,[1] María-C. Garrido,[2] Enrique Mencía-Gutiérrez,[1] and Silvia Pérez-Trigo[1]

[1]*Ophthalmology Department, 12 de Octubre Hospital, Complutense University, 28041 Madrid, Spain*
[2]*Pathology Department, 12 de Octubre Hospital, Complutense University, 28041 Madrid, Spain*

Correspondence should be addressed to Enrique Mencía-Gutiérrez; emencia.hdoc@salud.madrid.org

Academic Editor: Stephen G. Schwartz

Purpose. To retrospectively describe the clinical characteristics, management, and outcomes of four cases of orbital solitary fibrous tumor (SFT). In one patient, we present an ultrasonic aspirator system for tumor removal. *Methods.* Four patients with orbital SFT were selected: one patient with orbital SFT, another patient with frontal and ethmoidal SFT and orbital affectation with high rates of recurrence, the third patient with frontal lobe SFT and orbital invasion with multiple recurrences, and the fourth case with a history of craniopharyngioma surgery and SFT located on the orbital apex. *Results.* All cases showed proptosis, eye movement restriction, and, in three cases, visual acuity alteration. Different treatments were applied: in three cases, excision was performed, one of them with an ultrasonic aspirator system, and in the remaining case, an exenteration was done (in two cases, radiosurgery treatment was also applied). The immunohistochemical study revealed SFT, similar to hemangiopericytomas (HPCs). No recurrence has been observed after surgical treatment. *Conclusion.* The SFT is a spectrum of different tumors with similar histopathological characteristics. The use of immunohistochemical markers is very helpful in the diagnosis. The main problem of orbital involvement is the risk of damaging important structures adjacent to the tumor during the surgical removal. The ultrasonic aspirator system allows elimination of the tumor without damaging other orbital structures.

1. Introduction

Solitary fibrous tumor (SFT) is a rare tumor which was first described in the visceral pleura in 1931 by Klemperer and Rabin [1]. In the literature, numerous cases are described and there are reviews of extrapleural SFTs; currently, they are thought to appear anywhere in the body [1, 2]. SFT was first described in the orbit in 1994 by Westra et al. [3], and since then, there have been published 150 cases in English literature [4]. They are usually benign, although there are specific malignant cases with frequent local recurrences and invasion of adjacent structures [5, 6]. Stereotactic radiosurgery (SRS) is described in the literature as an adjunctive treatment option when surgical resection is not complete or as a treatment for recurrences [2]. At present, the SFT spectrum includes lesions like hemangiopericytomas (HPCs), giant cell angiofibromas, and fibrous histiocytomas (FHs) [7].

We report four cases of orbital SFT with descriptions of clinical symptoms, immunohistochemical and histopathological details, and treatment. In one case, we also describe the use of SONOPET® (Stryker, Kalamazoo, MI, USA) ultrasonic aspirator system for the tumor excision postincisional biopsy. It is a surgical tool that uses low-frequency ultrasonic vibrations to fragment tissue while simultaneously irrigating and aspirating the surgical field [8].

2. Case 1

The first case is a 25-year-old woman with loss of visual acuity (VA) in the right eye (RE) for one year. The best-corrected visual acuity (BCVA) was 0.5 (decimal scale, Snellen) in the RE and 1.0 in the left eye (LE). In the RE, she also presented alteration of the external ocular movements with limitation to supraduction and abduction (Figures 1(a) and 1(b)),

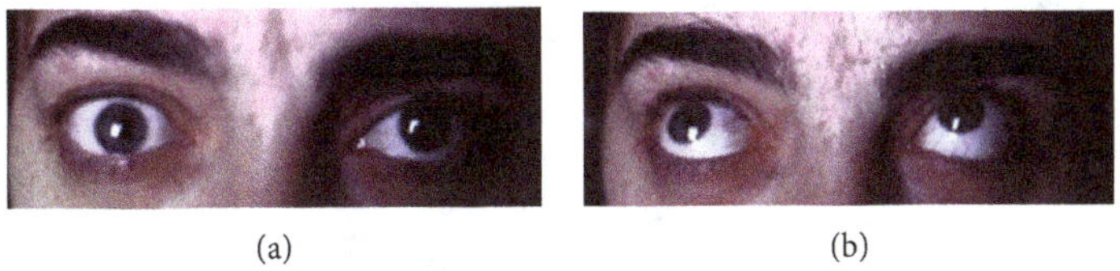

FIGURE 1: Case 1. (a, b) Clinical photograph shows alteration of the external ocular movements with limitation to supraduction and abduction.

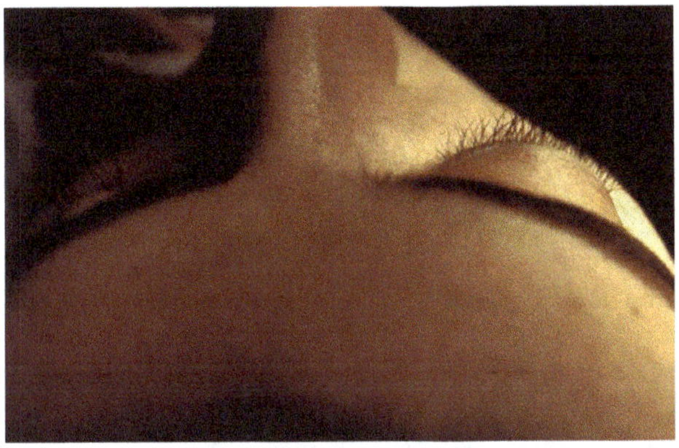

FIGURE 2: Case 1. Clinical photograph shows proptosis of 9 mm in the right eye.

proptosis of 9 mm (Figure 2), lagophthalmos of 3–4 mm, and a mass in the upper orbital region. The LE did not show any alteration. Orbital echography showed an extraconal superior mass with high density and an irregular pattern (Figure 3). In the magnetic resonance imaging (MRI), an extraconal, superior, and central orbital mass was observed; it measured 3.7 × 3.5 × 1.7 cm and extended up to the posterior third of the orbit, with hyperintensity on T2-weighted scans and hypointensity in T1-weighted scans (Figures 4(a) and 4(b)), compatible with cavernous angioma or meningioma. An upper orbitotomy was performed through the upper lid crease with dissection and removal of a compact, depressible pink lesion, which is well defined and without nutrient vascularization (Figure 5). Microscopically, the tumor was composed of a proliferation of spindle cells arranged in an irregular manner with a focal storiform pattern, bland cytology, and vascular proliferation with an HPC-like grown pattern. Immunohistochemistry was positive for CD34, CD99, BCL2, vimentin, and myoglobin (Figures 6(a)–6(d)). The tumor was negative for AE1-AE3 cytokeratin, epithelial membrane antigen (EMA), S100 protein, smooth muscle actin (SMA), and desmin. Mitotic activity showed a low mitosis index (<1–4 high-power fields (HPF)). There was no evidence of hemorrhage, necrosis, or infiltrative borders nor architectural signs of malignancy. After 15 years of follow-up, there has been no evidence of recurrence.

3. Case 2

The second case is a 74-year-old woman who had been receiving follow-up monitoring in otorhinolaryngology for 8 years for a frontal and ethmoidal SFT located on the right side; the SFT had been operated on five times for multiple recurrences despite complete resections. At the last visit, the patient was assessed by ophthalmology because of a 4 mm exophthalmos (Figure 7), with inferior and external displacement of the RE, and limitation to adduction and supraduction. The BCVA was 0.7 (decimal scale, Snellen) in the RE and 0.9 in the LE. Magnetic resonance imaging (Figure 8(a)) and computed tomography (CT) imaging (Figure 8(b)) with contrast showed a 2.2 cm mass that captured contrast; it was located in the right ethmoid sinus with medial invasion into the orbit with infiltration of the medial rectus muscle and minimal posterior extension to the sphenoid (Figure 8(c)). The patient was treated with a lateral orbitotomy to shift the eye, and then, through a transcaruncular approach, the tumor was located. First, samples were taken for histopathological and immunohistochemical study, and then, with the SONOPET® ultrasonic aspirator system, the tumor was completely aspirated.

Gross examination revealed a tan-colored tumor. Microscopically, the tumor showed a fibroblastic proliferation with hypo- and hypercellular areas alternating with each other and bands of sclerotic collagen fibers. The arrangement of the cells varied from area to area in the same tumor. In some areas, the cells were arranged in short ill-defined fascicles, with a storiform pattern, whereas in others they were arranged randomly in what is called a "patternless" pattern. In the most cellular phase of the tumor, tightly packed fusiform cells were arranged around a ramifying vascular network. Commonly, the vessels, particularly the large ones, showed a thick coat of collagen. There was no significant cellular atypia and mitosis was 1–4/10 HPF (Figures 9(a) and 9(b)). On immunohistochemistry, the tumor cells had typically strong and diffuse positivity for vimentin and BCL2, focal positivity for CD34, and weak diffuse positivity for CD99 but negativity for cytokeratins AE1–AE3, actin HHF35, actin 1A4, calponin, caldesmon, desmin, S-100 protein, and collagen IV (Figures 9(c) and 9(d)). With these findings, a final diagnosis of SFT was made. Treatment consisted of 35 Gy at a fractionation of 5 weekly sessions of 5 Gy, by 4 fields shaped static at an energy of 6 MV by multilamines. After this treatment, the patient presented great improvement in right supraversion and abduction with significant reduction in size. No recurrence was observed after 4 years of follow-up. The patient died of a stroke.

4. Case 3

The third case is a 78-year-old woman in follow-up by neurosurgery for an SFT at the base of the right frontal lobe which had been operated on eight times for multiple recurrences despite resections. In those operations, part of the lateral and upper wall of the right orbit had been resected due to

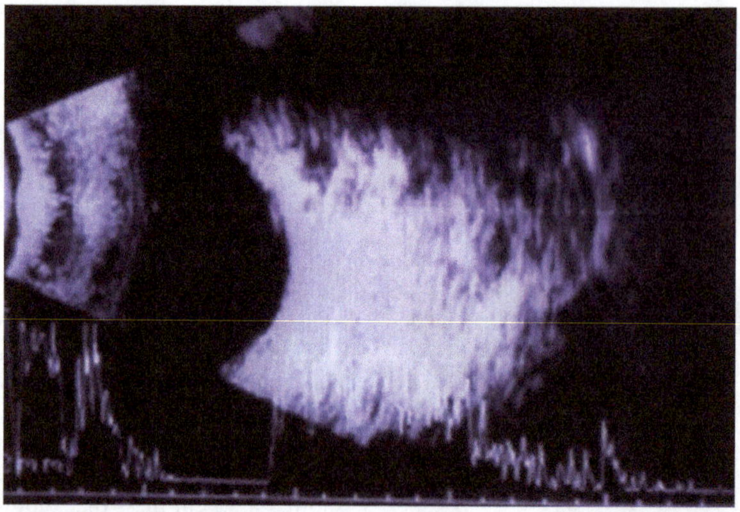

FIGURE 3: Case 1. Orbital echography shows a superior extraconal mass with high density and irregular pattern.

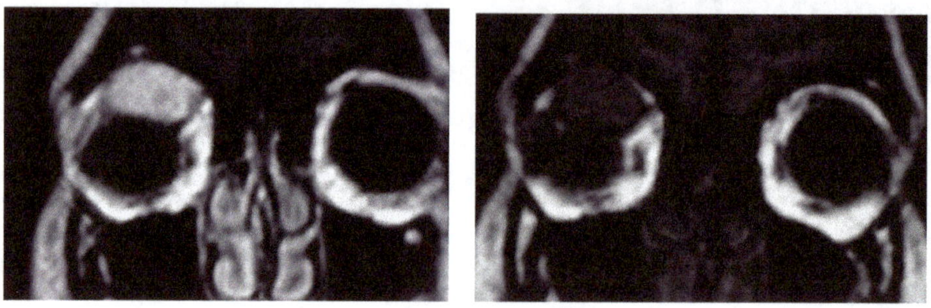

(a) (b)

FIGURE 4: Case 1. (a) Magnetic resonance imaging (MRI) in coronal image showing T2-weighted extraconal tumor based on superior and central orbital, which measures 3.7 cm in the greatest axis and hyperintensity image. (b) T1 weighted with hypointensity image.

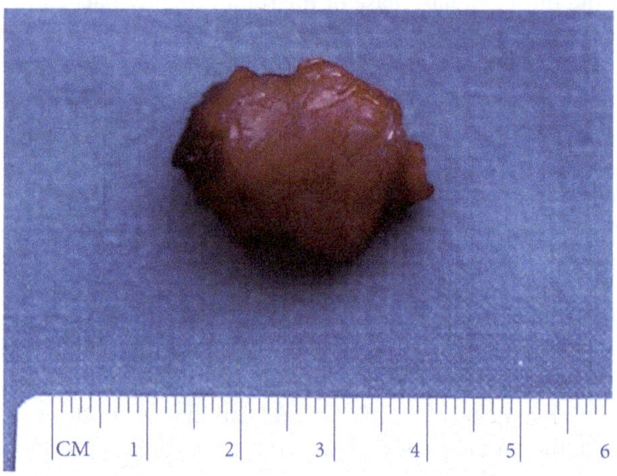

FIGURE 5: Case 1. Gross examination demonstrated a pink, indurated, well-circumscribed, and encapsulated appearance.

tumor invasion. The new recurrence was located on the left orbital apex. It was rounded and well defined with a diameter of 16 mm (Figures 10(a)–10(c)). The BCVA in the LE was 0.4 (decimal scale, Snellen), and there was amaurosis in the RE (the eye had been blind for 2 years) with painless exophthalmos and eye movement limitation. Due to the aggressive nature of the tumor, exenteration and reconstruction of the left orbit with a temporal muscle flap were performed (Figures 11(a) and 11(b)). The immunochemical study showed positive markers like vimentin, CD34 (positive focal), BCL2, CD99, S-100 protein, and MIB-1 (low positivity) and negative markers like actin, calponin, AE1–AE3 cytokeratins, caldesmon, desmin, and collagen IV. Cellular atypia and mitosis were >10 HPF. The histopathology confirmed SFT, which is HPC type. After the pathological confirmation and due to the high rate of recurrences of the tumor, SRS was indicated as adjunctive treatment. No recurrence has been observed after 5 years of follow-up.

5. Case 4

The fourth case is a 44-year-old woman with a history of craniopharyngioma surgery due to neurosurgery at 9 and 12 years of age. She showed proptosis in the right side, which had begun one week previously. She had amaurosis in the RE and BCVA in the LE 0.8 (decimal scale, Snellen). She had iatrogenic secondary panhypopituitarism due to previous neurosurgery and epilepsy (absence-type seizures with right frontal epileptiform focus). Given the suspicion of a possible recurrence, a CT scan was performed; it showed a lesion of $24 \times 24 \times 26$ mm with a rounded, hyperdense

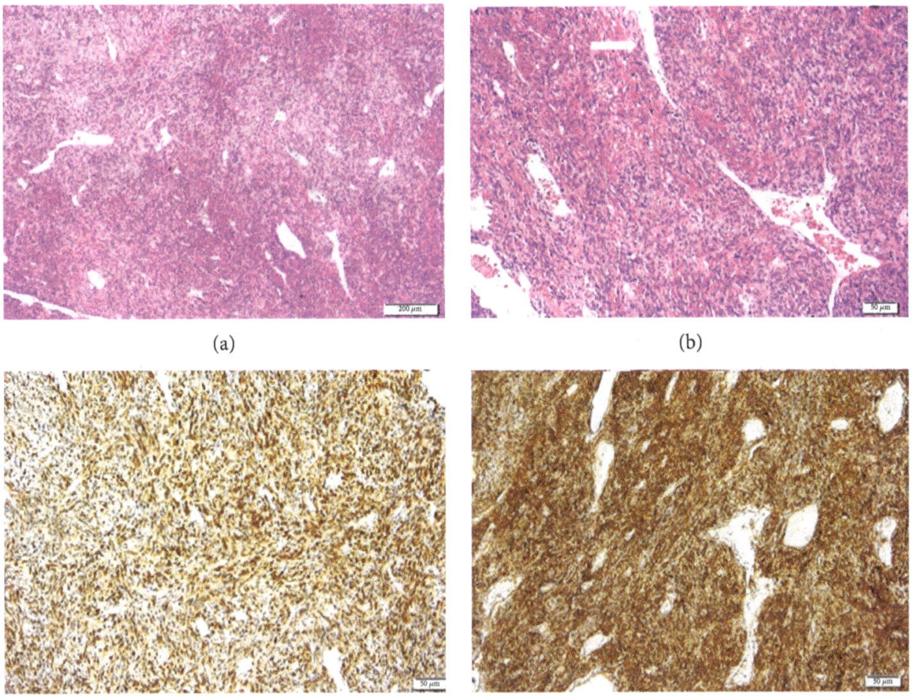

(a) (b) (c) (d)

Figure 6: Case 1. (a, b) Microscopic appearance of the tumor, composed of a proliferation of spindle cells arranged in an irregular manner with a focal storiform pattern, bland cytology, and vascular proliferation with a hemangiopericytoma-like growth pattern (arrow in (b)). (H&E, ×40 and ×100 magnification.) Positivity of the tumor for (c) BCL2 and (d) CD34. (Bar is indicated in μm, down and to the right).

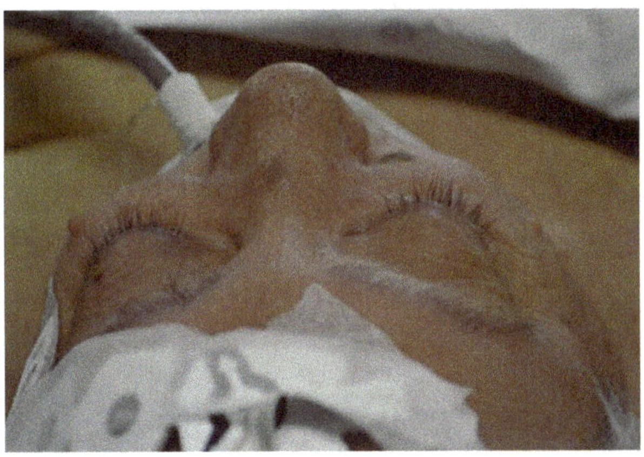

Figure 7: Case 2. Clinical photograph shows proptosis of 4 mm in the right eye.

morphology, located in the medial intraconal region of the right orbit. The lesion imprinted on the back of eyeball, as well as the optic nerve and internal rectus muscle, with direct contact with the external rectus muscle. Due to the previous neurosurgery, there was residual frontal cerebral lobe basal hypodensity, as well as hypodensities in white matter of both convexities in the frontal and temporal vertebral lobes (Figure 12(a)). In the MRI, the lesion presented isodensity with the extraocular muscles in T1- and T2-weighted sequences. After the introduction of intravenous contrast, an intense enhancement was observed except for a small hypocaptant focus in its anterior part. There was bone remodeling of the medial orbital wall and involvement of the optic nerve due to contiguity. In the cranial study, areas of signal hyperintensity were evident in T2 and FLAIR sequences in the bilateral frontobasal white substance (Figures 12(b) and 12(c)), bilateral temporobasal substance, and both internal capsules, all related to residual ischemic events/gliosis. A debulking was performed through a lateral orbitotomy. Microscopic study showed a moderate-highly cellular neoplastic proliferation, constituted by cells of mesenchymal-type morphology that were arranged forming bundles. The cells were spindle shaped, with oval nuclei, scarcely pleomorphic and without nucleolus; cytoplasms were eosinophilic and poorly defined. The mitotic index was 1/10 HPS. Some areas of the lesion were less cellular, showing a myxoid stroma, while in other areas the stroma was dense with a collagenous aspect. There were also numerous vascular clefts "in deer antler." Necrosis or hemorrhage foci were not observed (Figures 13(a) and 13(b)). In the immunohistochemical study, tumor cells showed positivity for CD34, CD99, and BCL2 and negativity for EMA, protein S100, and glial fibrillary acidic protein. There was negativity for CD31 except in the vascular endothelium (Figures 13(c) and 13(d)). A diagnosis for FST, HPC type, was made. No recurrence was observed after 2 years of follow-up. The patient died from infectious pericarditis and pneumonia.

6. Discussion

SFT is a rare fusocellular benign tumor that is more common in the visceral pleura [1] but can appear in extrapleural locations including the pericardium, mediastinum,

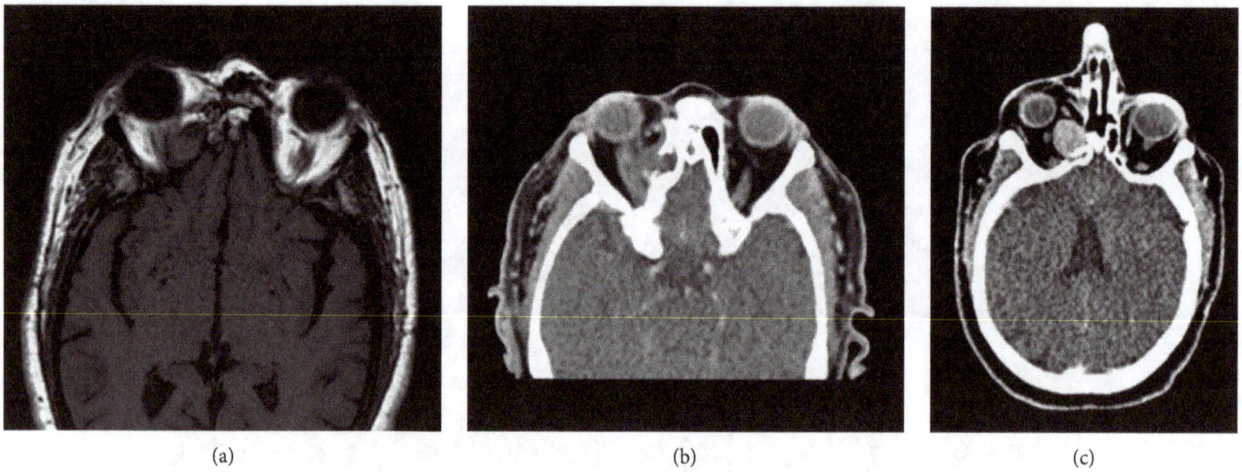

FIGURE 8: Case 2. (a) MRI in axial view showing the initial large, well-defined round mass over the superior and posterior orbits. Axial computed tomography (CT) imaging showing (b) the third recurrence which includes ethmoidal invasion 3 years later (c) and a fifth recurrence 5 years later.

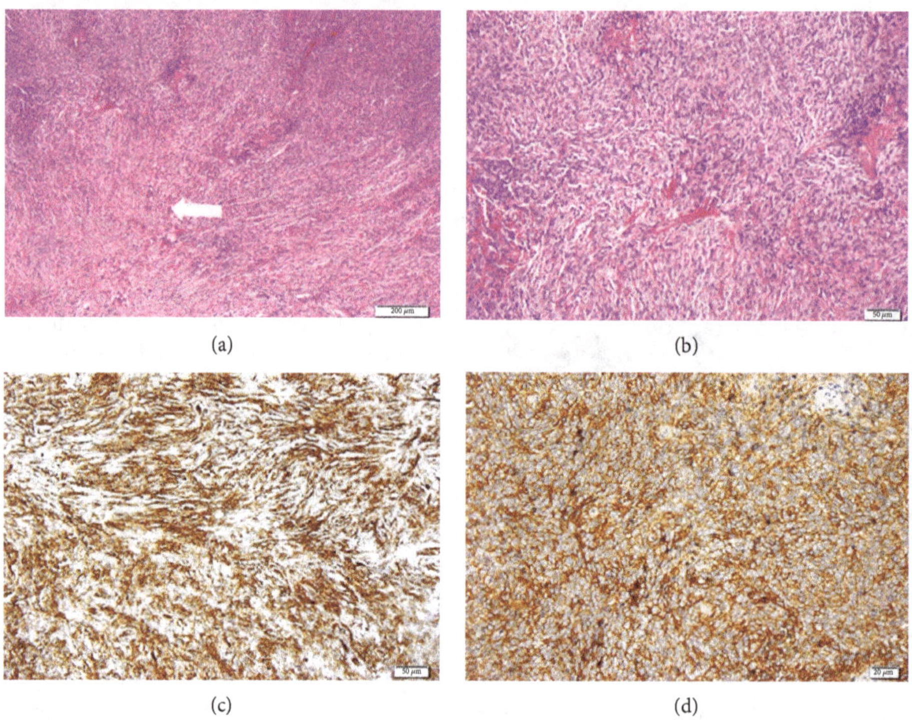

FIGURE 9: Case 2. (a) Microscopically, the tumor reveals fibroblastic proliferation with hypo- and hypercellular areas alternating with each other and bands of sclerotic collagen fiber networks (arrow points at the more hypocellular area) (H&E, ×40 magnification). (b) Higher magnification demonstrates the cellular phase of the tumor with tightly packed fusiform cells arranged around a ramifying vascular network (H&E, ×100 magnification). Positivity of the tumor for (c) CD34 and (d) CD99. Bar is indicated in μm, down and to the right.

peritoneum, paranasal sinuses, and orbit [9, 10]. After a systematic review, we found that 150 cases of orbital SFT have been described in the English literature [4]. Usually, orbital SFTs exhibit a benign course, but malignant forms with high rates of local recurrence have been reported [1]. The main orbital location is the upper and medial zone of the orbit, as in our four cases, but they have been described in many other locations [11].

This tumor appears mainly in the fifth decade of life, but it can appear any time from age 15 to over 89 [8]. All of our cases were adult patients (range: 25 to 78 years, mean: 55). In our study, all cases of SFT were in female patients, but the literature shows that there is no gender-based predilection [8, 12]. The most common form of clinical presentation is with unilateral painless proptosis, with slow growth; it may be associated with eyelid edema, visual alterations, the presence of a palpable mass, tearing, and ipsilateral ptosis [1, 11]. Our four cases showed unilateral painless exophthalmos and eye movement limitation. Three patients also showed loss of VA from the beginning,

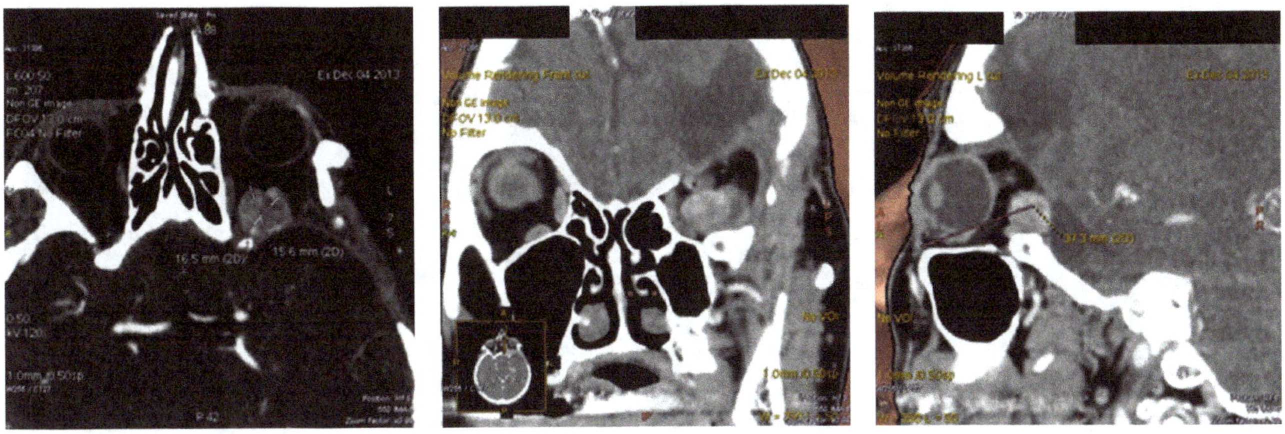

(a) (b) (c)

FIGURE 10: Case 3. (a) CT imaging showing a well-defined rounded lesion, in the left orbital apex. (b) Coronal view. (c) Sagittal view.

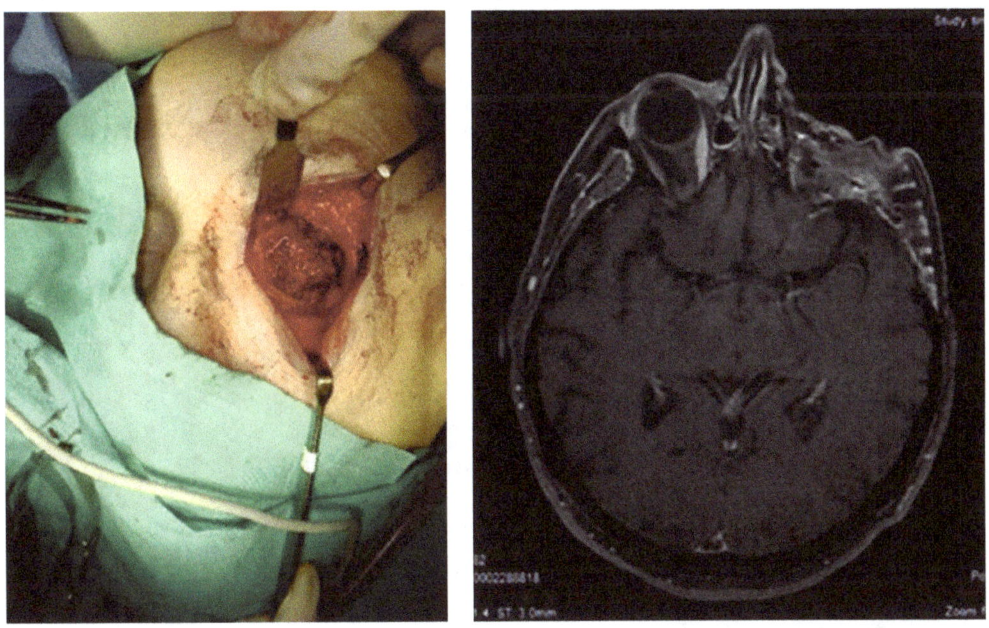

(a) (b)

FIGURE 11: Case 4. (a) Photograph of surgical exenteration. Temporal muscle fills the posterior part of the right orbit. (b) Axial view MRI postexenteration.

although the literature reveals that SFT does not often cause compression of the optic nerve [4].

In the radiological exam, SFT may be difficult to distinguish from other orbital lesions such as cavernous hemangioma, schwannoma, localized neurofibroma, varix, and orbital metastasis [4]. The computed tomography and MRI usually show a solitary well-defined soft tissue mass [4, 13] that can be located anywhere on the orbit but is more frequent in superior quadrants [4]. The pattern of contrast enhancement and washout on dynamic imaging may help to differentiate between cavernous hemangioma, SFT, and schwannoma [4]. Bone remodeling is present in cases of suspicious malignant transformation, but this is uncommon [13]. In our study, two cases show bone remodeling and high rates of recurrences, leading to suspicion of malignancy. The ultrasound shows a tumor that is well circumscribed, firm, or minimally compressible, variably vascular, with a regular internal structure and low to medium reflectivity [4].

The classic histopathological features of SFT are cells which are described as spindle shaped with a small cytoplasm and indistinct nucleoli, and the tumor matrix contains a distinctive thick "ropy" type of collagen between tumor cells [8, 14]. SFT should be differentiated from other spindle-shaped cell orbital tumors, such as fibrous histiocytoma, HPC, meningioma, and schwannoma [14]. The use of immunohistochemical markers is very helpful in diagnosing SFT. In the literature, there is great controversy about the diagnosis of

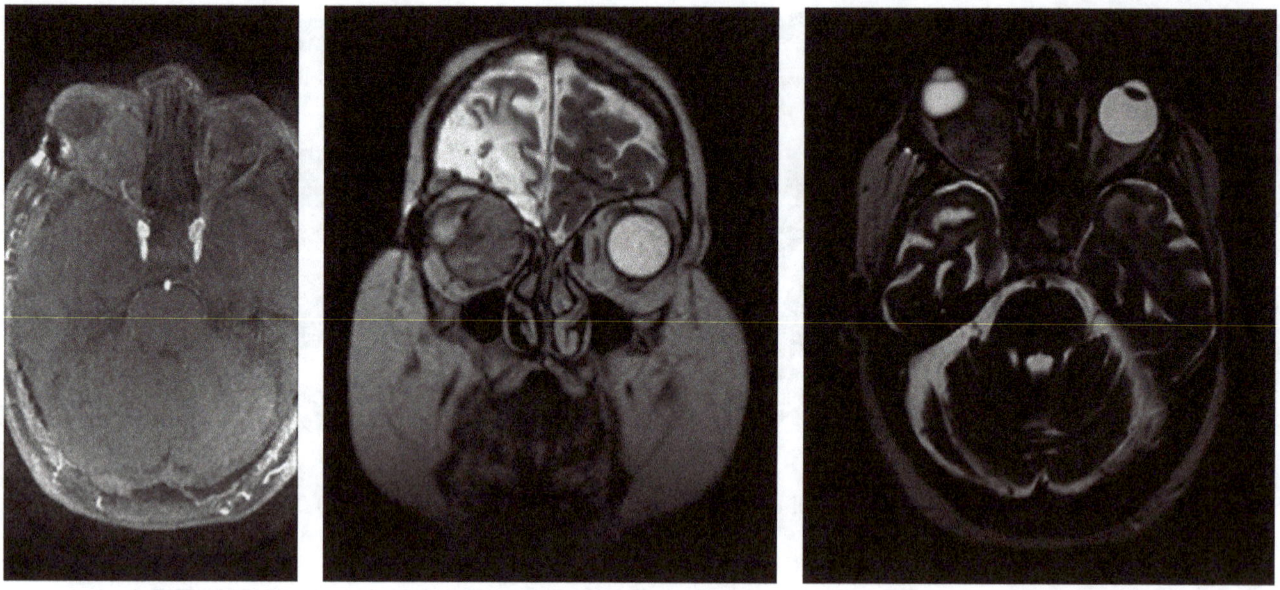

(a) (b) (c)

FIGURE 12: Case 4. (a) CT imaging with a great lesion, hyperdense morphology appears in the right intraconal region. The lesion imprints on the back of the globe, as well as the optic nerve and internal rectus muscle, with close contact with the external rectus muscle. (b, c) MR imaging, coronal view, presents lesion isodensity in T1- and T2-weighted sequences.

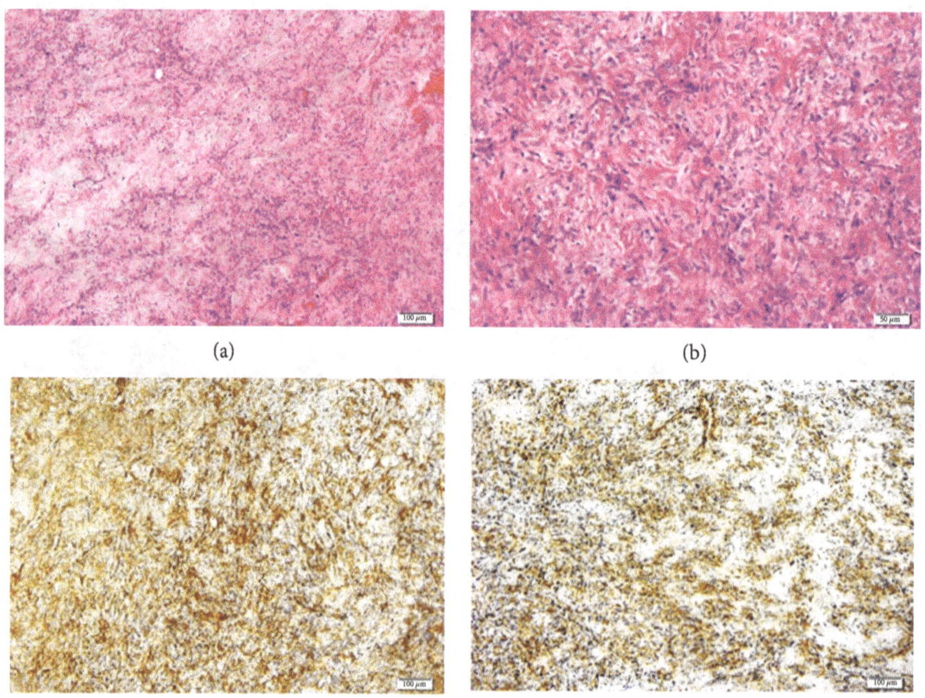

(c) (d)

FIGURE 13: Case 4. (a) It shows the histological appearance of a moderately fibroblastic neoplasia with a mostly storiform pattern. The tumor is composed of bland and uniform oval to spindle cells dispersed along thin parallel collagen bands with hypocellular areas (H&E, ×100 magnification). (b) Hypercellular areas (H&E, ×200 magnification). Positivity for (c) CD34 and (d) BCL2. Bar is indicated in μm, down and to the right.

SFT and HPC since they have similar morphological and immunohistochemical characteristics and there has been a great deal of discussion regarding whether or not they are the same clinical entity.

SFTs show strong and diffuse positivity with CD34 (90–100%) [8–10, 13], vimentin, BCL2, and CD99 [15, 16] and negativity with keratin, cytokeratin, EMA, S100, SMA, and desmin [14]. The CD34 protein is a transmembrane protein that is expressed in vascular and hematopoietic tissue. Smooth muscle tumors such as leiomyoma and leiomyosarcomas show strong positivity for actin and desmin and negativity for S100, BCL2, and CD34. Neural tumors such as schwannoma and neurofibroma can show focal positivity for BCL2 and CD34 and strong positivity for S100 protein. SFT, FH, and HPC all show positive reactivity with vimentin, BCL2, and CD34 [14]. A new classification, published in 2015, includes them in the same entity [3, 17]. Although they are currently included in the same entity, several subtypes of SFT have been differentiated, FH, HPCs, and another lipomatous type [18]. The HPC is originated in the pericytes of blood vessels and usually shows a rich vascular component. HPC cells show high reactivity against vimentin and CD34 but lack immunoreactivity for EMA [9]. FH shows that histiocytes are positive for CD68 but show some variation in CD34 reactivity [9]. CD34 is fairly sensitive for SFT, but it is relatively nonspecific [4]. Recently, NAB2-signal transducer and activator of transcription 6 (STAT6) gene inversion at 12q13 may be identified with an immunohistochemical antibody and it has high sensitivity and specificity for SFT [4, 19, 20].

SFT is a tumor classified as benign, but it can exhibit aggressive behavior with invasion of adjacent and distant tissues and the potential to become malignant. In these cases, high cellularity, mitotic activity > 4/10 HPF (high-power fields), nuclear pleomorphism, necrosis, and large tumors are usually found, although cases in which they did not show these characteristics but have recurrences are also described [10, 11].

For this reason, the treatment of choice for SFT, HPC, and FH is a complete excision of the tumor and careful follow-up in order to prevent recurrences and progression. In HPC, the histopathological features do not always correlate with biological behavior, including malignant potential [9, 21]. Our first case was treated with complete surgical excision of the tumor. In the second case, we used the SONOPET® ultrasonic aspirator system. This is a surgical tool that uses low-frequency ultrasonic vibrations to fragment tissue for tumor excision while simultaneously irrigating and aspirating the surgical field [8]. This device works by ultrasound and has been used previously in brain tumors. It is the first case that we have found in the literature in which it has been used for ophthalmological surgery. It proved to be very useful because it allowed a complete excision of the tumor reaching the ethmoid bone, without damaging adjacent structures. This was possible due to the higher water content and lower collagen and elastin content of the tumor tissues, compared to that of healthy tissues. Because SONOPET® destroys and aspirates the tumor, samples must be taken before the surgery so that a pathological study can be performed. In this case, although the tumor was completely removed, we treated this patient with SRS because of the previous high rate of recurrence.

The third case was treated with exenteration because of the high rate of recurrence and the great orbital affectation; SRS treatment was also implemented. All cases were carefully monitored with no recurrences during this time of follow-up.

The fourth case is a patient with a history of craniopharyngioma surgery in pediatric age; the tumor was resected due to a possible recurrence [22].

7. Conclusion

Orbital SFT is a rare benign tumor with a high rate of recurrence and sometimes with malignancy. Orbital location hinders complete surgical removal of the tumor, and this increases the risk of recurrence. By using the SONOPET® ultrasonic aspirator system, it is possible to perform a more complete removal of the tumor without damaging orbital structures adjacent to the tumor, thus increasing surgical success and patient survival.

Consent

Consent for the publication and consent of ophthalmic images were obtained from the patients.

References

[1] A. Genc, Z. Toktas, C. Azman, S. Uyar Bozkurt, and T. Kilic, "Solitary fibrous tumor of the orbit: a case report and review of the literature," *Turkish Neurosurgery*, vol. 25, no. 6, pp. 984–987, 2014.

[2] A. Tata, O. Cohen-Inbar, and J. P. Sheehan, "Treatment of orbital solitary fibrous tumour with gamma knife radiosurgery and systematic review of literature," *BMJ Case Reports*, vol. 2016, 2016.

[3] W. H. Westra, W. L. Gerald, and J. Rosai, "Solitary fibrous tumor. Consistent CD34 immunoreactivity and occurrence in the orbit," *The American Journal of Surgical Pathology*, vol. 18, no. 10, pp. 992–998, 1994.

[4] N. W. Blessing, J. A. Bermudez-Magner, M. P. Fernandez, A. E. Rosenberg, S. R. Dubovy, and T. E. Johnson, "Solitary fibrous tumor of the orbit: a case series with clinicopathologic correlation and evaluation of STAT6 as a diagnostic marker," *Ophthalmic Plastic & Reconstructive Surgery*, vol. 36, no. 2, pp. 164–171, 2020.

[5] D. A. O'Donovan, J. M. Bilbao, M. Fazl, and O. M. Antonyshyn, "Solitary fibrous tumor of the orbit," *Journal of Craniofacial Surgery*, vol. 13, no. 5, pp. 641–644, 2002.

[6] S. Hayashi, H. Kurihara, J. Hirato, and T. Sasaki, "Solitary fibrous tumor of the orbit with extraorbital extension: case report," *Neurosurgery*, vol. 49, no. 5, pp. 1241–1245, 2001.

[7] S. C. Smith, W. E. Gooding, M. Elkins et al., "Solitary fibrous tumors of the head and neck: a multi-institutional clinicopathologic study," *The American Journal of Surgical Pathology*, vol. 41, no. 12, pp. 1642–1656, 2017.

[8] Á. Bengoa-González, A. Galindo-Ferreiro, E. Mencía-Gutiérrez, H. Sánchez-Tocino, A. Martín-Clavijo, and M.-D. Lago-Llinás, "Deep Lateral Wall Partial Rim-Sparing Orbital Decompression with Ultrasonic Bone Removal for Treatment of Thyroid-Related Orbitopathy," *Journal of Ophthalmology*, vol. 2019, Article ID 9478512, 10 pages, 2019.

[9] S. K. Jung, J. S. Paik, G. S. Park, and S.-W. Yang, "CD34 + tumours of the orbit including solitary fibrous tumours: a six-case series," *BMC Ophthalmology*, vol. 17, no. 1, 2017.

[10] E. S. Tam, E. C. Chen, N. Nijhawan, J. T. Harvey, D. Howarth, and J. H. Oestreicher, "Solitary fibrous tumor of the orbit: a case series," *Orbit*, vol. 27, no. 6, pp. 426–431, 2008.

[11] J. Shen, H. Li, S. Feng, and H. Cui, "Orbital solitary fibrous tumor: a clinicopathologic study from a Chinese tertiary hospital with a literature review," *Cancer Management and Research*, vol. 10, pp. 1069–1078, 2018.

[12] C. D. M. Fletcher, "The evolving classification of soft tissue tumours - an update based on the new 2013 WHO classification," *Histopathology*, vol. 64, no. 1, pp. 2–11, 2014.

[13] N. Hayat, M. M. Afzal, and V. Dembra, "A solitary fibrous tumor of the eyelid," *Pakistan Journal of Medical Sciences*, vol. 35, no. 6, pp. 1745–1748, 2019.

[14] H. J. Kim, H.-J. Kim, Y.-D. Kim et al., "Solitary fibrous tumor of the orbit: CT and MR imaging findings," *American Journal of Neuroradiology*, vol. 29, no. 5, pp. 857–862, 2008.

[15] F. Bernardini, C. de Conciliis, S. Schneider, R. Kersten, and D. Kulwin, "Solitary fibrous tumor of the orbit: is it rare? Report of a case series and review of the literature," *Ophthalmology*, vol. 110, no. 7, pp. 1442–1448, 2003.

[16] R. B. Brunnemann, J. Y. Ro, N. G. Ordonez, J. Mooney, A. K. El-Naggar, and A. G. Ayala, "Extrapleural solitary fibrous tumor: a clinicopathologic study of 24 cases," *Modern Pathology*, vol. 12, no. 11, pp. 1034–1042, 1999.

[17] S. Rizzo, A. A. Giunta, and A. Pennacchi, "Tumore fibroso solitario nasosinusale e rinofaringeo: un caso clinico e una revisione della letteratura," *Acta Otorhinolaryngologica Italica*, vol. 35, no. 6, pp. 455–458, 2015.

[18] C. H. Hsu, Y. H. Wei, Y. Peng, and S. L. Liao, "Orbital hemangiopericytoma in an Asian population," *Journal of the Formosan Medical Association*, vol. 113, no. 6, pp. 356–363, 2014.

[19] G. Leoncini, V. Maio, M. Puccioni et al., "Orbital solitary fibrous tumor: a case report and review of the literature," *Pathology Oncology Research*, vol. 14, no. 2, pp. 213–217, 2008.

[20] G. Broggi, L. Salvatorelli, M. Reibaldi et al., "Solitary fibrous tumor of the orbital region: report of a case with emphasis on the diagnostic utility of STAT-6," *Pathologica*, vol. 112, no. 4, pp. 195–199, 2020.

[21] M. Mitamura, S. Kase, Y. Suzuki et al., "Solitary fibrous tumor of the orbit: a clinicopathologic study of two cases with review of the literature," *In Vivo*, vol. 34, no. 6, pp. 3649–3654, 2020.

[22] P. Yang, H.-C. Liu, E. Qiu et al., "Factors for postoperative recurrence of orbital solitary fibrous tumor: an analysis of long-term clinical follow-up results from a Chinese tertiary hospital," *BMC Ophthalmology*, vol. 21, no. 1, 2021.

21

Autologous Platelet-Rich Fibrin in the Treatment of Refractory Macular Holes

Arif Koytak, Fadime Nuhoglu, Havvanur Bayraktar, Rukiye Ercan, and Hakan Ozdemir

Bezmialem Vakif University, Faculty of Medicine, Department of Ophthalmology, Istanbul, Turkey

Correspondence should be addressed to Arif Koytak; akoytak@yahoo.com

Academic Editor: Cristiano Giusti

Purpose. To describe a novel method for the treatment of refractory macular holes. *Methods.* Two case reports on the use of autologous platelet rich fibrin (PRF), followed by sulfur hexafluoride gas tamponade to facilitate closure of refractory macular holes. *Results.* Macular holes were succesfully closed within a week in both cases. Best corrected Snellen visual acuities improved from counting fingers to 0.16 in the first case, and from 0.05 to 0.2 in the second case. No complication occurred during or after the procedures. *Conclusion.* The use of autologous PRF seems to be a safe and effective alternative method for the treatment of refractory macular holes. Further experience and studies are required to assess the value of autologous PRF in the management of challenging macular hole cases of different etiologies. To the best of our knowledge, this is the first use of autologous PRF in the treatment of macular holes.

1. Introduction

Full thickness macular holes (FTMH) are not infrequent and more than 90% of them are successfully treated with a single surgery [1]. Current surgical technique of choice consists of pars plana vitrectomy and internal limiting membrane (ILM) peeling, followed by air-gas exchange and postoperative face-down positioning. However, 5–10% of FTMHs which fail to close with a single surgery require further interventions [2].

Repeat air-gas exchange, sometimes with a longer acting gas, is the first option in the management of refractory macular holes. However, only 46.7% of these FTMHs are found to be closed following reoperation [3]. Success rates in chronic and large holes are even lower.

Several surgical techniques are developed and tried for the management of refractory macular holes. These include relaxing retinotomy, free and inverted ILM flaps, posterior lens capsular flap, autologous neurosensorial retinal flap, and foveal hydrodissection. Autologous blood products such as simple blood clot and platelet rich plasma, [4–6] as well as several tissue glues comprising nonautologous blood products and synthetic molecules are also tried for facilitating hole closure [7–12].

Platelet rich fibrin (PRF) is a leukocyte and platelet rich concentrate obtained from venous blood through a simple and inexpensive technique developed by Choukroun et al. which provides a strong and elastic fibrin matrix. In contrast to other autologous blood products, this concentrate is produced without any anticoagulants or gelifying agents [13, 14].

Here, we describe the closure of two refractory macular holes with the use of PRF. To the best of our knowledge, this is the first use of PRF in the treatment of FTMH.

2. Case 1

A 68-year-old woman had a history of pars plana vitrectomy with ILM peeling and silicone oil tamponade for the treatment of concommitant rhegmatogenous retinal detachment and FTMH in her left eye before 6 years. She had her retinal detachment repaired, but the macular hole persisted despite long term tamponade with silicone oil. A year after the initial one, she had a second surgery using short term gas tamponade with sulfur hexafluoride gas (SF_6), but the hole failed to close. A third attempt to close the macular hole was carried out a year after, with carbon hexafluoride gas (C_3F_8). Despite her strict obedience to face down positioning, the hole failed to close.

After three operations that failed, the patient did not prefer to have further interventions and remained on regular

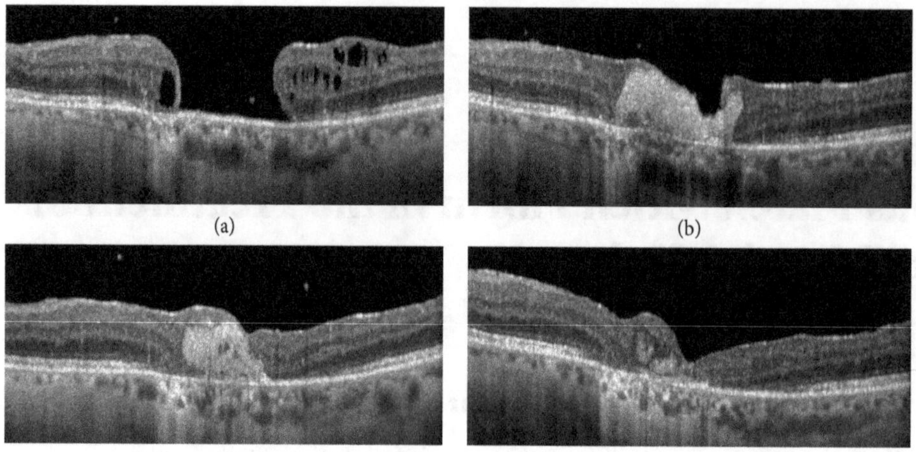

(a) (b) (c) (d)

FIGURE 1: Optical coherence tomographic images of the Case 1 before the operation (a), and one week (b), one month (c), and 3 months (d) after the operation.

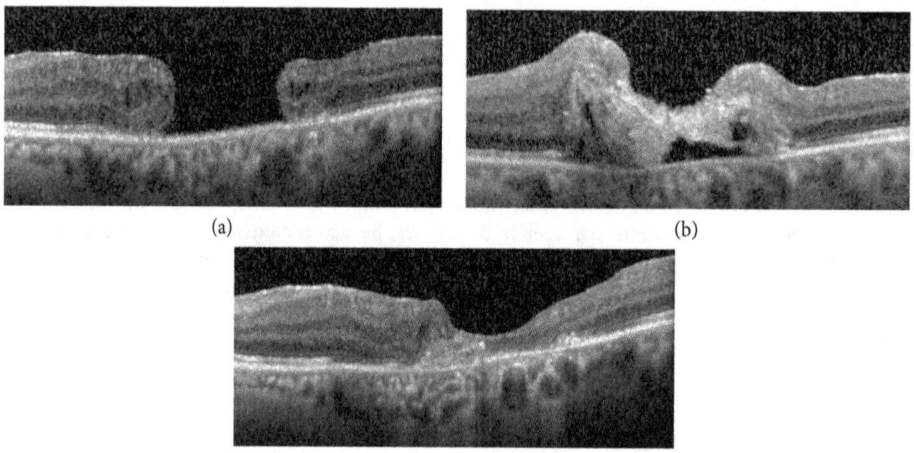

(a) (b) (c)

FIGURE 2: Optical coherence tomographic images of the Case 2 before the operation (a), and one week (b), and 3 months (c) after the operation.

follow-up visits for about 4 years. During this time period no significant anatomical and functional change occurred in her left eye.

In her last visit, she had a best corrected visual acuity (BCVA) of counting fingers (CF) in her left vitrectomized eye which had a chronic large macular hole with a base daimeter of 1697 micrometers. Upon proposal, she has accepted a fourth surgery with autologous PRF application.

The surgical technique included four ports pars plana approach for the application of a round button of PRF to the macular hole, followed by fluid-air and air-SF_6 gas exchange. The patient was ordered to have face down positioning for three days following the operation.

The PRF button was cut with scissors from a PRF membrane which was prepared with Choukrun's procedure described elsewhere [7, 8]. In short, this procedure consisted of centrifuge of autologous blood drawn immediately before the operation, followed by removal of the fibrin clot from the test tube and its compaction with a metal press board. The PRF button was slightly larger than the macular hole, permitting complete plugging of the hole (see video, Supplementary material 1, which summarizes surgical steps).

The week after the operation, the hole was shown to be completely sealed by the PRF button on optical coherence tomographic (OCT) images. The button was resorbed slowly until the third postoperative month, and replaced by neuroglial proliferation which closed the hole completely (Figure 1).

Despite the chronic course of the pathology and low initial visual acuity, the Snellen BCVA improved to 0.16 in the last control visit. No complication occurred during or after the procedure.

3. Case 2

A 79 years old woman with a FTMH in her left eye was treated with pars plana vitrectomy with ILM peeling and SF_6 gas tamponade. She had a Snellen BCVA of 0.05 in her left eye and the hole diameter was 1581 micrometers prior to the surgery. As the first operation failed to close the FTMH, she had a second operation consisting of four ports pars plana approach for the application of a round button of PRF to the macular hole, followed by fluid-air and air-SF_6 gas exchange. Three days strict face down positioning was ordered following the operation.

The week after the application of PRF, the hole was shown to be closed on OCT (Figure 2). The PRF button was slowly resorbed and the hole remained closed until the last visit at the fourth postoperative month. The Snellen BCVA improved from 0.05 to 0.2. The surgery and postoperative period was free of complications.

4. Conclusion

Pars plana vitrectomy with ILM peeling, followed by gas tamponade is the initial treatment of choice for the majority of uncomplicated macular holes and has been proven to be successful in more than 90% of cases. Large, highly myopic, [15] traumatic or chronic macular holes are less likely to close with a single procedure and several alternative methods are proposed for such refractory cases. The use of inverted or free ILM, posterior lens capsule, or autologous neurosensorial retinal flaps, relaxing retinotomy, foveal hydrodissection, and autologous serum are among alternatives suggested to be effective. Also, several blood products (autologous, allogeneic, or xenogeneic) and synthetic materials are studied as injectable tissue glues to seal retinal tears or macular holes in both animal experiments and human eyes [7–12]. Although most of these tissue glues are proven to be effective sealants, they gained limited popularity because of the complexity of their preparation and handling steps and their limited availability as expensive commercial products. Also, these glues which comprise nonautologous components such as allogeneic fibrinogen and thrombin, bovine thrombin, or synthetic molecules such as cyanoacrylate are suggested to carry risks of inflammation and/or retinal toxicity resulting in damage to adjacent healthy retina, epiretinal proliferation, retinal contraction, and subnormal visual recovery [7, 16–19].

Unlike all other injectable blood products that are studied for similar purposes, autologous PRF is a solid and elastic membrane which is easy to procure and manipulate at almost no cost. It acts as a resorbable plug, rather than a tissue glue. It is readily absorbed and totally replaced by the neuroglial tissue. And because it does not contain any nonautologous molecule, it seems not to provoque any unwanted inflammatory or toxic reactions. Autologous PRF, besides providing a dry medium and a solid framework for healing, acts as a slow-release fibrin matrix which contains several growth factors and cytokines as well as mesenchymal stem cells which are believed to promote healing process [20].

Our experience with two refractory large macular hole cases which achieved complete closure revealed a new alternative for the management of macular holes. During the follow-up period, we did not encounter any complication or adverse reaction related to the procedure. Anatomical restoration and functional improvement was achieved in both cases. To our knowledge, this is the first report about the use of autologous PRF in the treatment of FTMH.

The use of autologous PRF could be seen as a safe and effective alternative method for the treatment of challenging large, highly myopic, chronic, traumatic, recurrent, or pediatric macular hole cases. PRF buttons could also be helpful as temporary plugs in the surgical management of optic pits. Further experience and studies are required to assess the value of PRF in the management of each specific entity mentioned above.

Additional Points

We report two successful cases on the use of autologous platelet rich fibrin (PRF) to facilitate closure of refractory macular holes. The use of autologous PRF seems to be a safe and effective alternative method for the treatment of refractory macular holes.

References

[1] K. Kumagai, M. Furukawa, N. Ogino, A. Uemura, S. Demizu, and E. Larson, "Vitreous surgery with and without internal limiting membrane peeling for macular hole repair," *Retina*, vol. 24, no. 5, pp. 721–727, 2004.

[2] H. L. Brooks Jr., "Macular hole surgery with and without internal limiting membrane peeling," *Ophthalmology*, vol. 107, no. 10, pp. 1939–1948, 2000.

[3] M. J. J. D'Souza, V. Chaudhary, R. Devenyi, P. J. Kertes, and W.-C. Lam, "Re-operation of idiopathic full-thickness macular holes after initial surgery with internal limiting membrane peel," *British Journal of Ophthalmology*, vol. 95, no. 11, pp. 1564–1567, 2011.

[4] M. Paques, C. Chastang, A. Mathis et al., "Effect of autologous platelet concentrate in surgery for idiopathic macular hole: results of a multicenter, double-masked, randomized trial. Platelets in macular hole surgery group," *Ophthalmology*, vol. 106, pp. 932–938, 1999.

[5] A. Konstantinidis, M. Hero, P. Nanos, and G. D. Panos, "Efficacy of autologous platelets in macular hole surgery," *Clinical Ophthalmology*, vol. 7, pp. 745–750, 2013.

[6] M. S. Figueroa, A. Govetto, and P. Arriba-Palomero, "Short-term results of platelet-rich plasma as adjuvant to 23-G vitrectomy in the treatment of high myopic macular holes," *European Journal of Ophthalmology*, vol. 26, no. 5, pp. 491–496, 2016.

[7] I. Nasaduke and G. A. Peyman, "The use of autogenous rabbit fibrin sealant to plug retinal holes in experimental detachments," *Annals of Ophthalmology*, vol. 18, no. 11, pp. 324–327, 1986.

[8] D. J. Coleman, B. C. Lucas, J. A. Fleischman et al., "A biologic tissue adhesive for vitreoretinal surgery," *Retina*, vol. 8, no. 4, pp. 250–256, 1988.

[9] C. E. Gilbert, I. Grierson, and D. McLeod, "Retinal patching: a new approach to the management of selected retinal breaks," *Eye (London, England)*, vol. 3, no. 1, pp. 19–26, 1989.

[10] M. A. Tilanus and A. F. Deutman, "Full-thickness macular holes treated with vitrectomy and tissue glue," *International Ophthalmology*, vol. 18, no. 6, pp. 355–358, 1995.

[11] M. S. Blumenkranz, E. Ohana, S. Shaikh et al., "Adjuvant methods in macular hole surgery: intraoperative plasma-thrombin mixture and postoperative fluid-gas exchange," *Ophthalmic Surgery and Lasers*, vol. 32, no. 3, pp. 198–207, 2001.

[12] M. Tyagi and S. Basu, "Glue-assisted retinopexy for rhegmatogenous retinal detachments (GuARD): a novel surgical technique for closing retinal breaks," *Indian Journal of Ophthalmology*, vol. 67, no. 5, pp. 677–680, 2019.

[13] J. Choukroun, F. Adda, C. Schoeffler, and A. Vervelle, "An opportunity in paro-implantology: PRF," *Implantodontie*, vol. 42, pp. 55–62, 2001.

[14] D. M. Dohan Ehrenfest, L. Rasmusson, and T. Albrektsson, "Classification of platelet concentrates: from pure platelet-rich plasma (P-PRP) to leucocyte- and platelet-rich fibrin (L-PRF)," *Trends in Biotechnology*, vol. 27, no. 3, pp. 158–167, 2009.

[15] T.-T. Wu and Y.-H. Kung, "Comparison of anatomical and visual outcomes of macular hole surgery in patients with high myopia vs. non-high myopia: a case-control study using optical coherence tomography," *Graefe's Archieve for Clinical and Experimental Ophthalmology*, vol. 250, no. 3, pp. 327–331, 2012.

[16] E. Margalit, G. Y. Fujii, J. C. Lai et al., "Bioadhesives for intraocular use," *Retina*, vol. 20, no. 5, pp. 469–477, 2000.

[17] T. W. Olsen, P. Sternberg Jr., A. Capone Jr. et al., "Macular hole surgery using thrombin-activated fibrinogen and selective removal of the internal limiting membrane," *Retina*, vol. 18, no. 4, pp. 322–329, 1998.

[18] P. M. Shanmugam, "Commentary: fibrin sealant for temporary retinopexy," *Indian Journal of Ophthalmology*, vol. 67, no. 5, pp. 682–683, 2019.

[19] K. Anshuman and D. Ratra, "Commentary: fibrin glue in rhegmatogenous retinal detachment repair-are we there yet?" *Indian Journal of Ophthalmology*, vol. 67, no. 5, pp. 683–684, 2019.

[20] J. Choukroun, A. Diss, A. Simonpieri et al., "Platelet-rich fibrin (PRF): a second-generation platelet concentrate. Part IV: clinical effects on tissue healing," *Oral Surgery, Oral Medicine, Oral Pathology, Oral Radiology, and Endodontics*, vol. 101, no. 3, pp. e56–e60, 2006.

22

A Case Report Illustrating the Postoperative Course of Descemetorhexis without Endothelial Keratoplasty with Topical Netarsudil Therapy

Pimpiroon Ploysangam[1] **and Sangita P. Patel**[1,2]

[1]*Ross Eye Institute, Department of Ophthalmology, Jacobs School of Medicine and Biomedical Sciences, State University of New York at Buffalo, Buffalo, NY, USA*
[2]*Research and Ophthalmology Services, Veterans Administration of Western New York Healthcare System, Buffalo, NY, USA*

Correspondence should be addressed to Sangita P. Patel; sppatel@buffalo.edu

Academic Editor: Claudio Campa

Fuchs endothelial corneal dystrophy (FECD) is the most common indication for corneal transplantation in the United States. Recently, descemetorhexis without endothelial keratoplasty (DWEK) or Descemet's stripping only (DSO) has become an attractive alternative to corneal transplantation for these patients. DSO circumvents the challenges associated with cadaveric donor corneal transplantation by tapping into the potential of the patient's own corneal endothelium to repair defects. Outcomes have been variable with emerging knowledge on predictive factors for success. Our case describes a 51-year-old patient with visually significant confluent central guttae from FECD who underwent a successful DSO with immediate post-operative use of the Rho-associated protein kinase (ROCK) inhibitor (netarsudil). We report the preoperative and post-operative slit lamp images, specular microscopy data, and corneal topography, thickness, and densitometry data. These represent a unique data set for this new surgical treatment option for FECD. Despite a small descemetorhexis, we show the improvement in corneal thickness and opacity extends beyond the boundaries of the descemetorhexis. Early initiation of a ROCK inhibitor was a successful treatment for this patient.

1. Introduction

Fuchs endothelial corneal dystrophy (FECD) is the most common endothelial dystrophy, with its pathology characterized by the presence of deposits (guttae) in the basement membrane (Descemet's membrane) of the corneal endothelium and decreased endothelial cell density [1]. Treatment for advanced FECD is by corneal transplantation, and FECD accounts for more than 17,000 corneal transplants in the United States annually [2]. All of these surgical interventions for FECD require cadaveric donor tissue and carry the associated risks of graft rejection and failure. Transplantation options include penetrating keratoplasty (PKP), Descemet stripping endothelial keratoplasty (DSEK), and Descemet membrane endothelial keratoplasty (DMEK) [3, 4]. Cell therapy with Rho kinase (ROCK) inhibitors and cultured donor corneal endothelial cells has also recently been described [5]. Rho kinase halts progression of corneal endothelial cells through the cell cycle; inhibition leads to proliferation, attachment to substrate, and suppression of apoptosis in corneal endothelial cells [6].

Although it was thought that corneal endothelial cells were arrested in the cell cycle, recent cases show that descemetorhexis with removal of the diseased Descemet's membrane and endothelium can promote cell repopulation [7, 8]. The guttae microenvironment itself affects endothelial cell behavior. Large guttae stimulate apoptosis of corneal endothelial cells and increase markers of cell stress [9]. Descemet's stripping only (DSO), also known as Descemetorhexis without endothelial keratoplasty (DWEK), has thus emerged as a new alterative to corneal transplantation. DSO involves removing the central area of diseased Descemet's membrane and corneal endothelial cells via a descemetorhexis in order to allow peripheral corneal endothelial cells to repopulate the central corneal endothelial monolayer. DSO has the benefit of bypassing a need for donor tissue altogether, removing the risks associated with graft rejection and failure. Much is still unknown regarding this procedure including factors that would predict success [10]. While there are multiple case series on DSO, our case report details the pre- and postoperative course and associated clinical imaging of a patient with FECD undergoing DSO. This patient was also placed on ROCK inhibitor therapy immediately postoperatively, which currently has only been used in patients with nonclearing corneas after DSO [11].

2. Case Presentation

Our patient is a 51-year-old Caucasian female with history of FECD who presented with gradually worsening vision over the past year. She had noted fluctuating vision, photophobia, difficulty reading, and glare with oncoming headlights while driving. Her ocular history was remarkable for ocular rosacea with inspissated meibum and eyelid margin vascularization and glaucoma suspect due to cup to disc asymmetry. Ocular medications included intermittent use of artificial tears and sodium chloride 5% ointment.

Her eye exam revealed a corrected Snellen visual acuity of 20/40 (right; −0.75 +3.00×100) and 20/30 (left; −0.75 +2.75×085). Her corneas had central confluent endothelial guttae in both eyes measuring 4.0×4.0 mm (right) and 3.8×4.0 mm (left) with associated stromal haze in both eyes (Figure 1(a)). The peripheral corneas in both eyes were relatively spared of guttae. There was no clinically apparent corneal edema on slit lamp exam. Ultrasound pachymetry (DGH 555 Pachette 3 Ultrasonic Pachymeter, DGH Technology, Inc., Exton, PA) showed a central corneal thickness of 608 μm (right) and 595 μm (left). She also had 1+ nuclear sclerotic cataract in both eyes. Dilated fundus exam was unremarkable. Specular microscopy imaging (Konan Specular Microscope Noncon Robo Series NSP-9900, Konan Medical Inc., Japan) was completed and showed central confluent guttae (unable to count endothelial cell density). The peripheral cornea showed scattered, nonconfluent guttae with cell densities of 1508–1550 cells/mm^2 in the left eye (Figure 2). The location of "peripheral" corneal endothelial imaging by the Konan Specular Microscope is not specified, but we suspect a mid-peripheral location based upon the distribution of guttae in the corresponding red-reflex image (Figure 1(a)). Scheimpflug tomography (Pentacam, Oculus, Inc., Arlington, WA) showed 2 diopters of regular with-the-rule astigmatism (Figure 3(a)). The minimum central thickness was 593 μm in the left eye and the decreased back surface elevation suggested the presence of subclinical corneal edema (Figure 3(b)).

The patient's visual symptoms were felt to be secondary to corneal changes from FECD and mild cataract. Surgical options were reviewed with her including cataract extraction with intraocular lens placement with or without DSEK or DSO. Patient decided to proceed with cataract extraction with intraocular lens placement and DSO for her left eye, with the understanding that she might need corneal transplant should her cornea fail to clear following DSO.

The patient underwent routine cataract surgery with phacoemulsification and intraocular lens placement under

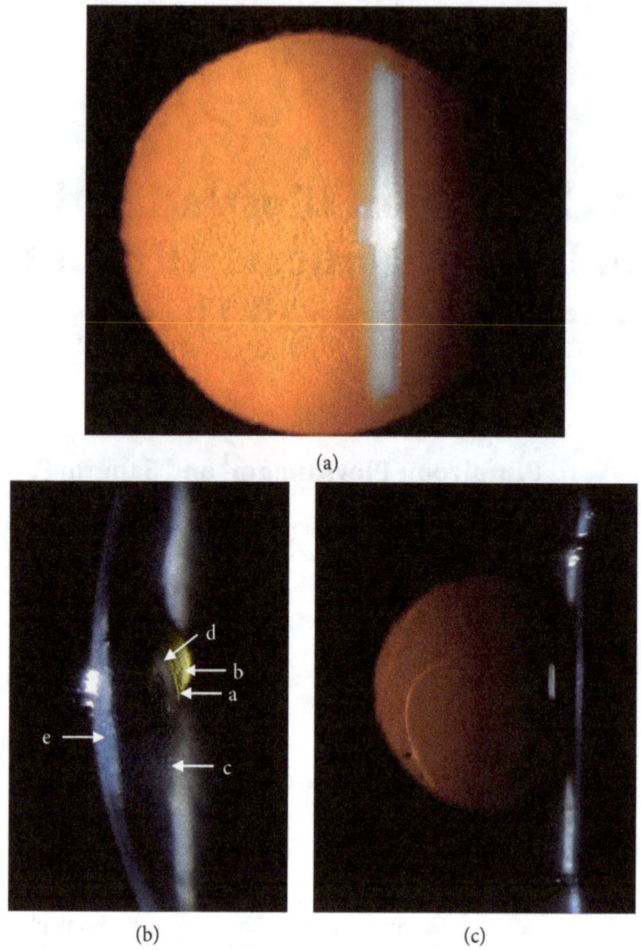

Figure 1: Slit lamp biomicroscopy photos pre- and post-DSO surgery for the left eye. (a) Preoperative red reflex photo with a dilated pupil shows confluent guttae in the visual axis, slightly greater in the inferior half of the visual axis compared to superior half. The peripheral cornea is relatively spared of guttae. (b) Slit photo through the central cornea at 1 week post-DSO surgery demonstrates a. the edge of the descemetorhexis; b. guttae outside the area of Descemet's stripping; c. reticular epithelial edema; d. peripheral ring of corneal clearing without edema in presumed area of endothelial healing; and e. corneal stromal edema. (c) One month postoperative red reflex photo shows inferocentral descemetorhexis with clear visual axis without guttae and peripheral nonconfluent guttae.

topical anesthesia. Following lens implantation, the central corneal area of densest guttae was marked at 4×4 mm with calipers on the corneal surface. While the eye was still filled with cohesive viscoelastic, a reverse sinskey hook was used to score and lift the Descemet's membrane/endothelium for approximately 1–2 clock hours in the marked region. Using the lifted edge of Descemet's membrane, a continuous descemetorhexis was pulled approximating the marked central region using utrata forceps. Viscoelastic was then removed from the anterior chamber, and the remainder of the case was completed per standard cataract surgery protocol.

On her postoperative day 1 visit, uncorrected vision in the left eye was 20/125 (pinhole to 20/60). Her cornea showed removal of greatest area of guttae in her left eye measuring 4 mm (vertical)×3.4 mm (horizontal), with slight inferior

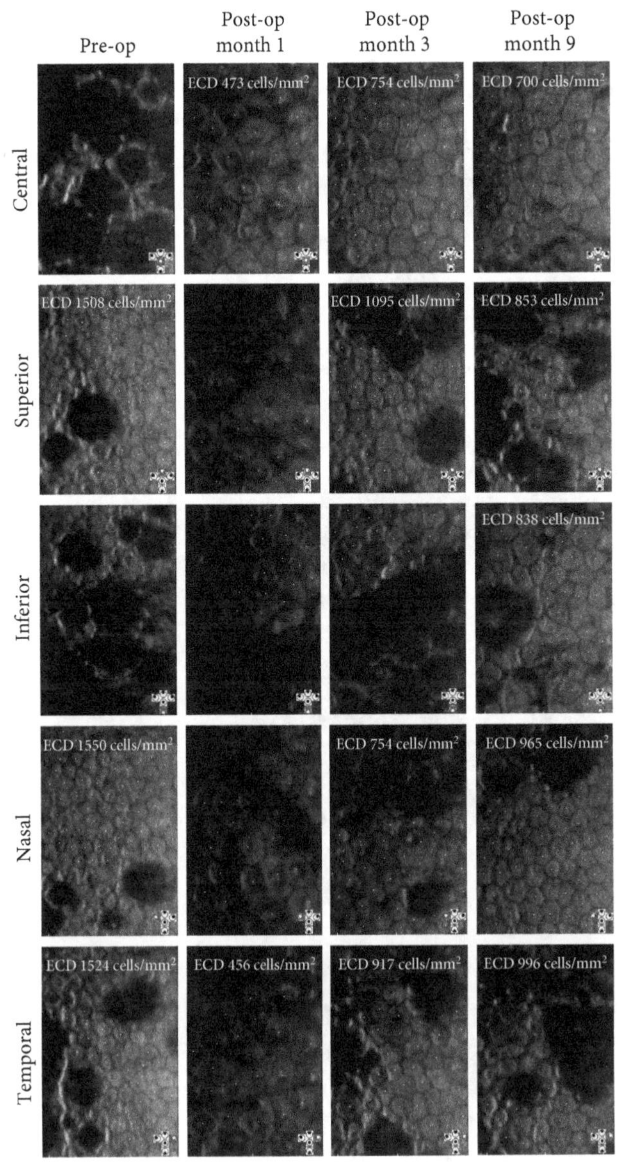

FIGURE 2: Specular microscopy imaging of the corneal endothelium pre- and post-DSO surgery for the left eye. The locations (central, superior, inferior, nasal, and temporal) are based upon the standard gaze positions of the Konan specular microscope. Endothelial cell density (ECD) is indicated when measurable.

displacement of area of stripping relative to the pupil, corresponding to the area with densest guttae preoperatively (Figure 1(a)). Ultrasound pachymetry was 936 μm. The anterior chamber was quiet, and posterior chamber intraocular lens was in proper position. The patient was started on the following eye drop regimen for the left eye: prednisolone acetate 1% 4x/day, polymyxin b sulfate-trimethoprim 4x/day, netarsudil at bedtime, and polymyxin B/neomycin/dexamethasone ointment at bedtime.

At postoperative week 1, her visual acuity in the left eye was 20/250 (pinhole to 20/100). Her cornea showed stromal and focal reticular epithelial edema in the left eye measuring 3 mm (vertical) × 2.8 mm (horizontal). Reticular edema has previously been noted with netarsudil use [12]. The area of stripping was clearly delineated and edges of this area were noted to be clearing (Figure 1(b)). The anterior chamber remained deep and quiet. Scheimpflug tomography imaging (Pentacam) showed inferocentral thickening and steepening in the area of Descemet's stripping (Figure 3(d)–3(f)). At this visit, the patient noted pain which was thought to be secondary to the corneal epithelial edema. Frequent application of artificial tears did not alleviate the pain. A bandage soft contact lens was placed for 1 week. All eye medications were continued except for the polymyxin B / neomycin/dexamethasone ointment.

At the postoperative one-month visit, her uncorrected vision measured 20/150 (pinhole 20/50). The corneal edema had resolved, but she continued to have a central anterior stromal haze. Scheimpflug tomography (Pentacam) showed a minimum central thickness at 565 μm (Figure 3(i)). The endothelium could be imaged by specular microscopy (Konan) and showed central endothelial cell counts of approximately 473 cells/mm^2. The polymyxin B sulfate-trimethoprim and netarsudil eye drops were stopped, and the prednisolone acetate 1% eye drop was tapered off over the next 3 weeks.

Her vision continued to improve at postoperative month two, with her best corrected vision at 20/40 (right; −0.75 +3.00 x 100 OD) and 20/25 (left; −1.50 +2.25 × 080). Due to persistent pain, a bandage soft contact lens was again placed at the postoperative month two visit for one more week, and the patient was started on fluorometholone eye drops 2x/day in the left eye. Pain has been reported as a side effect of instillation of netarsudil eye drops; however, she had stopped using netarsudil eye drops 1 month prior [13].

At 3 months, vision remained stable from the prior month. Specular microscopy (Konan) showed a central cell density of 754 cells/mm^2 (Figure 2). Scheimpflug tomography (Pentacam) demonstrated decreased corneal thickness compared to all prior measurements for the left eye (Figures 3(l) and 4). In addition, evaluation of corneal opacity by Scheimpflug corneal densitometry showed improved (reduced) densitometry values from both the anterior and posterior corneal layers, and from the central and peripheral corneal zones compared to preoperatively (Figure 5). She continued to have pain in her left eye which did not respond to bandage contact lens placement but was alleviated with periodic use of fluorometholone 0.1% eye drops once daily as needed. The etiology of the pain was not evident on exam, thus we suspect a neuropathic component. Fluoromethalone eye drops were continued for an additional 2 months. At 9 months postoperatively, her left eye pain had resolved. Her central corneal endothelial cell density was 700 cells/mm^2 and corneal pachymetry was 555 μm (Figures 2 and 3). The cell density of the peripheral corneal endothelium was noted to be decreased from pre-operatively.

3. Discussion

Our patient had a successful outcome from DSO surgery with improved corneal thickness, densitometry, and visual acuity, and rapidly repopulated central corneal endothelium without guttae. The cell density of the central corneal endothelium

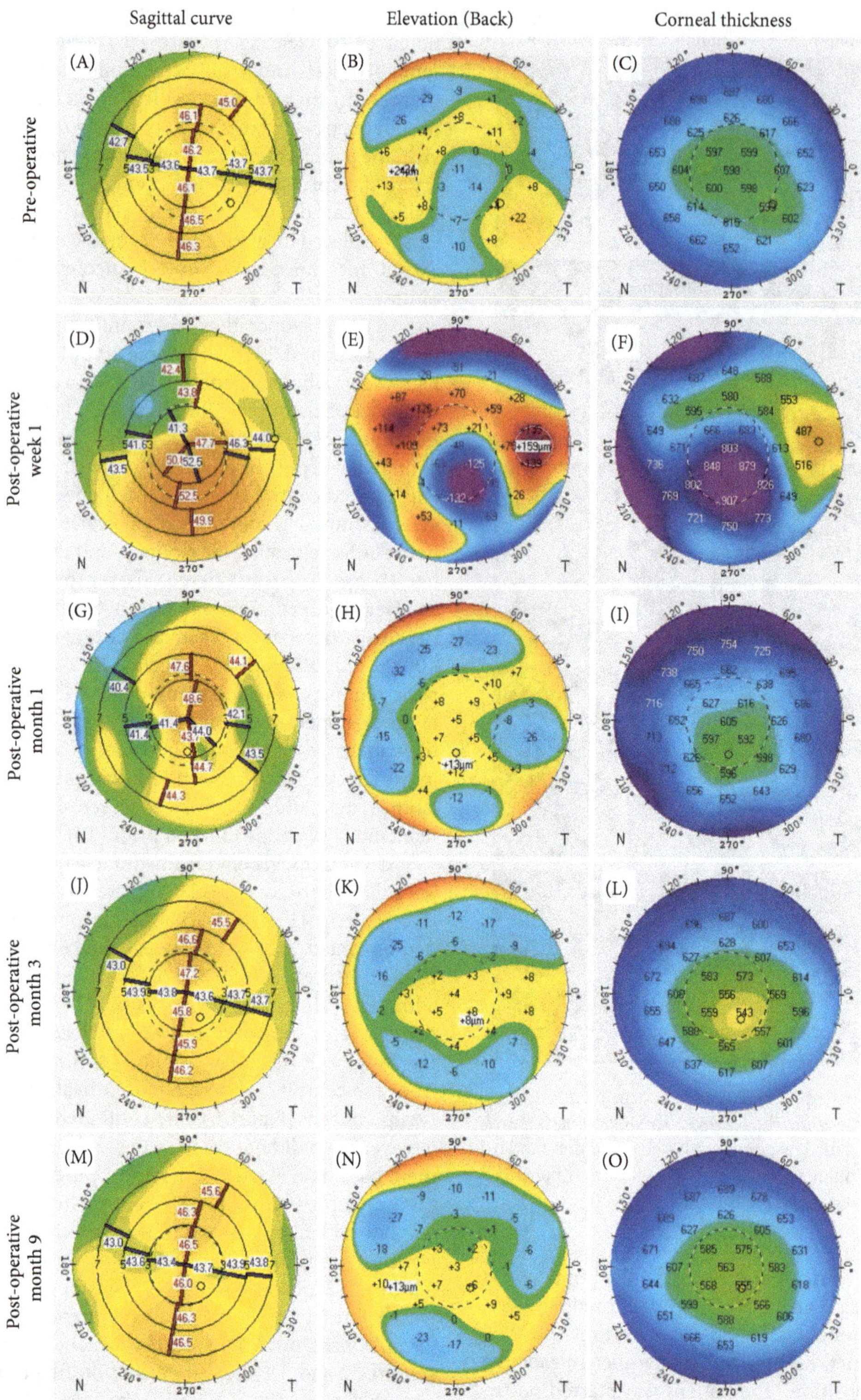

FIGURE 3: Sagittal corneal curvature, back surface elevation, and pachymetry maps pre- and post-DSO for the left eye.

could be measured by specular microscopy at 1 month after DSO surgery indicating healing of the endothelial monolayer and sufficient endothelial function to improve corneal edema to allow for imaging by that time point. Her visual acuity likely improved as a result of both cataract extraction and DSO. Although no clear predictive factors for success have been established for descemetorhexis [10], Moloney et al. have reported criteria for patient selection based on their successful pilot study; this includes visual symptoms from central guttae and not corneal edema, presence of healthy peripheral endothelial cell population, and symptoms disruptive enough to qualify for a graft otherwise [11]. Our patient met these

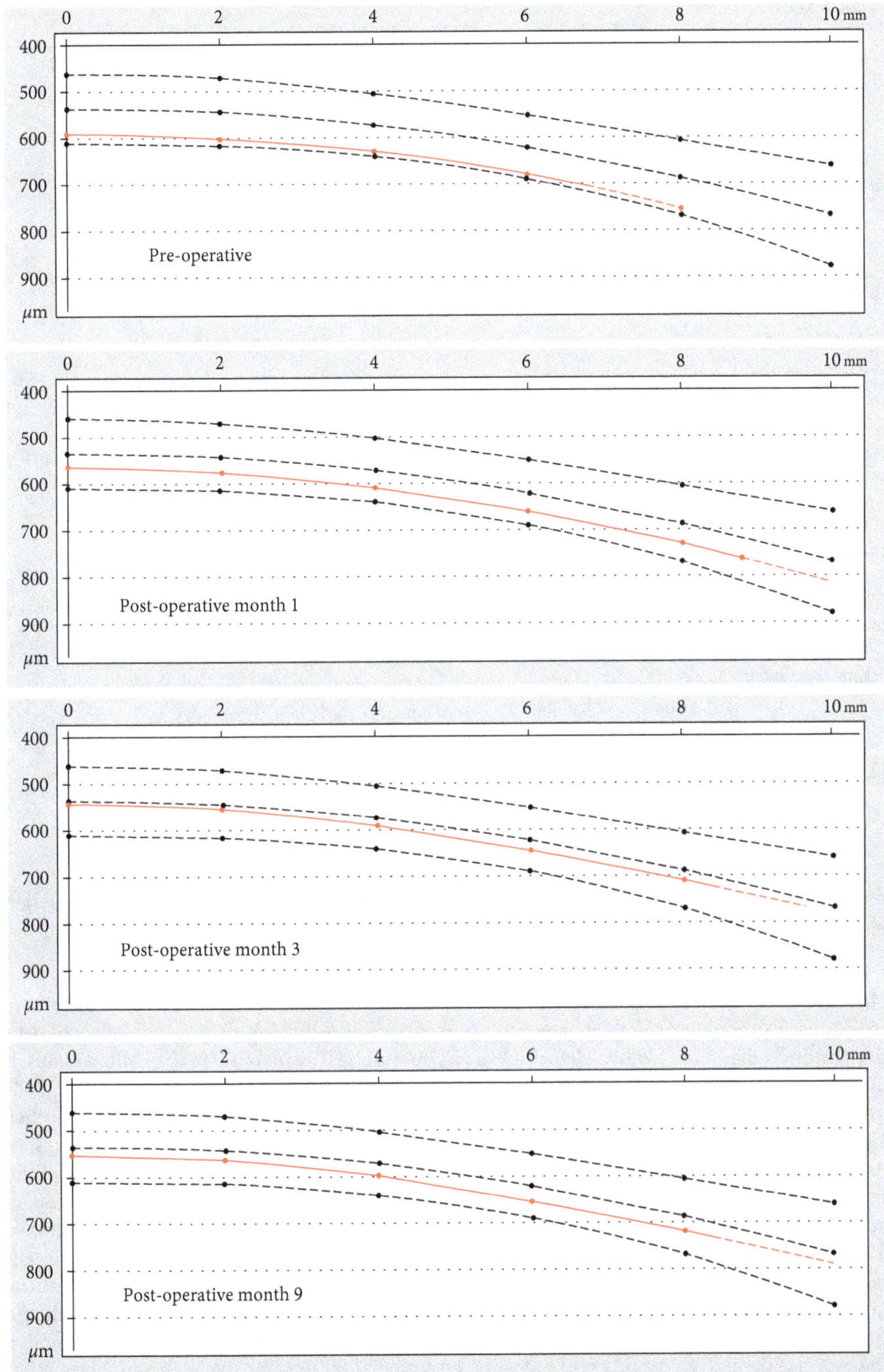

FIGURE 4: Corneal thickness spatial profile pre-and post-DSO for the left eye. The corneal thickness decrease following DSO is not limited to the central area of stripping but also extends to the peripheral cornea.

criteria. Successful outcomes of DSO have also been attributed to surgical technique, with continuous curvilinear descemetorhexis having better outcomes than descemetorhexis with 360° scoring [10]. For this patient, we used the successful continuous curvilinear descemetorhexis technique.

ROCK inhibitors have been used off-label for DSO surgery to promote corneal endothelial proliferation and clearing of the cornea when the corneal edema fails to resolve. Moloney et al. performed a series of successful DSO cases and used ROCK inhibitors in only the few cases that failed [11]. Two

Pre-operative

	0–2 mm	2–6 mm	6–10 mm	10–12 mm	Total
Anterior (120 μm)	19.8	17.4	23.6	40.1	23.7
Center layer	12.3	11.6	17.4	21.9	15.9
Posterior (60 μm)	14.8	11.9	17.2	22.4	15.9
Total	15.6	13.7	19.2	29.1	18.5

Post-operative month 1

	0–2 mm	2–6 mm	6–10 mm	10–12 mm	Total
Anterior (120 μm)	22.5	19.2	22.0	32.5	22.9
center layer	12.8	11.7	15.8	22.1	15.0
Posterior (60 μm)	12.0	11.4	15.4	21.7	14.6
Total	15.8	14.1	17.7	25.4	17.5

Post-operative month 3

	0–2 mm	2–6 mm	6–10 mm	10–12 mm	Total
Anterior (120 μm)	19.5	17.1	21.2	39.8	32.7
Center layer	12.2	11.3	15.4	23.7	14.9
Posterior (60 μm)	11.6	11.1	15.1	21.1	14.2
Total	14.4	13.1	17.2	28.2	17.3

Post-operative month 9

	0–2 mm	2–6 mm	6–10 mm	10–12 mm	Total
Anterior (120 μm)	19.1	16.9	21.4	34.1	21.6
Center layer	12.0	11.1	15.6	22.3	14.6
Posterior (60 μm)	10.9	10.5	14.9	20.8	13.8
Total	14.0	12.8	17.3	25.7	16.7

FIGURE 5: Corneal densitometries pre- and post-DSO for the left eye. Decrease in densitometry is noted not only in the posterior layer centrally (the region of Descemet's stripping), but also in the posterior layer peripherally and in the anterior layer throughout.

failed cases received the topical ROCK inhibitor ripasudil six times daily for two weeks, with subsequent complete resolution of cornea edema. In one failed case with a detached Descemet's membrane, topical compounded ROCK inhibitor Y-27632 failed to improved edema, and eventually the patient required endothelial keratoplasty [11]. The enhanced surgical success with ROCK inhibitor opens the possibility of extending descemetorhexis to previously borderline candidates [10]. Notably, our case describes one of the first to supplement DSO with netarsudil, and our post-operative course is similar to cases supplemented with other ROCK inhibitors, specifically ripasudil. Based upon our case report, we speculate that netarsudil can replicate the accelerated recovery noted with other ROCK inhibitors; however, we cannot verify this without a well-designed clinical trial.

In vitro studies on corneal endothelial wound healing with ROCK inhibitors show that cell cycle progression (i.e. corneal endothelial cell proliferation) is greatest closest to the wound edge and stops as soon as the wound is healed [14, 15]. These data suggest that the greatest benefit for enhancing corneal endothelial cell proliferation and future cell density would be immediately after surgery when the endothelial wound is open, rather than waiting later in the healing course. We therefore started our patient on a ROCK inhibitor (netarsudil) immediately following surgery. We selected netarsudil due to its commercial availability in the United States, its pharmacologic profile showing similar potency to Y-27632 for block of rho-kinase isoforms present in corneal endothelium [16] and its use in prior human clinical studies [17]. Given that results with DSOs have been highly variable and little is currently known regarding predictive factors for success, early initiation of ROCK inhibitor may help promote successful outcomes. In our patient, we noticed that the peripheral endothelial cell density decreased following DSO as the central cell density increased. This suggests that while netarsudil may be increasing corneal endothelial cell proliferation, repopulation of the endothelial monolayer likely also involves migration of cells from the peripheral cornea.

Interestingly, although the area of descemetorhexis for this patient was small, we noted improvement throughout the cornea. As expected from removal of guttae by descemetorhexis, corneal densitometry values decreased in the posterior corneal layer in the area of the descemetorhexis postoperatively. However, there was also a diffuse decrease in values across the whole cornea postoperatively, including in the anterior layers of the cornea and in the peripheral cornea outside the area of the descemetorhexis. Likewise, corneal pachymetry measurements decreased not only in the central area of stripping, but also in the peripheral cornea. These findings suggest that even a very small area of diseased Descemet's membrane removed during DSO surgery can have significant impact on the whole cornea.

4. Conclusion

Our study and published literature support DSO as a viable alternative to cadaveric corneal transplantation for a select group of FECD patients. The use of ROCK inhibitors may further extend this option to a larger group of patients. Additionally, based upon our patient data, a small descemetorhexis positively impacts corneal thickness and densitometry globally. This may prove helpful as a smaller descemetorhexis leaves a smaller area for healing, which may reduce the time for healing. Although our patient's outcome is promising, long-term outcomes data are still lacking for this procedure with or without ROCK inhibitors.

Consent

Patient consent to publish was obtained in writing.

Acknowledgments

This work was supported in part by and facilities and resources provided by the VA Western New York Healthcare System. The contents of this work do not represent the views of the Department of Veterans Affairs or the United States government.

References

[1] G. Vedana, G. Villarreal, and A. Jun, "Fuchs endothelial corneal dystrophy: current perspectives," *Clinical Ophthalmology*, vol. 10, pp. 321–330, 2016.

[2] Eye Bank Association of America, "Eye Banking Statistical Report," 2017, http://restoresight.org/wp-content/uploads/2017/04/2016_Statistical_Report-Final-040717.pdf.

[3] J. L. Güell, M. A. El Husseiny, F. Manero, O. Gris, and D. Elies, "Historical review and update of surgical treatment for corneal endothelial diseases," *Ophthalmology and Therapy*, vol. 3, no. 1-2, pp. 1–15, 2014.

[4] M. O. Price, P. Gupta, J. Lass, and F. W. Price, "EK (DLEK, DSEK, DMEK): new frontier in cornea surgery," *Annual Review of Vision Science*, vol. 3, no. 1, pp. 69–90, 2017.

[5] S. Kinoshita, N. Koizumi, M. Ueno et al., "Injection of cultured cells with a ROCK inhibitor for bullous keratopathy," *New England Journal of Medicine*, vol. 378, no. 11, pp. 995–1003, 2018.

[6] N. Okumura, S. Kinoshita, and N. Koizumi, "Application of Rho kinase inhibitors for the treatment of corneal endothelial diseases," *Journal of Ophthalmology*, vol. 2017, Article ID 2646904, 8 pages, 2017.

[7] M. J. Huang, S. Kane, and D. K. Dhaliwal, "Descemetorhexis without endothelial keratoplasty versus DMEK for treatment of Fuchs endothelial corneal dystrophy," *Cornea*, vol. 37, no. 12, pp. 1479–1483, 2018.

[8] B. Van den Bogerd, S. N. Dhubhghaill, C. Koppen, M.-J. Tassignon, and N. Zakaria, "A review of the evidence for in vivo corneal endothelial regeneration," *Survey of Ophthalmology*, vol. 63, no. 2, pp. 149–165, 2018.

[9] V. Kocaba, K. R. Katikireddy, I. Gipson, M. O. Price, F. W. Price, and U. V. Jurkunas, "Association of the gutta-induced microenvironment with corneal endothelial cell behavior and demise in Fuchs endothelial corneal dystrophy," *JAMA Ophthalmology*, vol. 136, no. 8, pp. 886–892, 2018.

[10] E. Davies, U. Jurkunas, and R. Pineda, "Predictive factors for corneal clearance after descemetorhexis without endothelial keratoplasty," *Cornea*, vol. 37, no. 2, pp. 137–140, 2018.

[11] G. Moloney, C. Petsoglou, M. Ball et al., "Descemetorhexis without grafting for Fuchs endothelial dystrophy - supplementation with topical ripasudil," *Cornea*, vol. 36, no. 6, pp. 642–648, 2017.

[12] M. M. Fernandez, "Reticular epithelial edema in edematous corneas treated with netarsudil," *Ophthalmology*, vol. 125, no. 11, p. 1709, 2018.

[13] L. Dasso, T. Al-Khaled, S. Sonty, and A. A. Aref, "Profile of netarsudil ophthalmic solution and its potential in the treatment of open-angle glaucoma: evidence to date," *Clinical Ophthalmology*, vol. 12, pp. 1939–1944, 2018.

[14] N. Okumura, Y. Okazaki, R. Inoue et al., "Effect of the rho-associated kinase inhibitor eye drop (ripasudil) on corneal endothelial wound healing," *Investigative Opthalmology & Visual Science*, vol. 57, no. 3, pp. 1284–1292, 2016.

[15] N. Okumura, N. Koizumi, E. D. P. Kay et al., "The ROCK inhibitor eye drop accelerates corneal endothelium wound healing," *Investigative Opthalmology & Visual Science*, vol. 54, no. 4, pp. 2493–2502, 2013.

[16] C.-W. Lin, B. Sherman, L. A. Moore et al., "Discovery and preclinical development of netarsudil, a novel ocular hypotensive agent for the treatment of glaucoma," *Journal of Ocular Pharmacology and Therapeutics*, vol. 34, no. 1-2, pp. 40–51, 2018.

[17] J. B. Serle, L. J. Katz, E. McLaurin et al., "Two phase 3 clinical trials comparing the safety and efficacy of netarsudil to timolol in patients with elevated intraocular pressure: Rho kinase elevated IOP treatment trial 1 and 2 (ROCKET-1 and ROCKET-2)," *American Journal of Ophthalmology*, vol. 186, pp. 116–127, 2018.

23

Successful Photorefractive Keratectomy in a Case of Wilson's Disease

Saeed Shokoohi-Rad and Hamid-Reza Heidarzadeh

Eye Research Center, Mashhad University of Medical Sciences, Mashhad, Iran

Correspondence should be addressed to Hamid-Reza Heidarzadeh; dr.hamidreza.heidarzade@gmail.com

Academic Editor: Nicola Rosa

Purpose. To report a female with a history of Wilson's disease who underwent a successful photorefractive keratectomy (PRK) for myopic correction. *Case Presentation.* A twenty-year-old female with a history of Wilson's disease and D-penicillamine use was referred to our clinic for myopic refractive surgery. Her best-corrected visual acuity (BCVA) was 20/20 for both eyes with a refraction of -1.25-0.5 * 75° and -1.25-0.25 * 55° for the right and left eyes. The slit examination showed a prominent Kayser-Fleischer ring (K-F ring) in both eyes. She underwent a successful myopic PRK surgery, and her BCVA became 20/20 with no significant refraction. *Conclusions.* In this report, we report a successful PRK surgery for myopic correction in a case of Wilson's disease with prominent K-F rings in both eyes.

1. Introduction

Photorefractive keratectomy (PRK) is a Food and Drug Administration- (FDA-) approved refractive surgery for the correction of myopia, hyperopia, and astigmatism which employs a 193 nm argon fluoride excimer laser to ablate the anterior corneal stroma [1].

Wilson's disease is an autosomal recessive genetic disorder of copper metabolism caused by a mutation of the ATP7B gene, leading to copper accumulation in many tissues, mainly the liver, brain, cornea, and kidney [2]. The ocular manifestations include the Kayser-Fleischer ring (K-F ring) and sunflower cataract [3]. There has been no report that considers Wilson's disease a contraindication for refractive surgery, and this is the second case report of refractive surgery in a patient with Wilson's disease up to now.

Here, we describe a case of Wilson's disease with a prominent K-F ring who underwent a successful PRK for myopic correction.

2. Case Presentation

A twenty-year-old female with a history of Wilson's disease was referred to our clinic for refractive surgery. She was under treatment with D-penicillamine, an anticopper drug. Her best-corrected visual acuity (BCVA) was 20/20 for both eyes with a refraction of -1.25-0.5 * 75° in the right eye and -1.25-0.25 * 55° in the left eye. Keratometry was 43.25 * 40°/43.5 * 130° in the right eye and 43 * 5°/43.5 * 95° in the left eye. Her present glass and cycloplegic refractions were the same as BCVA. Slit-lamp examination showed prominent circumferential K-F ring in both eyes with clear lenses without any other pathologies. Intraocular pressure was 12 mm Hg without antiglaucoma medications in both eyes. Indirect ophthalmoscopy showed a 0.3 cup to disc ratio in both eyes without any other pathologies.

Corneal imaging studies performed and corneal topography (Orbscan II-Bausch & Lomb and Oculus-Pentacam) showed prolate corneal profile with a round pattern and enantiomorphism in both eyes. Pachymetry examination (Oculus-

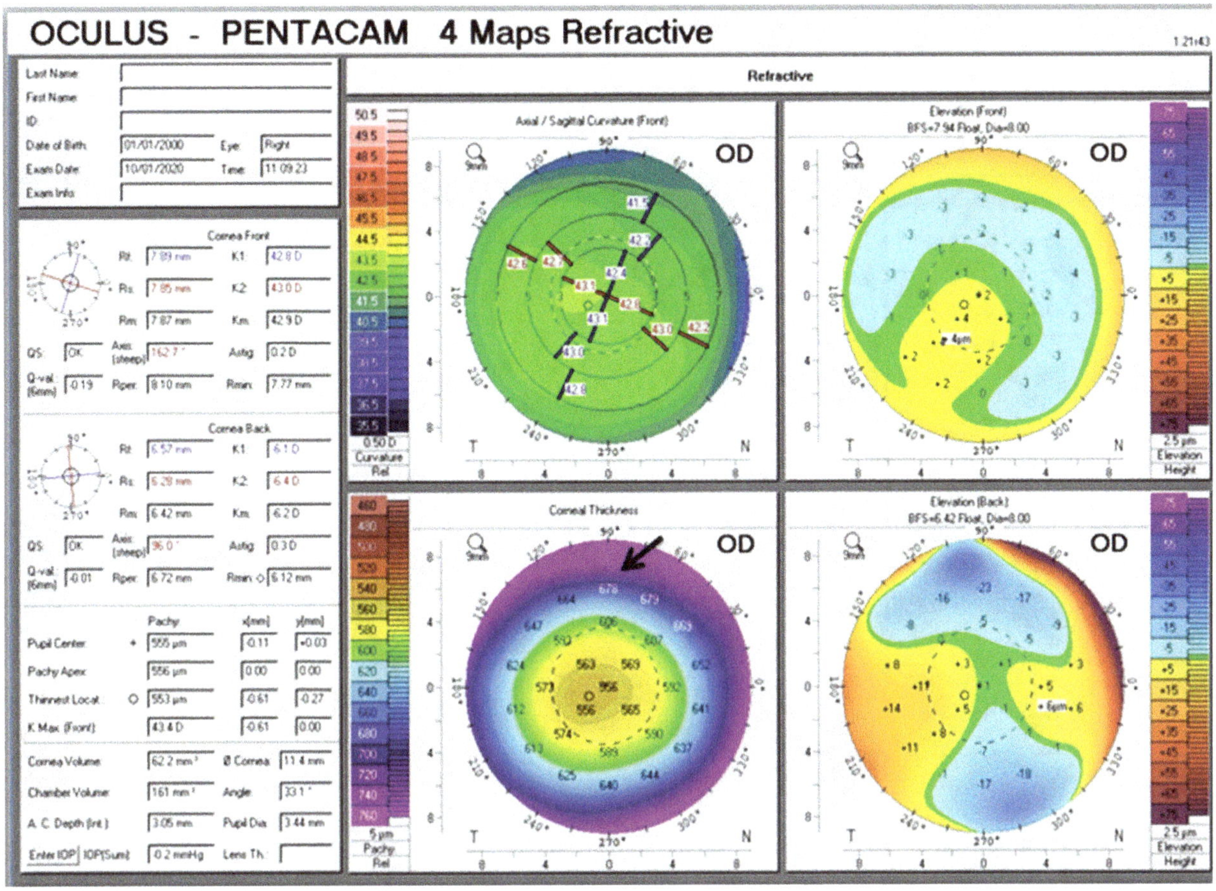

(a)

Figure 1: Continued.

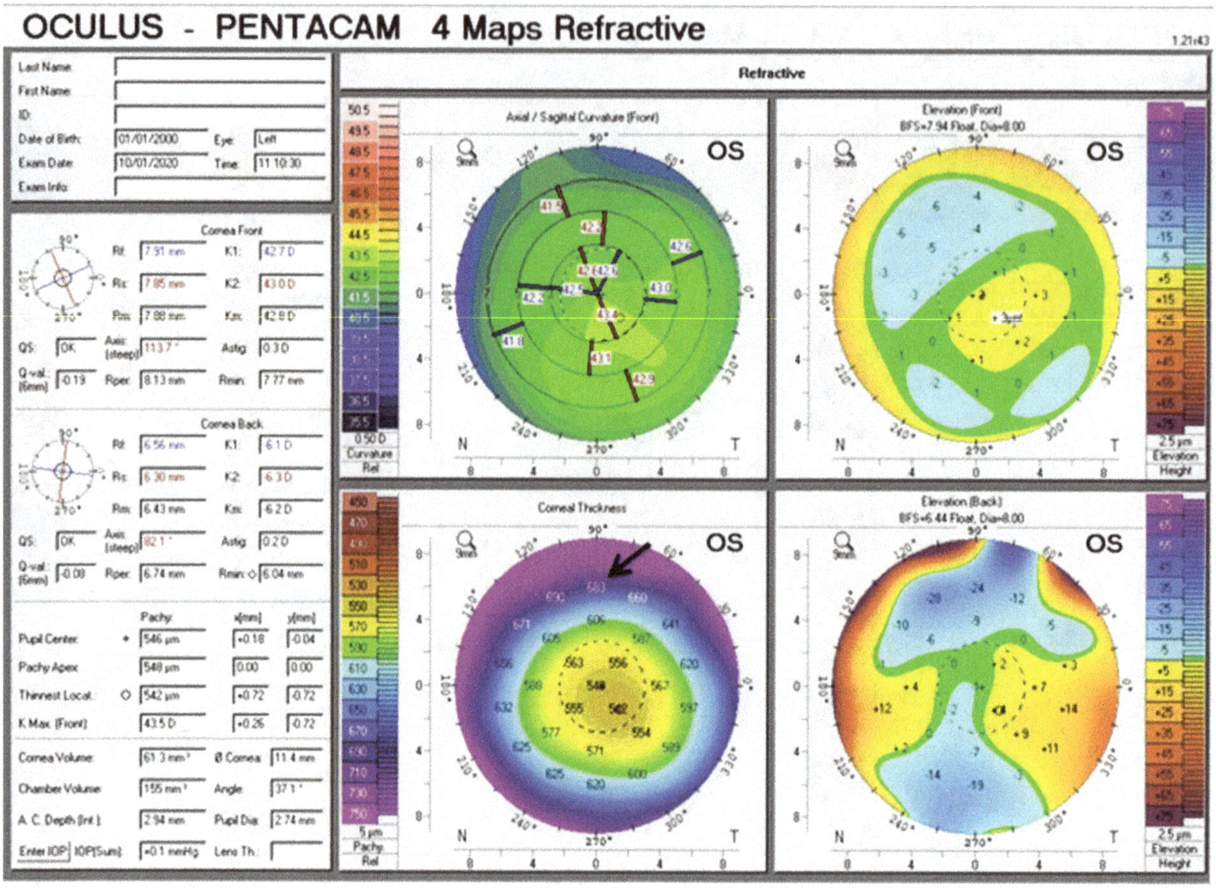

(b)

FIGURE 1: Corneal topography printouts of the right (a) and the left (b) eyes (Oculus-Pentacam). Corneal thickness maps show increased superior peripheral corneal thickness in both eyes due to copper deposition in Descemet's membrane (black arrows).

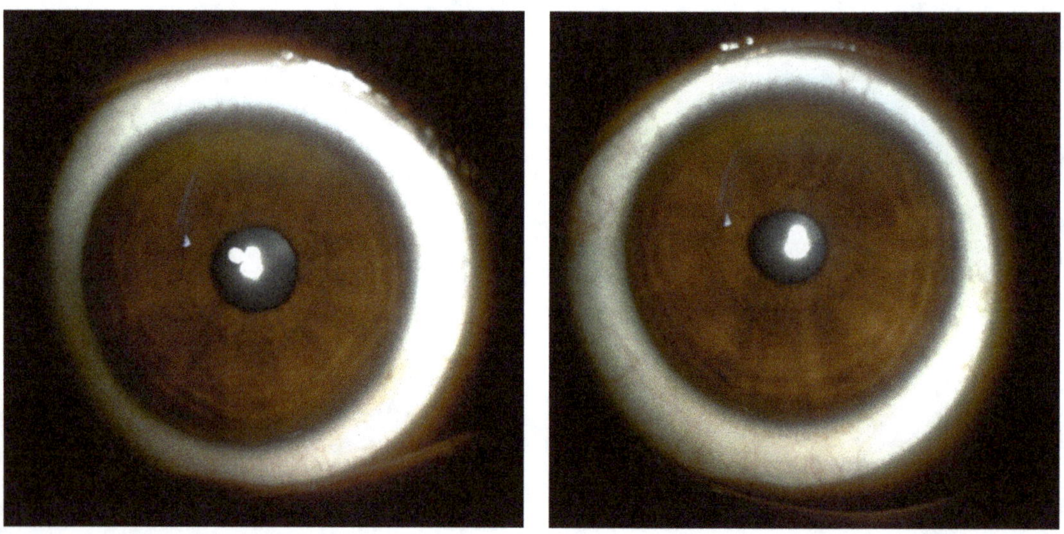

(a) (b)

FIGURE 2: Slit-lamp photograph of the right eye (a) and the left eye (b) postoperation shows K-F ring in peripheral cornea, and the central area is clear.

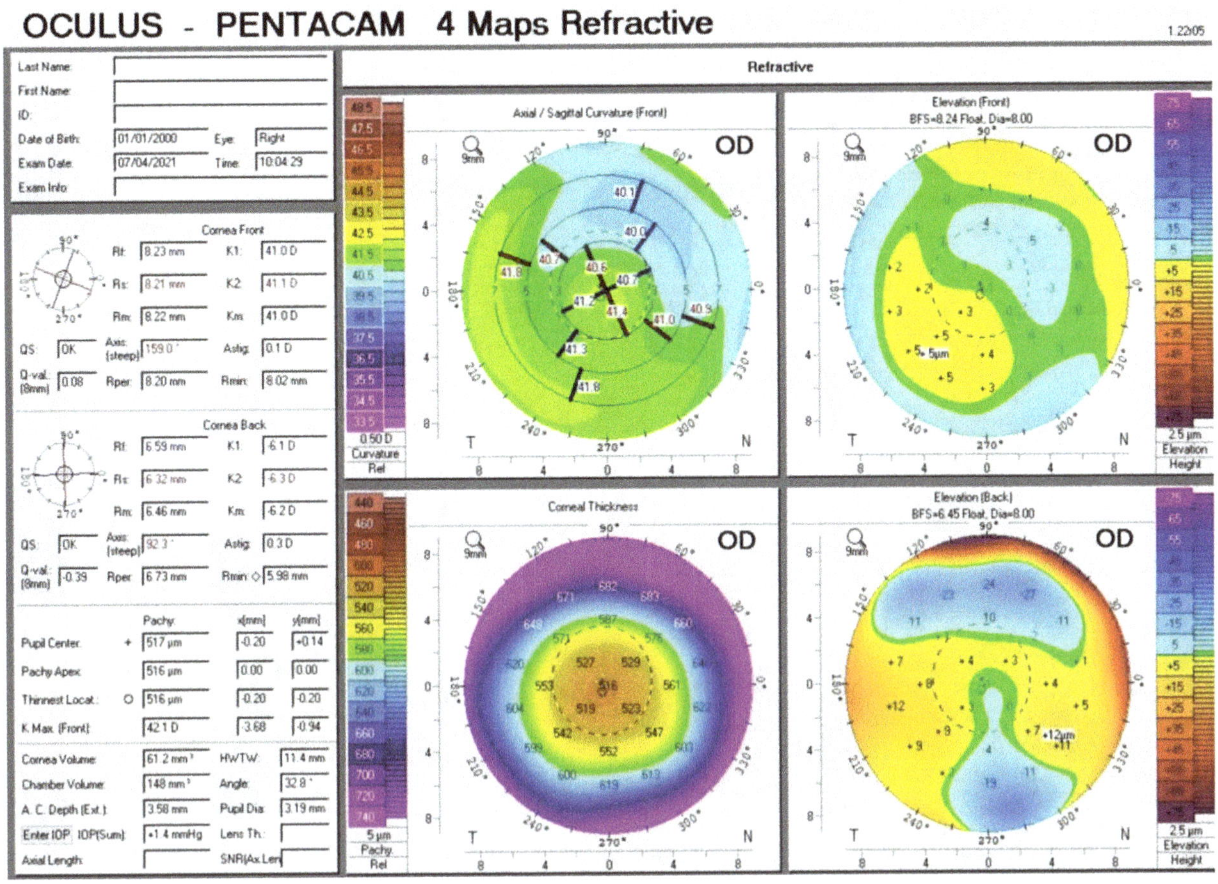

(a)

Figure 3: Continued.

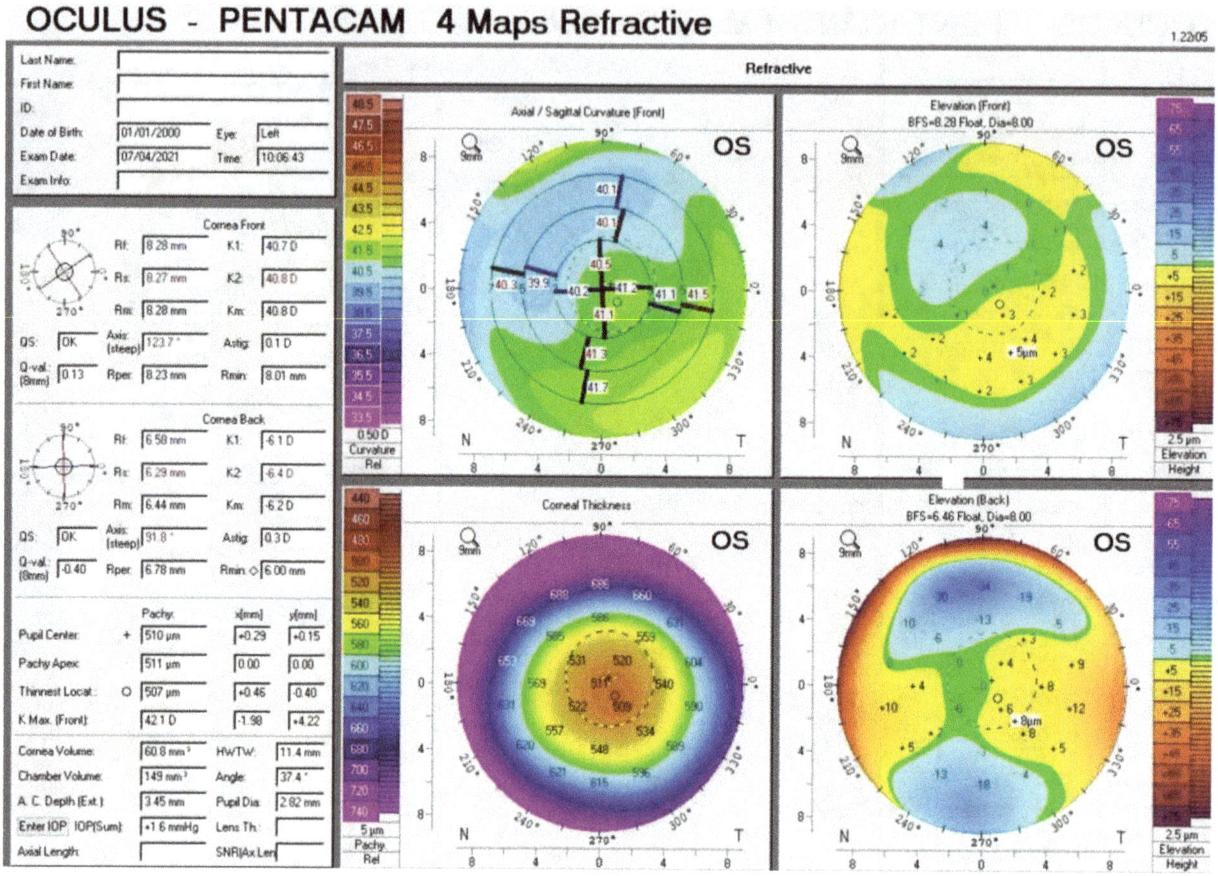

(b)

FIGURE 3: Postoperative corneal topography printouts of the right (a) and the left (b) eyes show no sign of corneal ectasia (Oculus-Pentacam).

Pentacam) revealed the central corneal thickness to be 555 μm in the right eye and 546 μm in the left eye (Figure 1). There was no sign of keratoconus in patient corneal topography and tomography studies. In aberrometry imaging (Bausch & Lomb Zywave aberrometer), there was a central comma in both eye higher-order aberration (HOA), and predicted phoropter refraction (PPR) was -1.03-0.69 * 83° in the right eye and -1.21-0.41 * 83° in the left eye.

The PRK was performed using Technolas Perfect Vision GmbH (Bausch & Lomb). After topical anesthesia, under sterile conditions, a 7 mm diameter mark centered on the pupil was performed on the corneal surface. The epithelium was removed mechanically with a blunt scraper. The correction was preset at -2-0.5 * 75° for the right eye and -2.25 – 0.25 * 55° for the left eye in the PROSCAN treatment mode. Maximum ablation was 52 μm in the right eye and 55 μm in the left eye within the treatment areas of 8.54 * 8.2 mm in the right eye and 8.51 * 8.67 mm in the left eye. After the procedure, levofloxacin solution was used and a therapeutic contact lens (TCL) was placed on both eyes. Betamethasone, levofloxacin single dose, and artificial tear drops were prescribed for the patient.

Seven days later, the patient visited for a follow-up. Corneal epithelium resurfacing was completed with no corneal haziness and TCL removed. Her uncorrected visual acuity was 20/20 in both eyes.

In 1 and 6 months after procedure follow-ups, her BCVA was 20/20 in both eyes with no significant refraction or residual refractive errors and her cornea showed no complication.

Nine months later, her BCVA was 20/20 in both eyes with no significant refraction. The slit-lamp examination showed a prominent circumferential K-F ring in both eyes, and the cornea center was clear (Figure 2). In aberrometry imaging, there was a central comma in both eye HOA, and PPR was +0.37-0.38 * 92° in the right eye and +0.57-0.19 * 86° in the left eye. The Zernike root mean square was 0.13 μm in the right eye and 0.15 μm in the left eye, which shows that PRK did not induce HOA. In the Pentacam imaging, the central corneal thickness postoperation was 516 μm in the right eye and 507 μm in the left eye, and there was no sign of corneal ectasia in both eyes (Figure 3).

3. Discussion

PRK is a safe and effective refractive surgery option for correction of myopia up to -12 diopter (D), astigmatism up to 6 D, and hyperopia up to 5 D which use a 193 nm argon fluoride excimer laser to ablate the anterior corneal stroma [4].

Absolute contraindications of PRK are significant cataract, unstable glaucoma, corneal ectasias, thinning, edema, interstitial or neurotrophic keratitis, and extensive vascularization. Also, patients with active systemic connective tissue diseases such as systemic lupus erythematosus and rheumatoid arthritis have a contraindication for PRK due to the risk of corneal hazing and melting [1, 5].

PRK is relatively contraindicated in pregnant women, nursing mothers, functional monocularity, ocular conditions that limit visual function, excessively steep or flat corneas, abnormal corneal topography, significant irregular astigmatism, inadequately controlled dry eye, uveitis, glaucoma, history of herpes simplex keratitis, uncontrolled diabetes, and taking medications with a high risk of ocular side effects like isotretinoin and amiodarone [1, 5].

Typical ocular manifestations of Wilson's disease are K-F ring and sunflower cataract [3]. The K-F ring was described by the German ophthalmologists Bernhard Kayser and Bruno Fleischer [6]. At least 50% of patients and all patients with neurological disorder have this sign [7]. The extracellular copper depositions in Descemet's membrane of the cornea, which is called K-F ring, are almost bilateral and start primarily in the superior peripheral cornea, then inferior and later became circumferential [6]. Free copper loosely bound to albumin enters the aqueous humor, and the peripheral deposition in Descemet's membrane is attributed to the direction of the aqueous humor [8]. The K-F ring is reported to fade with anticopper therapy [9]. Theoretically, due to the depth and peripheral place of the K-F ring, it should not affect the laser beam, and the laser ablation zone is placed in the corneal central zone.

There is limited understanding of the safety of refractive surgery in patients with Wilson's disease. There has been just one report on PRK in a patient with Wilson's disease which was about undercorrection after PRK in a patient who had a prominent K-F ring like our patient, and it showed that PRK was performed safe and without any complication in that patient [10].

In conclusion, PRK showed to be a safe and effective refractive surgery for correction of myopia with no complication in our patient with a prominent K-F ring in both eyes due to Wilson's disease.

Consent

Consent was not applicable.

Authors' Contributions

All the authors contributed significantly to this report, and all authors agree to be accountable for all aspects of the work. All authors read and approved the final manuscript.

References

[1] S. N. Somani, M. Moshirfar, and B. C. Patel, "Photorefractive keratectomy," in *StatPearls*, StatPearls Publishing, Treasure Island (FL), 2021.

[2] J. Liu, J. Luan, X. Zhou, Y. Cui, and J. Han, "Epidemiology, diagnosis, and treatment of Wilson's disease," *Intractable & Rare Diseases Research*, vol. 6, no. 4, pp. 249–255, 2017.

[3] S. Goel, P. Sahay, P. K. Maharana, and J. S. Titiyal, "Ocular manifestations of Wilson's disease," *BML Case Reports*, vol. 12, no. 3, article e229662, 2019.

[4] R. Stein, "Photorefractive keratectomy," *International Ophthalmology Clinics*, vol. 40, no. 3, pp. 35–56, 2000.

[5] K. S. Bower and F. Woreta, "Update on contraindications for laser-assisted in situ keratomileusis and photorefractive keratectomy," *Current Opinion in Ophthalmology*, vol. 25, no. 4, pp. 251–257, 2014.

[6] J. C. Suvarna, "Kayser-Fleischer ring," *Journal of Postgraduate Medicine*, vol. 54, no. 3, pp. 238–240, 2008.

[7] T. Veharanta and P. Immonen, "Hepatolenticular degeneration, Wilson's disease," *Duodecim*, vol. 97, no. 11, pp. 743–745, 1981.

[8] J. Harry and R. Tripathi, "Kayser-Fleischer ring. A pathological study," *The British Journal of Ophthalmology*, vol. 54, no. 12, pp. 794–800, 1970.

[9] B. Esmaeli, M. A. Burnstine, C. L. Martonyi, A. Sugar, V. Johnson, and G. J. Brewer, "Regression of Kayser-Fleischer rings during oral zinc therapy: correlation with systemic manifestations of Wilson's disease," *Cornea*, vol. 15, no. 6, pp. 582–588, 1996.

[10] Y.-S. Lee, Y. M. Su, and H. C. Lin, "Undercorrection after photorefractive keratectomy in Wilson's disease," *Taiwan Journal of Ophthalmology*, vol. 4, no. 3, pp. 133–136, 2014.

Localized Bilateral Superior and Inferior Orbital Neurofibroma in the Absence of Neurofibromatosis

Daniela Rojas-Correa,[1] Álvaro Bengoa-González,[1] Enrique Mencía-Gutiérrez,[1] Aurelio Hernández-Laín,[2] Elena Salvador,[3] Agustín Martín-Clavijo,[4] Justino Jiménez-Almonacid,[2] and María-Dolores Lago-Llinás[1]

[1]*Ophthalmology Department, 12 de Octubre Hospital, Complutense University, 28041 Madrid, Spain*
[2]*Neuropathology Department, 12 de Octubre Hospital, Complutense University, 28041 Madrid, Spain*
[3]*Radiology Department, 12 de Octubre Hospital, Complutense University, 28041 Madrid, Spain*
[4]*Dermatology Department, Queen Elizabeth Hospital, Birmingham University, B15 2TH Birmingham, UK*

Correspondence should be addressed to Enrique Mencía-Gutiérrez; emencia.hdoc@salud.madrid.org

Academic Editor: Alexander A. Bialasiewicz

Localized or isolated neurofibromas are peripheral nerve sheath tumors. They are rare in the orbit and occur without a systemic neurofibromatosis. There are few cases of bilateral tumors reported but none affecting both supraorbital and infraorbital nerves. We report a 45-year-old female who presented an extraconal mass in the right orbit as an incidental finding in a head computer tomography, without ocular symptoms. Magnetic resonance image showed a well-defined oval mass in the right supraorbital and infraorbital nerves, of similar characteristics, as well as smaller masses in the left supraorbital and infraorbital nerves. A progressive increase in size of the left supraorbital and infraorbital tumor motivated their surgical excision. The histological result was compatible with a neurofibroma. These uncommon orbital tumors are slow growing and affect the sensory nerves of the trigeminal nerve. Neurofibromas usually present progressive symptoms due to the orbital mass, proptosis, or visual changes although not in this case. Surgical removal is the only definitive treatment.

1. Introduction

Neurofibromas are classified within the tumors that affect peripheral nerves. Localized or isolated neurofibromas are peripheral nerve sheath tumors and are rare in the orbit, representing less than 1% of orbital tumors [1, 2]. Unlike the relatively more common plexiform neurofibromas, localized neurofibromas tend to be well circumscribed and are not typically associated with type 1 neurofibromatosis (NF) [1, 3]. These tumors can be solitary but more frequently are multiple [1]. Solitary neurofibromas in the adult orbit, in the absence of systemic NF, are difficult to clinically differentiate from other orbital tumors [4]. They are composed of Schwann cells, perineural cells, and fibroblasts [5]. Most of the few reported cases were unilateral [6, 7] with 5 cases of bilateral tumors reported in the literature [8]. Herein, we report a case of neurofibromas affecting both supraorbital and infraorbital nerve bilaterally, without association with familiar NF, a combination not reported before.

2. Case Presentation

Three years ago, a 45-year-old female presented an extraconal mass in the right orbit as an incidental finding in a head computer tomography scan and magnetic resonance image (MRI) during investigations following two syncopal episodes.

On examination, she had a best corrected visual acuity (BCVA) of 1.0 (decimal scale) in both eyes with no exophthalmos nor diplopia and only a minimal asymmetry of the palpebral fold between both eyes. Extraocular muscle movement was normal. There were no alterations in fundoscopy, and the intraocular pressure was normal.

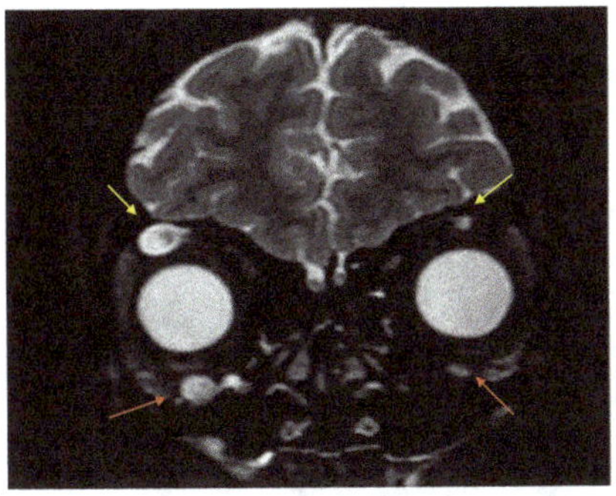

(a)

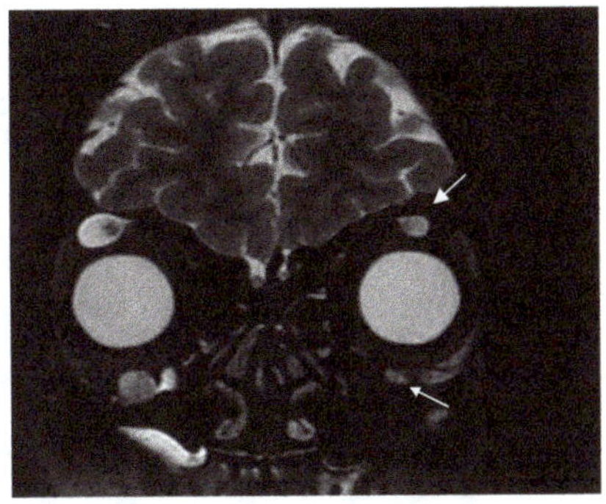

(b)

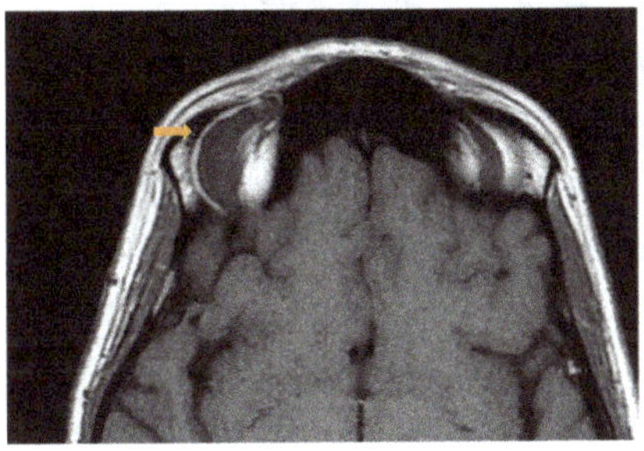

(c)

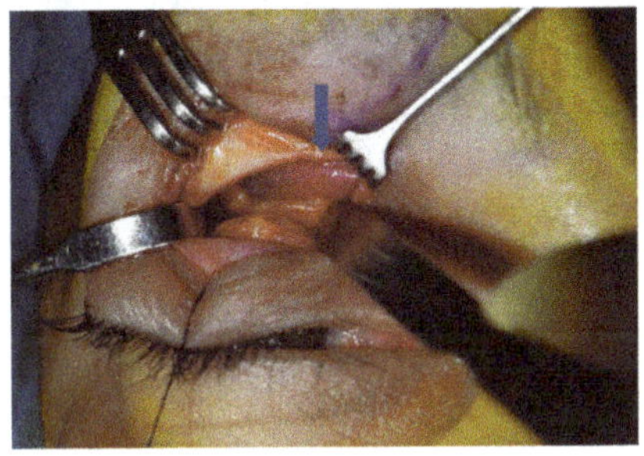

(d)

FIGURE 1: (a) Coronal MRI T2-weighted imaging showed bilateral hyperintense well-defined extraconal masses in the anterosuperior margin of both orbits (yellow arrows) (the greater one on the right side) corresponding to the supraorbital nerves. There was also another extraconal mass in the anteroinferior margin of the right orbit related to the infraorbital nerve, with similar appearance, and smaller on the left side (red arrows). (b) Growth of lesions in the left orbit (white arrows). (c) MRI axial T1-weighted imaging demonstrated the right anterosuperior tumor with isointensity relative to muscle with a fusiform morphology (orange arrow). (d) Intraoperative image of the lesion (blue arrow).

The MRI showed a well-defined hypodense oval mass in T1 and hyperintense in T2 sequencing. There was also an ill-defined area, appearing hypodense on T2 but of intermediate density in T1, measuring 24 × 9 mm (Figures 1(a) and 1(c)). The mass had very well-defined borders in the anterosuperior margin of the right orbit, probably corresponding to the supraorbital nerve. With this presentation, the initial differential diagnosis was of a vascular lesion or a schwannoma. An MRI angiogram showed no uptake of contrast, ruling out a vascular lesion, but showed a second mass in the right orbit, of similar characteristics, in the right infraorbital nerve, as well as smaller masses in the left supraorbital and infraorbital nerves (Figure 1(a)). Although the lacrimal glands and the extraocular muscles were not affected, the findings were suggestive of an IgG4-related disease; however, the serum IgG4 levels were within normal ranges.

As the masses were affecting several nerves and were asymptomatic, a watchful wait approach was adopted. During the 3 years of follow-up, MRI demonstrated the existence of similar lesions, located in the right supra- and infraorbital nerve as well as on the left side. However, there was a progressive increase in size and signal enhancement corresponding to the left supraorbital nerve during the last year, which also affected the left infraorbital nerve (Figure 1(b)), leading us to remove the tumor to make a definitive diagnosis.

An orbitotomy with access through the upper eyelid skin crease was performed, exposing a fusiform lesion, cystic in appearance, measuring approximately 3 cm in its major axis, protruding from the supraorbital nerve and extending deeply into the orbit (Figure 1(d)). The lesion was removed en bloc. There was no deficit in the ocular mobility postsurgically nor any reduction in BCVA; the patient only presented decreased sensation and numbness in the right frontal nerve distribution area; this decreased sensation in the right forehead has not completely recovered at the last visit. MRI follow-up demonstrated no recurrence of the excised tumor and a slight increase in size of the other lesions (Figure 2).

The microscopic analysis showed a lesion with a loose connective stroma, areas with spindle and oval cells with wavy nuclei, along with dense bundles of hyalinized collagen in the form of "shredded carrots" and others composed of concentric structures of Schwann cells around axons with an "onion bulb" appearance (Figures 3(a)–3(c)). Immunohistochemistry showed positivity with S100 protein in the Schwann cells; axons inside the lesion were positive for neurofilament protein, epithelial membrane antigen (EMA), and CD34 in cells around Schwann cells. The histological findings and the presence of all the cellular elements of the nerve were compatible with a diagnosis of neurofibroma (Figures 4(a)–4(c)). No inflammatory infiltrates, plasma cells, or other data suggestive of IgG4 disease were identified.

Further investigation showed an absence of axillary/inguinal freckling, cafe au lait spots, and Lisch nodules of the iris. No first- or second-degree relatives suffered from similar illness or had any such clinical stigmata. The patient had no other dysmorphic features or endocrine syndromes and no systemic stigmata indicative of familial NF, nor any compatible family history. Due to the benign appearances of the

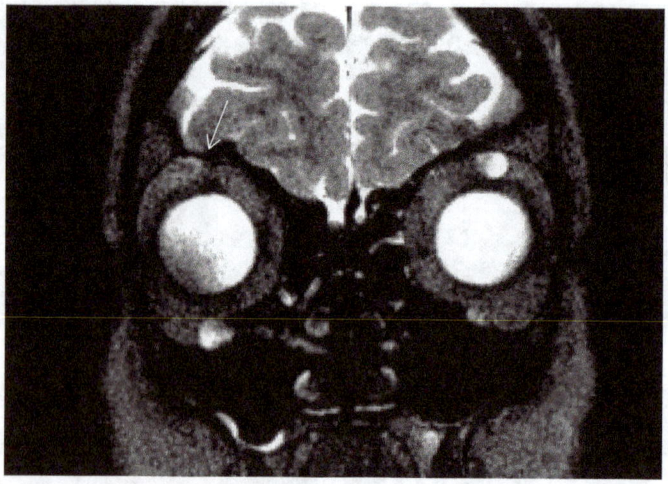

FIGURE 2: Postoperative coronal RMI T2-weighted imaging showed no recurrence in superior orbit right side (arrow). There was discrete increase in size of those located in the inferior right orbit and in the superior and inferior left orbit.

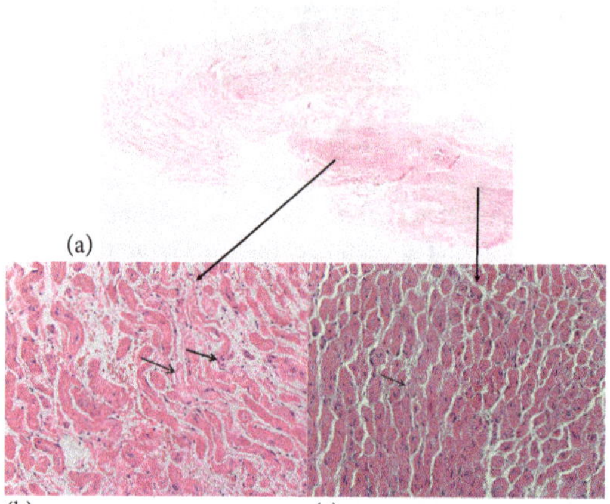

FIGURE 3: (a) Microscopic panoramic view of the lesion. Hematoxylin and eosin, 20x. (b) Heavy collagen bundles described as "shredded carrots" (thick arrow). Note the oval and wavy nuclei (thin arrow). Hematoxylin and eosin, 200x. (c) Whorls reminiscent of true onion bulbs (arrow). Hematoxylin and eosin, 200x.

lesion, it was decided, together with the patient, to restart the watchful wait and to intervene only if there was a significant change in size or functional deficits. None have been noted after 20 months of follow-up.

3. Discussion

Isolated neurofibromas of the orbit (also known as localized, solitary, or circumscribed) is the term used to refer to those neurofibromas of the orbit, which occur without a systemic diagnosis of NF1, previously known as von Recklinghausen disease [9]. Overall, neurofibromas are uncommon in adults, 1-3% of all space-occupying lesions of the orbit [2, 10]. The incidence of true isolated neurofibromas in the orbit is difficult to determine because of its relation to NF; it has been estimated that 10%-28% of all solitary neurofibromas are related to NF [6]. Some authors [6, 7, 11] described solitary neurofibromas in their series, but there is a paucity of reports of bilateral solitary neurofibromas in non-NF patients [8]. The case we present is the first to our knowledge affecting the supra- and infraorbital nerves bilaterally. As in other cases [12], our patient was middle-aged, and the tumors were slow growing, affecting the sensory nerves of the trigeminal nerve [4]. The location of tumors in the superior orbit in the distribution of the ophthalmic nerve (V1) is typical, but involvement of the maxillary nerve (V2) in the floor of the orbit, as in our case, is less frequent [1]. Garrity et al. noted multiple tumors in a single patient involving other nerves traversing the orbit [6].

Even though our patient was asymptomatic and the tumor was found as an incidental finding, patients with solitary neurofibromas usually present with a long history of progressive symptoms due to the orbital mass, a palpable mass, gradually progressing proptosis, visual changes, diplopia, hypoesthesia, or pain (although pain is less frequent) [4, 11, 12]. As a differential diagnosis, IgG4-related disease was considered [13] although the histological findings were not supportive. This illness affects primarily the lacrimal gland, but an increase in size can also be seen in other orbital structures such as the supraorbital and infraorbital nerves [14]. Suspicion of this disease arises when high serum levels of IgG4 are found. However, normal serum levels (as was our case) do not rule out the diagnosis. Other differential diagnoses included cavernous hemangioma, hemangiopericytoma, orbital varix, neurilemmoma, and fibrous histiocytoma, among others [1]. Differential diagnosis of a peripheral nerve sheath tumor encompasses schwannoma, neurofibroma, perineurioma, granular cell tumor, benign hybrid tumors, and malignant peripheral nerve sheath tumors [4, 15].

We were able to rule out familial NF. The diagnostic criteria require the presence of 2 or more of the following criteria [15]:

(i) Six or more cafe au lait macules over 5 mm in their greatest diameter in prepubertal individuals and over 15 mm in postpubertal individuals

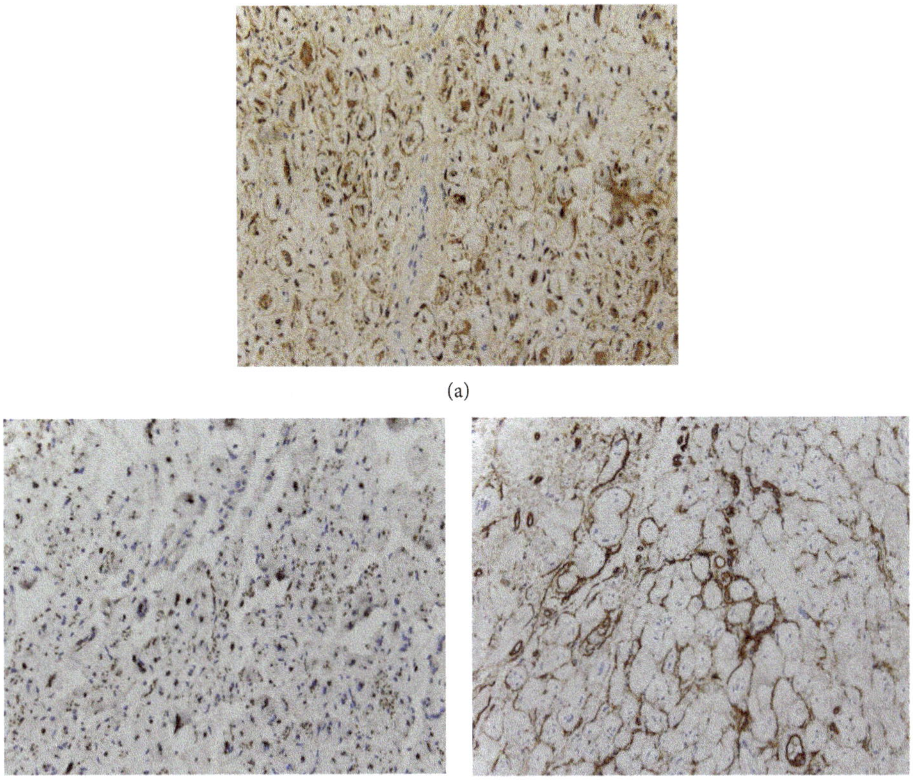

(a)

(b) (c)

Figure 4: (a) S100 protein immunoreactivity showed Schwann cells. (b) Immunochemistry with neurofilaments was positive in axons. (c) Intermixed cells CD34 positive were observed.

Table 1: Pathologic and immunophenotypic features useful in the differential diagnosis of Schwann cell neoplasms [15].

	Neurofibroma	Schwannoma	MPNST
Cytology			
Nuclear size	+	++	++/+++
Nuclear hyperchromasia	+	++	+++
Wavy nuclei	+++	+	++
Histology			
"Shredded carrot" type collagen	+++	−	−/+
Capsule	−	+++	−
Hyalinized vessels	−/+	+++	−
Fascicular growth pattern	−/+	++	+++
Mitotic activity	−/+	−/+	+++
Necrosis	−	−/+	+++
Immunohistochemistry marker			
S100 protein	++/+++	+++	+/++
Collagen IV	++/+++	+++	+/++
EMA	+	−(capsular)	−
CD34	+++	+++	++
Neurofilament protein	++	+(capsular rare intratumoral axons)	+/+++
Podoplanin	+	++	+
Calretinin	+	+++	NA
Sox10	+++	+++	+/++

MPNST: malignant peripheral nerve sheath tumor; EMA: epithelial membrane antigen; NA: not applicable.

(ii) Two or more neurofibromas of any type or one plexiform neurofibroma

(iii) Freckling in the axillary or inguinal region

(iv) Optic glioma

(v) Two or more Lisch nodules (iris hamartomas)

(vi) A distinctive osseous lesion such as sphenoid dysplasia or thinning of long bone cortex with or without pseudarthrosis

(vii) A first-degree relative (parent, sibling, or offspring) with NF1 by the above criteria

Several imaging features, including multiplicity, multilobulation, ring-configured contrast enhancement, and MRI signal intensity heterogeneity, may point to the diagnosis of localized neurofibroma [4]. MRI can help with preoperative planning and selecting the best surgical approach should surgery become necessary [4]. Surgical resection may be the only way to arrive at a definitive diagnosis [12].

The orbital mass was biopsied via anterior orbitotomy by eyelid crease approach.

Ultrastructural studies showed that this tumor was composed of a mixture of three cell types: Schwann cells, perineural cells, and fibroblasts [7, 16]. Immunohistochemistry showed immune reactivity in EMA and S100 protein (Figures 4(a)–4(c)) in perineurioma and neurofibroma, respectively [17, 18]. Immunohistochemistry in our case was compatible with neurofibroma [15] (Table 1).

The importance of the localized neurofibroma is that the tumor can be easily removed leading to a complete surgical cure. In cases where the tumor was not completely excised, no recurrences requiring further surgery were found after long follow-up periods [7, 11]. Patients with localized neurofibromas usually see a return to normal globe position, visual acuity, and sensation after surgery. However, there is a risk for postoperative anesthesia, reported in 72% of patients with neurofibromas, likely attributable to damage to the involved sensory nerves during removal [12].

4. Conclusion

Neurofibromas without associated NF rarely occur in the orbit. In addition, the peculiarity of our case lies in the bilateral involvement of the supra- and infraorbital nerves not previously described in medical literature.

References

[1] D. R. Meyer and J. L. Wobig, "Bilateral localized orbital neurofibromas," *Ophthalmology*, vol. 99, no. 8, pp. 1313–1317, 1992.

[2] J. A. Shields, B. Bakewell, J. J. Ausburger, and J. C. Flanagan, "Classification and incidence of space-occupying lesions of the orbit," *Archives of Ophthalmology*, vol. 102, no. 11, pp. 1606–1611, 1984.

[3] S. Takeuchi, K. Wada, K. Nagatani, and H. Nawashiro, "Localized neurofibromas in the bilateral orbits," *Indian Journal of Surgery*, vol. 75, no. 5, pp. 407-408, 2013.

[4] S. R. Tripathy, S. S. Mishra, R. C. Deo, I. Mohanta, D. Das, and M. C. Satapathy, "Trochlear Nerve Neurofibroma in a Clinically NF-1-Negative Patient; A Case Report and Review of Literature," *World Neurosurgery*, vol. 89, pp. 732.e13–732.e18, 2016.

[5] D. M. Skovronsky and J. C. Oberholtzer, "Pathologic classification of peripheral nerve tumors," *Neurosurgery Clinics of North America*, vol. 15, no. 2, pp. 157–166, 2004.

[6] J. A. Garrity and J. W. Henderson, "Tumors of peripheral nerve sheath origin," in *Henderson's Orbital Tumors*, Lippincot Williams and Wilkins, Philadelphia, PA, USA, 4th edition, 2007.

[7] H. M. Alkatan, "Solitary neurofibroma in the absence of neurofiromatosis," *Canadian Journal of Ophthalmology*, vol. 42, no. 4, pp. 628-629, 2007.

[8] K. M. Alshomar, H. M. Alkatan, and A. H. Alsuhaibani, "Bilateral orbital isolated (solitary) neurofibroma in the absence of neurofibromatosis - a case report," *Saudi Journal of Ophthalmology*, vol. 32, no. 1, pp. 83–85, 2018.

[9] S. P. Braich, J. C. Donalson, G. S. Bajat, and W. H. Bearden, "Isolated neurofibroma of the orbit: case report and literature review," *Ophthalmic Plastic and Reconstructive Surgery*, vol. 34, no. 1, pp. 1–6, 2018.

[10] L. R. Lee, J. W. Gigantelli, and M. C. Kincaid, "Localized neurofibroma of the orbit," *Ophthalmic Plastic and Reconstructive Surgery*, vol. 16, no. 3, pp. 241–246, 2000.

[11] G. E. Rose and J. E. Wright, "Isolated peripheral nerve sheath tumours of the orbit," *Eye*, vol. 5, no. 6, pp. 668–673, 1991.

[12] J. J. Evans, M. J. Wilkinson, and C. S. Specht, "Solitary orbital neurofibroma presenting as a cystic mass," *Canadian Journal of Ophthalmology*, vol. 47, no. 6, pp. e39–e41, 2012.

[13] Y. S. Song, H.-H. Choung, S.-W. Park, J.-H. Kim, S. I. Khwarg, and Y. K. Jeon, "Ocular adnexal IgG4-related disease: CT and MRI findings," *British Journal of Ophthalmology*, vol. 97, no. 4, pp. 412–418, 2013.

[14] M. Takahira, Y. Ozawa, M. Kawano et al., "Clinical Aspects of IgG4-Related Orbital Inflammation in a Case Series of Ocular Adnexal Lymphoproliferative Disorders," *International Journal of Rheumatology*, vol. 2012, Article ID 635473, 5 pages, 2012.

[15] F. J. Rodriguez, A. L. Folpe, C. Giannini, and A. Perry, "Pathology of peripheral nerve sheath tumors: diagnostic overview and update on selected diagnostic problems," *Acta Neuropathologica*, vol. 123, no. 3, pp. 295–319, 2012.

[16] M. Zamecnik and M. Michal, "Perineurial cell differentiation in neurofibromas. Report of eight cases including a case with composite peurineurinoma-neurofibroma features," *Pathology, Research and Practice*, vol. 197, no. 8, pp. 537–544, 2001.

[17] C. P. Leung, E. Chan, H. Y. J. Ng, and T. C. S. Ko, "Novel case of hybrid perineurioma-neurofibroma of the orbit," *Canadian Journal of Ophthalmology*, vol. 54, no. 6, pp. e283–e285, 2019.

[18] J. J. Mulvihill, D. M. Parry, J. L. Sherman, A. Pikus, M. I. Kaiser-Kupfer, and R. Eldridge, "Neurofibromatosis 1 (Recklinghausen disease) and neurofibromatosis 2 (bilateral acoustic neurofibromatosis)," *Annals of Internal Medicine*, vol. 113, no. 1, pp. 39–52, 1990.

25

Treatment of Recurrent Primary Cutaneous Mucinous Carcinoma of the Eyelid with Modified Wide Local Excision

Stephanie M. Tillit[1] **Siva S. R. Iyer**[2] **Eric J. Grieser**[2] **and John T. LiVecchi**[2]

[1]*College of Medicine, University of Florida, Gainesville, FL, USA*
[2]*Department of Ophthalmology, University of Florida, Gainesville, FL, USA*

Correspondence should be addressed to John T. LiVecchi; jlivecchi@ufl.edu

Academic Editor: Maurizio Battaglia Parodi

Primary cutaneous mucinous carcinoma (PCMC) is a rare, low-grade malignant neoplasm of the sweat gland, whose history has been controversial regarding eccrine versus apocrine origin. This case report describes a 53-year-old male who presented to the University of Florida, Gainesville, ophthalmology clinic and was referred to the oculoplastics service with a painless, subcentimeter mass on the lateral right upper eyelid including the canthus, consistent with recurrent primary cutaneous mucinous carcinoma of the eyelid. Four years prior, the patient had undergone excisional biopsy of the lesion in a clinic, which revealed residual tumor, but the patient deferred further surgery at the time. The patient underwent surgical excision of the mass with reconstruction without operative complications and with negative surgical margins. PCMC is difficult to diagnose clinically due to its rarity and requires a histopathological examination for confirmation of the diagnosis. This report presents the first case in the literature of primary cutaneous mucinous carcinoma in a patient with human immunodeficiency virus (HIV). With this case report, we aim to raise awareness of primary cutaneous mucinous carcinoma as a potential part of the differential diagnosis for malignant eyelid lesions, including those present in patients with HIV.

1. Introduction

Carcinomas of the sweat gland are known to be rare malignancies with locally aggressive features and high rates of recurrence [1]. These have been traditionally subdivided into the groups of eccrine, apocrine, mixed origin (eccrine and apocrine) and other unclassifiable sweat gland tumors [1]. There is a lack of consistent immunohistochemical markers identified in these, as well as histological similarities to other malignancies, which can make diagnosis difficult. For example, primary cutaneous mucinous carcinomas (PCMCs) may resemble mucinous carcinomas found elsewhere in the body (e.g., breast, lung, gastrointestinal-type tumors) [2]. For this reason, one must rule out the possibility of metastatic lesions and correlate clinically. Herein, we report the case of a 53-year-old male with recurrent primary cutaneous mucinous carcinoma of the right upper eyelid, including diagnosis, management, and follow-up. This is the first case of PCMC in a patient with human immunodeficiency virus (HIV) reported in the literature.

2. Case

A 53-year-old male presented to the ophthalmology clinic for a right upper eyelid mass that had been subjectively growing over the last year. Past medical history was significant for hypertension and human immunodeficiency virus (HIV). Past ocular history was significant for primary cutaneous mucinous carcinoma of the right upper eyelid and bilateral senile nuclear sclerosis.

Four years prior, the patient had presented to the University of Florida, Gainesville, ophthalmology clinic for a painless right upper lid mass, which initially was diagnosed as a chalazion. The mass failed to improve with conservative therapy, and excision of the lesion was performed in a clinic, with pathology showing histologic features compatible with mucinous carcinoma. The tumor cells were immunoreactive for Cytokeratin 7 and Gross Cystic Disease Fluid Protein 15 (GCDFP-15) and negative for Cytokeratin 5/6 and p63. The mucin infiltrated and dissected through the fibrotic stroma and appeared to extend to the deep resection margin. Metastatic workup, including CT of the chest, abdomen, and pelvis, was negative for other disease. Though the patient was counseled on the high likelihood of recurrence, he declined any further surgery at the time. The patient followed up for one year after excisional biopsy but was subsequently lost to follow-up.

Three years later, he presented to the oculoplastics clinic with a 4 mm × 5 mm mass on the lateral right upper eyelid including the canthus, which had subjectively gradually grown over the last year per the patient, without any soreness or drainage of the lesion (Figures 1(a)–1(c)). Slit lamp exam showed a right upper lid lesion, bilateral blepharitis, bilateral pigmentation and pinguecula of the conjunctiva, and bilateral senile nuclear sclerosis. A diagnostic incisional biopsy of the lesion in clinic revealed recurrent mucinous carcinoma.

The patient subsequently underwent surgical excision of the mucinous carcinoma of the right upper lid with reconstruction. There is currently no standard of care for the surgical treatment of PCMC, and interventions range from standard excision to wide local excision and Mohs surgery. [3] Herein, we describe our modified wide local excision technique to avoid significant morbidity in this patient with lid margin and lateral canthal involvement.

The right upper eyelid was inspected, and a pentagonal wedge of tissue including the carcinoma lesion was excised using an 11 blade and Westcott scissors. The lesion measured approximately 15 mm × 10 mm and was labelled as the "main" specimen with the medial aspect marked with a single suture. Margin procurement was completed with the aim of achieving satisfactory disease-free margins while retaining adequate postsurgical function. Initial full-length margins 2.5 mm wide were excised medially, temporally, superiorly, and deep. These were followed by a second set of additional excisions 5 mm wide medially, temporally, superiorly, and deep, making the total margin taken at least 7.5 mm. The outermost, or second excised, margins were sent to pathology labelled with their respective location.

The tarsus was reapproximated using a double-armed 6-0 Vicryl suture in a horizontal mattress suture. A single interrupted 6-0 Vicryl suture was used to reapproximate the anterior border of the tarsus. A lateral canthotomy was performed using Stevens scissors to make the lateral lid more mobile for closure. The superior tarsus and remaining skin defects were closed using 6-0 plain gut. Adequate hemostasis was obtained, and there was minimal loss of blood with no immediate postoperative complications.

A histological description of the specimen is provided in Figure 2. Furthermore, tumor cells were immunoreactive for Cytokeratin 7 and GCDFP-15 and negative for Cytokeratin 5/6. Pathologic evaluation revealed negative margins around the site of excision medially, temporally, superiorly, and deep. At his one-week follow-up appointment, the patient had some trace swelling of the right upper eyelid with mild inflammation-induced ptosis and scabbing but reported neither changes in visual acuity nor discomfort. Six months after surgical excision with negative margins, the patient remained asymptomatic with no evidence of local recurrence.

3. Discussion

Sweat gland tumors are characterized by their locally aggressive behavior and high rate of recurrence [1]. The subset of eccrine carcinomas accounts for less than 0.01% of diagnosed cutaneous malignancies, with mucinous carcinoma being only one of the many subtypes of malignant entities [1]. Primary cutaneous mucinous carcinoma is a rare low-grade malignant neoplasm that was originally believed to be only of eccrine origin. It is now known that these tumors demonstrate apocrine-type differentiation as well, which indicates that the traditionally used term "mucinous eccrine carcinoma" is actually a misnomer [3].

PCMCs predominantly affect males and most often occur in the seventh decade of life but can be seen earlier [3]. Clinically, these are slow growing and may arise on a variety of locations, including the face (with a predominance of the eyelids), axilla, scalp, and trunk [3]. A 2014 systematic review and meta-analysis by Kamalpour et al. noted approximately 215 cases of PCMC reported in the literature, with 79 (36.7%) of these involving the eyelid/canthus/brow area [3]. Per Rismiller et al. in their 2019 population-based data analysis, there were 411 cases of PCMC reported in the National Cancer Institute's Surveillance, Epidemiology, and End Results (SEER) database from 1972 to 2013, with 159 (38.7%) of these involving the eyelid as the primary site [4].

The histopathological features of primary cutaneous mucinous carcinoma include the presence of nests and strands of epithelial cells imbedded in abundant pools of mucin, separated from each other by thin fibrous septa. Positivity for markers such as GCDFP-15 and human milk fat globulin supports an apocrine lineage, which debunked previous schools of thought [5]. Due to the rarity of these lesions, they are difficult to diagnose and are clinically confused with other lesions such as basal cell carcinoma, epidermoid cysts, Kaposi sarcoma, neuromas, lacrimal sac tumors, squamous cell carcinoma, granulomatous tumors [6], sebaceous gland carcinoma, Merkel cell carcinoma, and metastatic adenocarcinoma. In order to differentiate PCMC from metastasis of mucinous carcinoma, a thorough clinical and imaging assessment must be completed; however, some features that may suggest a primary cutaneous origin include location on head/neck region and presence of an in situ component. A proposed precursor to PCMC is endocrine mucin-producing sweat gland carcinoma (EMPSGC), which is differentiated from PCMC by demonstrating little mucin deposition extracellularly [5].

With regard to the eyelid specifically, a large retrospective study completed by Kersten et al. assessed the accuracy of clinical diagnoses of cutaneous eyelid lesions and concluded that malignant eyelid lesions can masquerade as a number of different clinically benign conditions. Such conditions include melanocytic nevus, hidrocystoma, chalazion, molluscum contagiosum, amyloidosis, capillary hemangioma, cavernous hemangioma, syringoma, telangiectasia, xanthelasma, dermal fibrosis, trichoepithelioma, sebaceous hyperplasia, sebaceous adenoma, sarcoid, pyogenic granuloma, papilloma, seborrheic keratoses, verrucae, fibroepithelial polyp, and the aforementioned epidermoid cyst. This study established that histologic

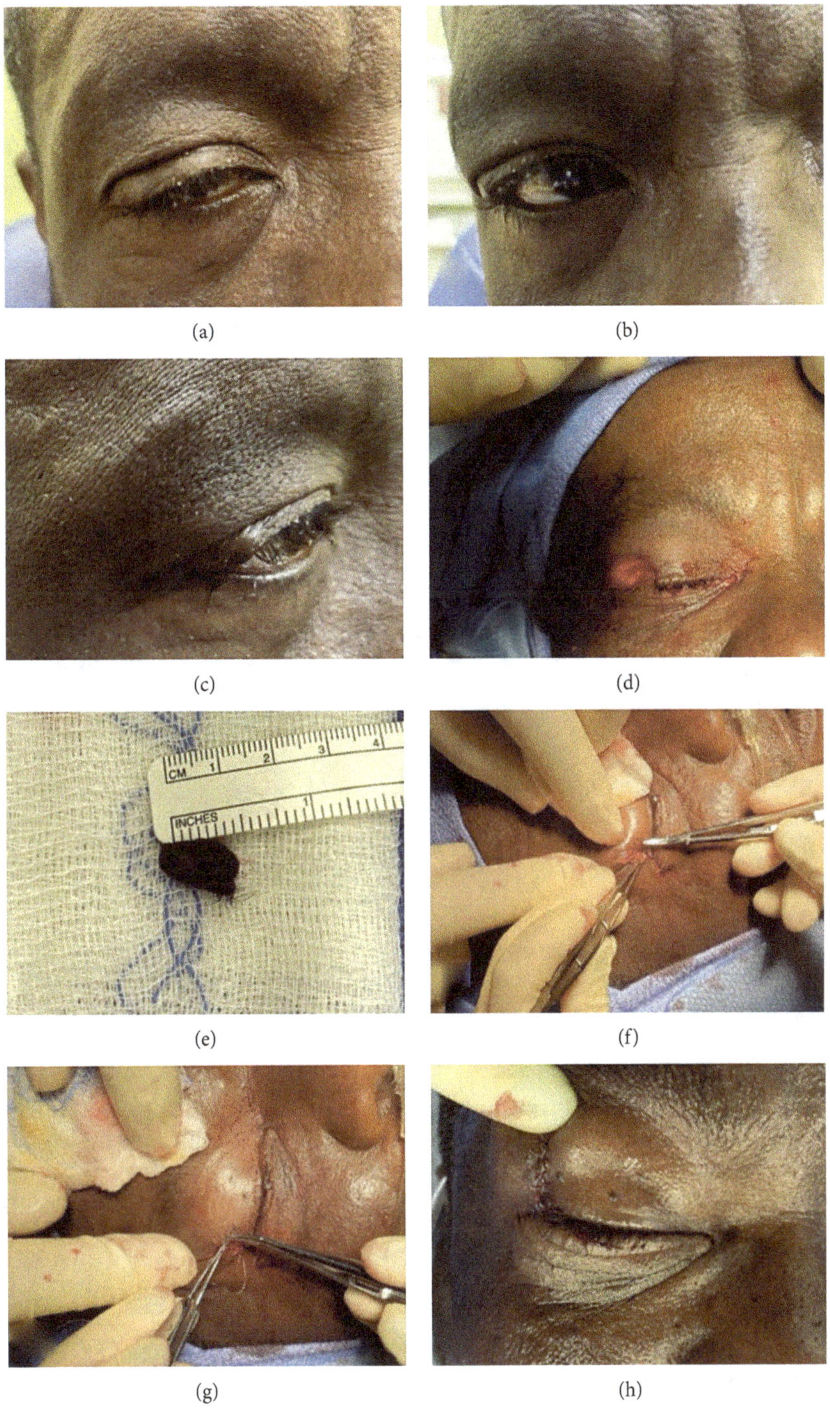

FIGURE 1: Preoperative, perioperative, and postoperative images: (a–c) preoperative photographs of patient's right upper eyelid lesion; (d) site of surgical excision postremoval of visible tumor (e) and margins; (f, g) reconstruction of excisional site including performing undermining of the two sides of the excisional site creating a sliding flap; (h) repaired site of surgical excision immediately postoperation.

confirmation is essential, because it is not possible to obtain complete accuracy in diagnosing eyelid lesions on clinical grounds alone. Repeat biopsy was recommended if the initial histopathologic evaluation did not agree with the malignant clinical diagnosis [7].

The majority of patients seem to have only local disease [4], and morbidity of PCMC is associated with incomplete resection [8, 9]. This statement is further supported by this case, in which initially, the tumor extended to the deep resection margin of the original excisional biopsy. Unfortunately, because the patient was opposed to further surgery at the time, this was most likely the nidus for the recurrence of the lesion. Tumor size over 1.5 cm is associated with increased risk of regional disease, but eyelid tumors are more likely to present with distant disease compared to other locations on the head and neck [4]. Even though the age-adjusted

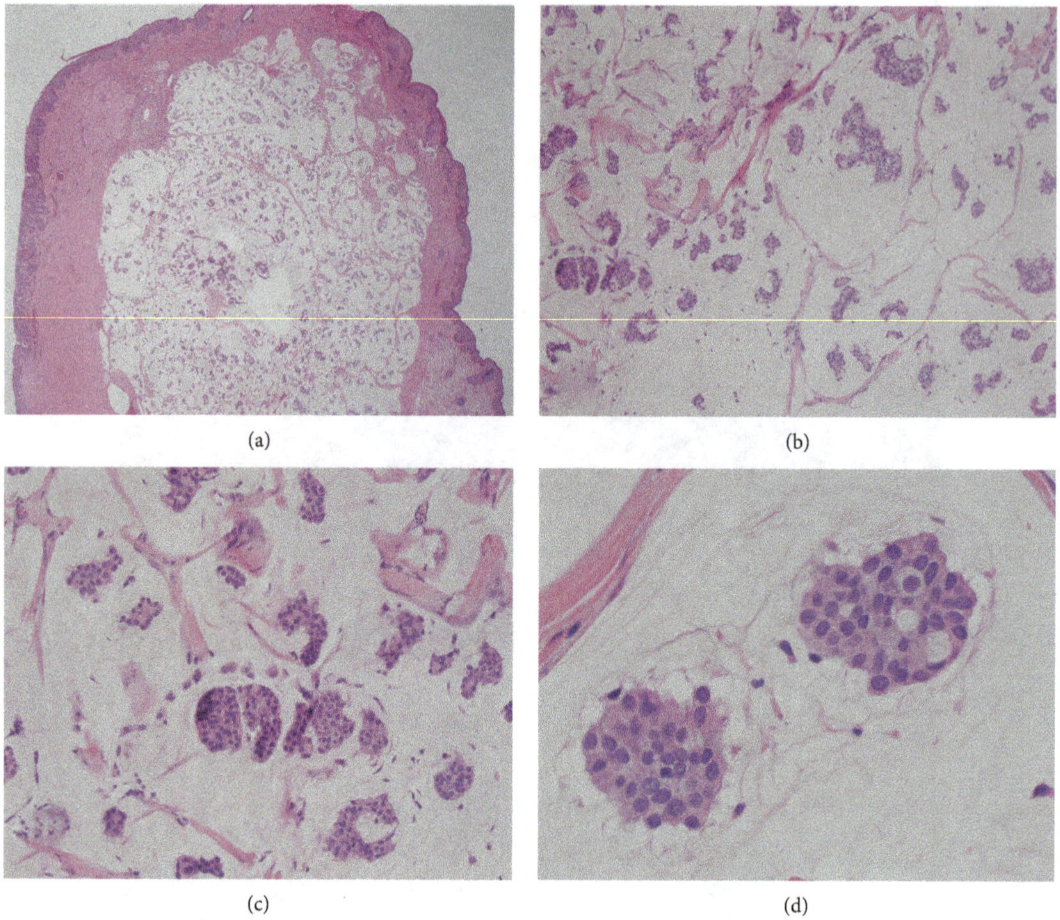

FIGURE 2: Histologic examination of the surgical specimen. Histology slide analysis was consistent with cutaneous mucinous carcinoma, including large pools of basophilic mucin with islands of relatively bland epithelioid cells with abundant cytoplasm. The cells were arranged in nests and duct/glandular-like patterns and could be seen floating within the mucin. Mitotic figures were rare. (a) 2x, (b) 10x, (c) 40x, and (d) 60x.

incidence of PCMC is 2.4-fold higher in blacks than Caucasians, PCMC-specific mortality is independent of many factors such as sex, age, race, primary site, histologic tumor grade, tumor size, tumor stage, or treatment [4].

As previously acknowledged, there is currently no standard of care for the surgical treatment of cutaneous mucinous carcinoma. Specific descriptions of local excisions, especially regarding margins in particular, have not been well-described in the literature. The SEER database analysis described wide excision versus nonwide excision as ≥1.0 cm and <1.0 cm, respectively [4]. Some sources have recommended wider margins of at least 10 mm for procedures without intraoperative frozen section control, but no studies have confirmed this as a standard margin that prevents recurrence. Location of the lesion and impact on function must also be taken into account, as taking such large margins in the periorbital area can add significant morbidity and be cosmetically disfiguring. Complications of upper eyelid repair may include and are not limited to notching, trichiasis, conjunctivalization, entropion, retraction, ptosis, and ectropion [10].

Eyelid tumors of this kind are less likely to undergo wide local excision and are more frequently treated with Mohs micrographic surgery [4], most likely due to the aforementioned potential complications. Intervention with Mohs surgery or excision with frozen section control usually reports better outcomes with only 7% recurrence rate [11]. There is a 30-40% recurrence rate with surgical removal without intraoperative evaluations of surgical margins [11]. However, the type of surgery used does not correlate with survival [4]. Long-term follow-up is essential due to the recurrent nature of PCMC, with the SEER database analysis reporting an average follow-up length of 88.2 months [4].

4. Conclusion

In the age of combination antiretroviral therapy, patients with HIV have a decreased incidence of AIDS-defining cancers; however, the same cannot be said about melanoma and nonmelanoma skin cancers [12]. Non-AIDS-defining cancers are usually treated according to the standard of care [13]. In this patient with a non-AIDS-defining cancer, the first reported in the literature with PCMC, the lack of a standard of care regarding management of this lesion is evident. Due to the rarity of PCMC, there have been no randomized control trial studies to directly compare the effects of wide local excision with or without frozen section control versus Mohs surgery on recurrence rates, nor to determine a definite desired clear margin length. In this case, a modified wide local excision, in the context of involvement of the lid margin and lateral canthus, was performed with adequate safety margins of at least 5 mm resulting in the preservation of function and avoidance of postsurgical morbidity. In this patient with a relatively small tumor, who had previously deferred Mohs surgery, modified wide local excision was a viable alternative which achieved clear margins and prevented recurrence up to six months after excision. Due to the favorable margins obtained in this case, there is hopeful resolution of this recurrent primary cutaneous mucinous carcinoma of the eyelid; however, long-term follow-up will be necessary.

Authors' Contributions

S.T. was responsible for conceptualization, data analysis, writing, editing, and revising the manuscript. S.I. was responsible for conceptualization, editing, and revising the manuscript. E.G. was responsible for editing and revising the manuscript. J.L. was responsible for conceptualization, editing, and revising the manuscript.

Acknowledgments

The authors acknowledge Jena Auerbach, DO, dermatopathologist at University of Florida, Gainesville, for courteously providing pathology slides (Figure 2). This study was funded by an unrestricted grant from Research to Prevent Blindness.

References

[1] H. Kaseb and H. M. Babiker, *Cancer, an overview of eccrine carcinoma*, StatPearls, 2020, https://www.ncbi.nlm.nih.gov/books/NBK541042/.

[2] K. K. Gowda, P. Agarwal, and A. Bal, "Mucinous eccrine carcinoma of the eyelid: re-emphasizing the need for awareness of rare lesions," *Dermatology Reports*, vol. 6, no. 1, p. 5498, 2014.

[3] L. Kamalpour, R. T. Brindise, M. Nodzenski, D. Q. Bach, E. Veledar, and M. Alam, "Primary cutaneous mucinous carcinoma: a systematic review and meta-analysis of outcomes after surgery," *JAMA Dermatology*, vol. 150, no. 4, pp. 380–384, 2014.

[4] K. P. Rismiller, D. R. Crowe, and T. J. Knackstedt, "Prognostic factors, treatment, and survival in primary cutaneous mucinous carcinoma: a SEER database analysis," *Dermatologic Surgery*, vol. 46, no. 9, pp. 1141–1147, 2020.

[5] J. C. Cardoso and E. Calonje, "Malignant sweat gland tumours: an update," *Histopathology*, vol. 67, no. 5, pp. 589–606, 2015.

[6] G. Marrazzo, R. B. Thorpe, and W. H. Black, "Primary mucinous carcinoma of the eyelid treated with Mohs micrographic surgery," *Cutis*, vol. 100, no. 5, pp. E7–E10, 2017.

[7] R. C. Kersten, D. Ewing-Chow, D. R. Kulwin, and M. Gallon, "Accuracy of clinical diagnosis of cutaneous eyelid lesions," *Ophthalmology*, vol. 104, no. 3, pp. 479–484, 1997.

[8] J. D. Wright and R. L. Font, "Mucinous sweat gland adenocarcinoma of eyelid: a clinicopathologic study of 21 cases with histochemical and electron microscopic observations," *Cancer*, vol. 44, no. 5, pp. 1757–1768, 1979.

[9] S. N. Snow and G. T. Reizner, "Mucinous eccrine carcinoma of the eyelid," *Cancer*, vol. 70, no. 8, pp. 2099–2104, 1992.

[10] B. A. O'Donnell and G. E. Mannor, "Oculoplastic surgery for upper eyelid reconstruction after cutaneous carcinoma," *International Ophthalmology Clinics*, vol. 49, no. 4, pp. 157–172, 2009.

[11] J. A. Papalas and A. D. Proia, "Primary mucinous carcinoma of the eyelid: a clinicopathologic and immunohistochemical study of 4 cases and an update on recurrence rates," *Archives of Ophthalmology*, vol. 128, no. 9, pp. 1160–1165, 2010.

[12] A. Latini, L. Alei, F. Magri, L. Eibenschutz, and C. Cota, "Non-melanoma skin cancer and melanoma in HIV-1-infected patients," *AIDS*, vol. 34, no. 10, pp. 1570–1572, 2020.

[13] R. Yarchoan and T. S. Uldrick, "HIV-associated cancers and related diseases," *The New England Journal of Medicine*, vol. 378, no. 11, pp. 1029–1041, 2018.

26

TAG (Tube and Graft) Sandwich Technique: A Novel Single-Stage Scleral Reinforcement and Aqueous Drainage Tube Implantation

Faisal Ahmed[1,2] **and Nada G. Mohamed**[3,4]

[1]*The Western Eye Hospital, Imperial College Healthcare NHS Trust, 153-173 Marylebone Rd, London, UK*
[2]*The Imperial College Ophthalmic Research Group (ICORG), Imperial College London, 153-173 Marylebone Rd, London, UK*
[3]*The Ophthalmology Department, Faculty of Medicine, Alexandria University, Champollion Street, Alexandria, Egypt*
[4]*Whipps Cross Hospital, Barts Health NHS Trust, Whipps Cross Rd, Leytonstone, London, UK*

Correspondence should be addressed to Faisal Ahmed; faisal.ahmed5@nhs.net

Academic Editor: Hsin Yi Chen

Purpose. Refractory glaucoma patients continue to require surgical intervention in the form of trabeculectomy surgery or glaucoma drainage device (GDD). Those patients that require a GDD but have thin sclera or scleromalacia present a challenge. *Methods*. In this article, we present a novel "TAG sandwich" single surgical procedure in which thinned sclera is reinforced with a pericardial patch graft ("bottom layer of the sandwich") allowing safe implantation of the GDD ("the tube sandwich filling") and then placing another patch graft on top of the tube part of the GDD ("top layer of the sandwich"). The surgery was performed on an open-angle glaucoma patient with a generalized thin sclera and uncontrolled intraocular pressure despite maximal topical medication and oral acetazolamide. *Results*. Reinforcing a compromised sclera with a pericardium patch graft allowed the safe implantation of a glaucoma drainage device. The patient's intraocular pressure was safely controlled at 7 mmHg almost 1-year postsurgery without intraocular pressure-lowering drops. *Conclusions*. This scleral strengthening procedure can be considered by readers in other ocular surgeries where there is a risk of scleral perforation, as well as part of a combined surgery where refractory glaucoma patients with thin sclera require scleral reinforcement to allow for safer implantation of a glaucoma drainage device.

1. Introduction

Glaucoma drainage devices (GDD) are increasingly utilized with a survey in the US reporting an increase from 7,788 in 2003 to 12,021 in 2012 (1). GDDs are used in patients with advanced refractory glaucoma (2, 3). In cases with thin sclera or anterior staphyloma, trabeculectomy surgery can be difficult with possible scleral melting; perforated flaps, and surgical failure (4). In these cases, implantation of a glaucoma drainage device (GDD) can be considered (2, 3). However, this does come with additional risk in patients who have pre-existing thin sclera.

The senior surgeon FA had already described a 2-stage scleral reinforcement with GDD implant, with the thin sclera reinforced in the first operation, and 1 month later, a GDD was implanted (5).

This short article describes a novel TAG sandwich technique to strengthen scleral thinning and implant glaucoma drainage device in a single-staged operation. Pericardial tutoplast (Innovative Ophthalmic Products, Costa Mesa, California, USA) was used for scleral reinforcement of thin sclera ("bottom layer of sandwich") followed by implantation of a GDD on top of the scleral reinforcement ("middle tube layer of sandwich") followed by gluing of another pericardial Tutoplast^{Tm} graft on top of the tube ("top layer of sandwich"), in a complex case of refractory primary open-angle glaucoma with generalized thin sclera.

2. Case Report

Our patient was a 29-year-old lady with Ehler-Danlos syndrome, with uncontrolled advanced open-angle glaucoma.

She had previously lost vision in the right eye after an unsuccessful retinal detachment repair. Her only seeing left eye had thinned blue sclera which was considered to be an ocular manifestation of Ehler-Danlos syndrome (6).

Other ocular features that were present in our case included bilateral microcornea, which was reported with Ehler-Danlos type VI but to a lesser extent than Keratoglobus (7). The patient also has pathological myopia which is also seen in Ehler-Danlos patients (8).

Despite maximum medical therapy, and attempted micropulse cyclophotocoagulation (to avoid intraocular surgery), her intraocular pressure remained uncontrolled. Her IOP maintained at 26 mmHg on full topical intraocular pressure-lowering drops, in addition to oral: acetazolamide 250 mg three times a day, and unfortunately, the patient was symptomatic with deteriorating visual fields and vision.

The patient's axial length in this eye was 29.84 mm, and horizontal corneal diameter as shown by white-to-white measurement was 9.83 mm. Her visual acuity preoperatively was 6/36, with a refraction of -11.75 sphere and -1.00 cylinder axis 95 degrees. Her central corneal thickness was 443 microns (thin cornea), and she had grade 4 on Van Herick and AC depth of 3.04 mm as evident from her biometry.

Other Ehler-Danlos-related systemic manifestations in our patient included mitral valve prolapse, which reduced her ASA (American Society of Anesthesiologists classification) rating. The decision was made to implant a glaucoma drainage device. However, scleral reinforcement was required as generalized blue sclera made tube implant challenging.

Although the senior author FA had already described a two-step procedure of scleral reinforcement with pericardial Tutoplast^{Tm} surgery initially with glaucoma tube implant as a second procedure 1 month later, this would have meant 2 anesthetics and delay in IOP control (5). Therefore, it was decided to perform a one surgery scleral strengthening and tube surgery—using the "TAG sandwich technique" under general anesthetic.

The first part of the procedure consisted of a superior peritomy, a 7/0 silk corneal traction suture was used to enhance visualization, and care on taking the suture was made to allow enough depth and not too much traction to avoid cheese wiring of the suture. Reinforcement of the existing thin sclera ("bottom layer of sandwich") from the limbus with a double layer of pericardial Tutoplast^{Tm} was then performed, and the Tutoplast^{Tm} was glued onto the sclera with Tisseel fibrin sealant (Baxter AG, Vienna, Austria). The sclera under the plate was also reinforced by gluing a single layer of pericardial Tutoplast^{Tm} to it as a precaution. The second part of the procedure was to place a (nonvalved) Baerveldt^{R} BG 101-250 (Abbot Medical Optics, Santa Ana, California, USA) GDD over the Tutoplast^{Tm} ("middle tube layer of sandwich"), and the plate was then sutured successfully to an area of sclera that did not show thinning on visualization using 9/0 Prolene suture on a spatulated needle. This was to ensure the plate was secured in place and minimize its movement. The tube was fixed to the Tutoplast^{Tm} to avoid perforating the sclera as the rest of the anterior sclera showed bluish discoloration and thinning. The GDD lumen was occluded via a 3/0 Supramid suture to avoid postoperative hypotony, and the tube was inserted into the anterior chamber through a superotemporal limbal tunneled incision. The free end of the Supramid suture was then tucked to the inferior fornix. Another double layer of pericardial Tutoplast^{Tm} was glued over the tube, and the conjunctiva was placed over the graft ("top layer of patch graft tube sandwich"). Conjunctival closure was achieved via suturing and gluing at the limbus only (Figure 1).

Postoperatively, the intraocular pressure was controlled by full topical intraocular pressure-lowering drops, in addition to systemic acetazolamide, until the Supramid suture was removed 6 weeks after the original surgery to allow for the formation of the fibrous capsule around the tube to avoid hypotony. This was performed by instilling topical anesthesia, making a small conjunctival incision with Westcott scissors at the free edge of the Supramid suture which was placed in the inferior bulbar conjunctiva. Once the free end of the Supramid was exposed, the whole suture was held with Moorfield forceps and pulled out. The patient has completed 11 months of follow-up, her intraocular pressure is controlled at 7 mmHg on no intraocular pressure-lowering medications, her pinhole vision was 6/36 in that eye before posterior subcapsular cataract started to develop, for which the patient underwent a cataract surgery about a year after her tube surgery, and her current best corrected vision is 6/24.

3. Discussion

Donor materials including pericardial Tutoplast™ have been used to cover the tube part of glaucoma drainage devices to prevent tube exposure and are performed by most tube surgeons routinely (9).

In this refractory glaucoma patient with thinned sclera who required a glaucoma drainage device to control her intraocular pressure, it was important to strengthen the sclera below the GDD to reduce the risk of scleral perforation.

Other possible solutions previously described for refractory glaucoma patients with thin sclera include strengthening the sclera with other materials such as fascia lata, (10) but in our patient, this would have required another surgical step to obtain fascia lata from the thigh with another surgical wound and longer anesthetic time in an already high risk patient. The use of endocyclophotocoagulation to reduce inflow was described by Rodrigues et al. in a case of scleromalacia and thus avoid the need for more challenging filtration surgery (11). However, we had already performed a micropulse diode laser which had made no impact on IOP control, and a second ciliary body modulating procedure including endocyclophotocoagulation was deemed to have minimal benefit and in our patient especially as they were a high risk phakic patient with abnormal ocular anatomy who had an axial length that was almost 30 mm and a microcornea.

Another solution to avoid the need for scleral reinforcement is to find areas of more normal sclera and thus change the usual supertemporal site of GDD implantation; however, inferior placed tubes carry increased risk of exposure, which may increase the risk of endophthalmitis (12). In particular, our patient had generalized scleral thinning, and there was no advantage to position the GDD elsewhere as scleral reinforcement was required wherever we had placed the GDD.

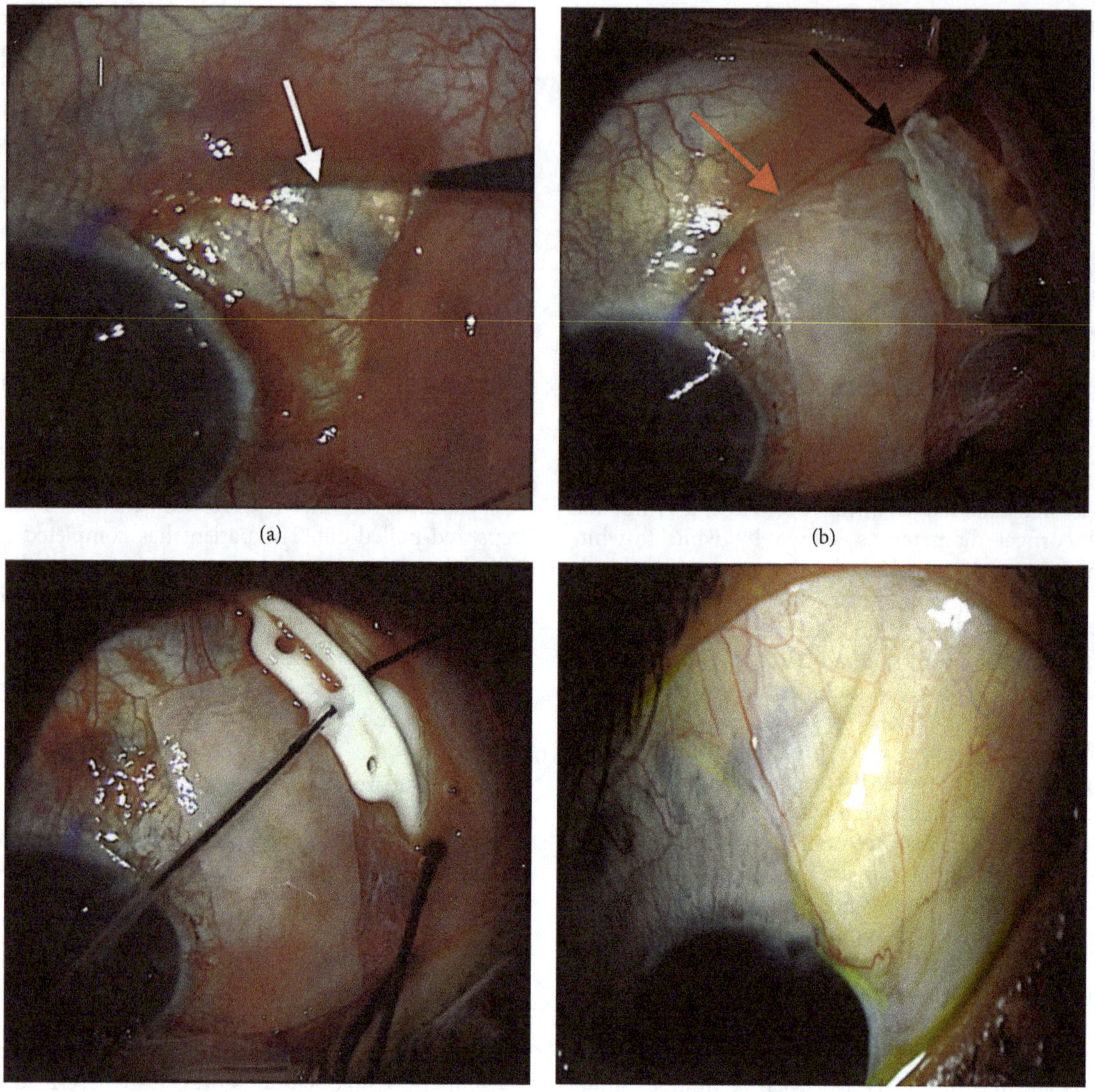

FIGURE 1: (a) shows scleral thinning evident after conjunctival dissection (white arrow). (b) shows Tutoplast^{Tm} in place covering the bed of the plate (black arrow) and the tube (red arrow). (c) shows the plate and the tube in place over the Tutoplast^{Tm}. (d) shows postoperative slit-lamp picture of the tube in place with over lying Tutoplast^{Tm}.

Our combined "TAG sandwich" technique allowed most of the suturing to be into the Tutoplast^{Tm} avoiding suturing directly into the sclera, ensuring safe plate fixation (13). A two-staged procedure was described earlier by the senior author FA in cases with scleral thinning, to achieve scleral strengthening (5).This novel combined procedure has the advantage of minimizing the number of procedures required under general anesthetic and implanting the GDD immediately for more timely intraocular pressure control.

4. Conclusion

We believe our combined "TAG sandwich" technique provides another option in high-risk refractory glaucoma patients with thin sclera or scleromalacia who require filtration surgery. This procedure allowed a safe and effective outcome for our young refractory glaucoma patient with generalized scleral thinning in one surgery, avoiding complications associated with multiple surgeries as well as systemic risks.

Consent

Patient's written consent was obtained for using photos, and case details in publication, and teaching.

References

[1] K. S. Arora, A. L. Robin, K. J. Corcoran, S. L. Corcoran, and P. Y. Ramulu, "Use of various glaucoma surgeries and procedures in Medicare beneficiaries from 1994 to 2012," *Ophthalmology*, vol. 122, no. 8, pp. 1615–1624, 2015.

[2] G. Marchini, P. Ceruti, G. Vizzari et al., "Long-term outcomes of a modified technique using the Baerveldt glaucoma implant for the treatment of refractory glaucoma," *Journal of Glaucoma*, vol. 25, no. 12, pp. 952–958, 2016.

[3] S. J. Gedde, J. C. Schiffman, W. J. Feuer et al., "Treatment outcomes in the tube versus trabeculectomy (TVT) study after five years of follow-up," *American journal of ophthalmology*, vol. 153, no. 5, pp. 789–803.e2, 2012.

[4] I. Coutinho, D. Silva, M. Mota, M. Lisboa, F. Trancoso Vaz, and I. Prieto, "Reconstruction of delayed scleral flap melting with bovine pericardium after trabeculectomy with mitomycin C," *GMS ophthalmology cases*, vol. 7, 2017.

[5] M. Bhalla, S. Luk, R. Jolly, and F. Ahmed, "Two-stage aqueous drainage tube implant with pericardial graft patch," *Eye*, vol. 33, no. 9, pp. 1509–1516, 2019.

[6] R. J. Wenstrup, S. Murad, and S. R. Pinnell, "Ehlers-Danlos syndrome type VI: clinical manifestations of collagen lysyl hydroxylase deficiency," *The Journal of pediatrics*, vol. 115, no. 3, pp. 405–409, 1989.

[7] J. A. Cameron, "Corneal abnormalities in Ehlers-Danlos syndrome type VI," *Cornea*, vol. 12, no. 1, pp. 54–59, 1993.

[8] M. Gharbiya, A. Moramarco, M. Castori et al., "Ocular features in joint hypermobility syndrome/Ehlers-Danlos syndrome hypermobility type: a clinical and in vivo confocal microscopy study," *American Journal of Ophthalmology*, vol. 154, no. 3, pp. 593–600.e1, 2012.

[9] T. Raviv, D. S. Greenfield, J. M. Liebmann, P. A. Sidoti, H. Ishikawa, and R. Ritch, "Pericardial patch grafts in glaucoma implant surgery," *Journal of Glaucoma*, vol. 7, no. 1, pp. 27–32, 1998.

[10] S. Egrilmez, A. Yagci, H. Ates, S. S. Azarsiz, and K. Andac, "Glaucoma implant surgery with autogenous fascia lata in scleromalacia perforans," *Ophthalmic Surgery, Lasers and Imaging Retina*, vol. 35, no. 4, pp. 338–342, 2004.

[11] I. As Rodrigues, D. Lindfield, M. R Stanford, and S. Goyal, "Glaucoma surgery in scleromalacia: using endoscopic cyclophotocoagulation where conventional filtration surgery or angle procedures are contraindicated," *Journal of current glaucoma practice*, vol. 11, no. 2, pp. 73–75, 2017.

[12] H. J. Kwon, N. M. Kerr, J. B. Ruddle, and G. S. Ang, "Endophthalmitis associated with glaucoma shunt intraluminal stent exposure," *Journal of current glaucoma practice*, vol. 10, no. 1, pp. 36-37, 2016.

[13] E. S. Novitskaya, L. Clifford, and A. J. Vivian, "Tutoplast pericardium patch graft for scleral thinning following strabismus surgery," *Eye*, vol. 27, no. 5, pp. 682-683, 2013.

27

Multifacet of Cornea Patch Graft in Anterior Segment Diseases

Prema Chendran, Yong Meng Hsien, and Wan Haslina Wan Abdul Halim

Department of Ophthalmology, University Kebangsaan Malaysia Medical Centre (UKMMC), Jalan Yaacob Latif, 56 000 Bandar Tun Razak, Kuala Lumpur, Malaysia

Correspondence should be addressed to Wan Haslina Wan Abdul Halim; afifiyad@yahoo.co.uk

Academic Editor: Sandra M. Johnson

Incidence of cornea melting or perforation is commonly seen in variety of cornea conditions. It can cause debilitating vision loss and impair patient's daily activity. Several techniques have been described to surgically treat cornea perforation and melting. In this article, a series of corneal diseases treated with corneal patch graft are highlighted to relate different approach of cornea patch graft surgery. Post-operative management and complications are discussed.

1. Introduction

Cornea patch graft has been advocated as the surgical procedure to treat variety of anterior segment pathologies. It involves patching the affected area with full thickness or partial thickness corneal donor tissue. The aim is to restore globe integrity and prevent further inflammation that could lead to devastating complications such as endophthalmitis. Cornea perforation and melting can occur in infectious keratitis, autoimmune diseases such as rheumatoid arthritis, ocular trauma and ocular surface disorder.

Patch graft materials are derived from cornea, sclera, pericardium and dura mater [1]. Scleral patch graft is commonly used in anterior segment pathologies because it is relatively cost effective and easy to preserve. However due to its avascular property it is often associated with progressive tissue necrosis or melting [2]. Pericardial graft is used as patch graft in glaucoma drainage devise (GDD) exposure prevention. It is commercially available, no need to be dependent on eye bank for its availability and has high sterility but has tendency to develop graft thinning and subsequent exposure of the GDD [3] besides being expensive.

Cornea patch graft has been indicated in cases of corneal perforation, cornea thinning [4], scleral thinning or as prophylaxis to prevent the exposure of GDD [1]. The advantages of cornea patch graft compared to others is that: it is translucent, less chances of graft melting and conjunctiva retraction [1]. It can provide good tectonic support for the ocular wall as the tissue has good strength and rigidity [1]. This case series of corneal diseases treated with corneal patch graft in UKMMC is presented. The author discuss about the post-operative management that was tailored individually to each patient.

2. Case History

2.1. Case 1. A 32-year-old gentleman, presented to eye casualty with sudden onset left eye redness and discomfort. He had history of foreign body entering into his left eye while hammering 1 week prior to that. Examination revealed deeply seated rust ring on the anterior cornea stroma. Failure to remove the rust ring completely resulted in corneal ulceration 1 week later. Topical antibiotics and lubricants were initiated. However, he started to develop cornea thinning. Despite being treated with intensive antibiotics and lubricants, the cornea thinning progressed to cornea perforation with flat anterior chamber (AC) (Figure 1(a)). He underwent series of nonsurgical (cornea glue, bandage contact lens (BCL) application) and surgical (AC reformation and cornea patch graft) intervention. He was able to regain his vision to 6/9 with presence of stable cornea patch graft during last review (Figure 1(b)).

2.2. Case 2. A 38-year-old gentleman with underlying diabetes mellitus (DM) type I, hypertension, end stage renal failure (ESRF), right eye pseudophakia presented with right eye blurring of vision associated with photophobia and watery eye for 1 month. Examination revealed right eye vision of 6/60

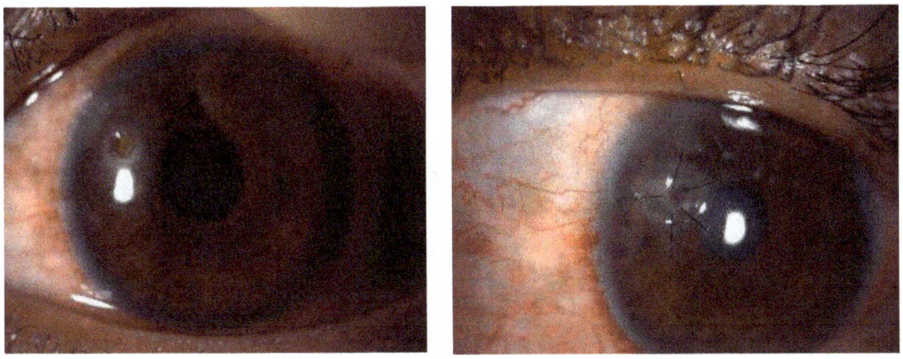

(a) (b)

FIGURE 1: (a) Presence of stromal ring infiltrate with central cornea perforation and shallow anterior chamber. (b) Cornea patch graft applied. Post-surgery 4 months.

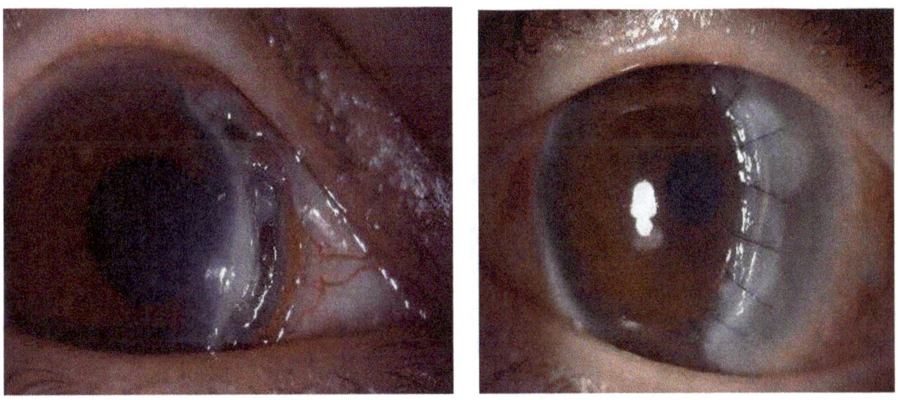

(a) (b)

FIGURE 2: (a) Peripheral cornea thinning from12 to 5 o'clock. (b) Post banana shaped corneal patch graft.

pinhole 6/36. He had a furrow cornea thinning from 12 to 5 o'clock with overhanging edge where there's only Descemet remaining. There's adjacent cornea epithelial defect but no cornea perforation seen (Figure 2(a)).

Systemic examination and blood investigations were normal. He was diagnosed having Mooren's ulcer. Topical corticosteroid and antibiotic, systemic immunosuppressant and collagenase inhibitor were commenced. He underwent conjunctival resection and cryotherapy twice and amniotic membrane patch graft once before a banana shaped corneal lamellar patch graft was performed (Figure 2(b)). His vision post operatively at 4 months improved to 6/18 pinhole 6/12. Post operatively he developed secondary open angle glaucoma secondary to chronic steroid usage and required topical anti-glaucoma.

2.3. Case 3. A 46-year-old Malay gentleman, without any comorbid, presented with progressively worsening left eye vision associated with pain and redness for 1 year duration. Symptoms started to appear 6 months post pterygium excision. His left eye vision on hand motion only. On examination, there was a crescent shape peripheral corneal thinning from 4 to 1 o'clock. The remaining cornea with its overhanging edge remains oedematous. Examination of fellow eye was normal.

He was investigated for underlying autoimmune or related diseases. A diagnosis of Mooren's ulcer were made and he was started on systemic and topical immunosuppression therapy. Despite this treatment, 3 months later, his eyes showed disease progression where there was continuous cornea melting to almost 360 degree (Figure 3(a)) for which he underwent conjunctival resection. However, the cornea keratolysis worsened and he was subjected to tectonic keratoplasty (cornea scleral patch graft) (Figure 3(b)). His cornea showed signs of activity stabilization 4 months post operatively.

2.4. Case 4. A 42-year old gentleman with underlying DM, hypertension with history of Steven Johnson Syndrome (SJS) 10 years ago presented with left progressive blurring of vision with occasional eye redness and discomfort. He had history of bilateral myopic laser refractory surgery done 3 years prior to this.

Examination revealed right eye vision 6/24 and left eye counting finger. Both eyes showed presence of extensive peripheral cornea thinning. Peripheral edge of left cornea had slow leak but with deep anterior chamber (Figure 4(a)). Other examinations were unremarkable.

Series of investigation were taken to rule out autoimmune related diseases. He was diagnosed as Mooren's ulcer. He was started on systemic immunosuppressant, collagenase inhibitor

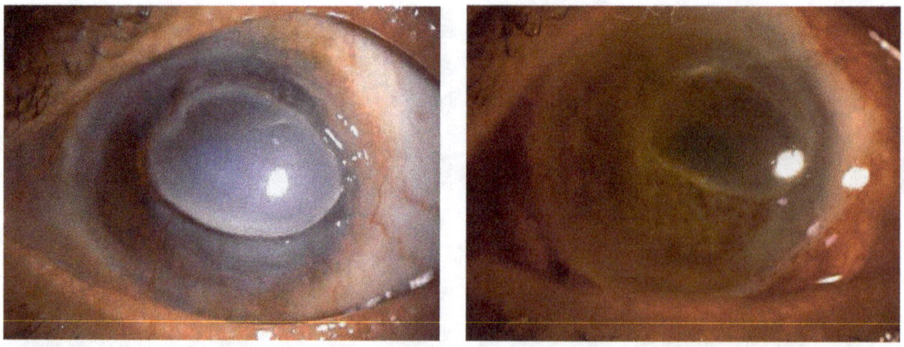

(a) (b)

FIGURE 3: (a) Showing progression of cornea melt to 360 degrees. (b) Whole cornea patch graft.

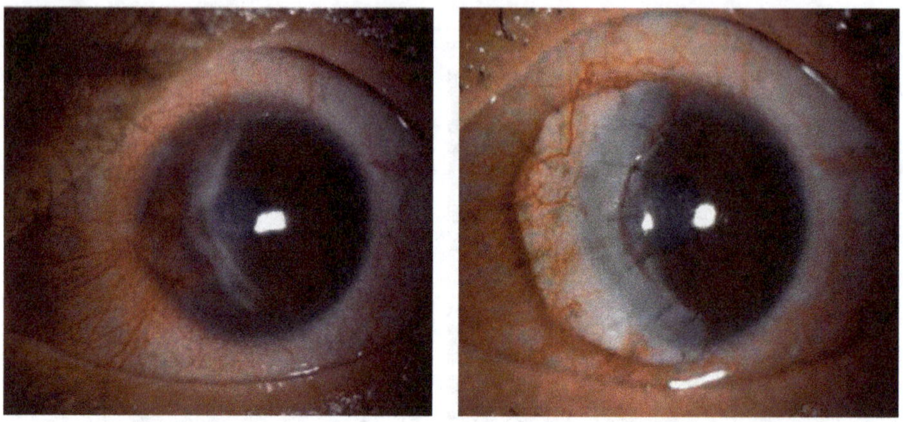

(a) (b)

FIGURE 4: (a) Peripheral cornea melting on left eye. (b) Post banana shaped corneal patch graft on left eye.

and topical corticosteroid and antibiotic. He was scheduled for left eye cornea banana-shaped patch graft (Figure 4(b)). Post operatively his vision improved to 6/18 at 3 months and it remains stable without any recurrence.

2.5. Case 5. A 32-year-old Myanmar lady, complained of right eye discomfort with recurrent eye redness for the past 2 years. The eye redness usually resolve temporarily with over the counter eye drop. She noticed the presence of bluish discoloration at the right nasal conjunctiva for the past 1 year which was increasing in size. Her vision on both eyes were 6/6. She had history of trauma to right eye during childhood.

Right eye examination showed two locations of scleral thinning with visible uveal tissue at inferonasal quadrant with adjacent cornea scarring (Figure 5(a)). Other ocular examination were normal. Her infectious and autoimmune disease screening were negative. She was given topical lubricants and topical antiglaucoma (prophylaxis).

She underwent cornea patch graft for the scleral thinning (Figure 5(b)). Post-operatively she was prescribed with topical antibiotic, topical and systemic corticosteroid. Two weeks post-operatively, her graft was melting, oral corticosteroid was stepped up, topical steroid and lubricants were continued and she was under close observation for every 2 weeks. Subsequently, no further melting was noted after 5 months post-operative period (Figure 5(c)).

2.6. Case 6. A 15-year-old boy with congenital right eye temporal limbal dermoid (Figure 6(a)) was seen in eye clinic. This child has been on regular follow up with refraction. He had amblyopia on right eye. The presence of limbal dermoid on his right eye didn't cross his visual axis.

He underwent excision of the limbal dermoid and corneal patch graft surgery (Figure 6(b)). Post-operatively, the graft looked stable. However his refraction noted to have high astigmatism for which he is being followed up.

3. Discussion

Cornea melting is a sequelae of progressive keratolytic process. Untreated cases can lead to cornea perforation. Application of corneal patch graft is another way to address this issue. Corneal patch graft use when the cornea defect is too large until the application of cyanoacrylate tissue adhesive is not recommended (perforation of >1 mm) [5] or when there is cyanoacrylate tissue adhesive application failure [5]. This technique will allow the perseverance of globe integrity, stabilize the eye while waiting for the systemic immunosuppressant effect to take place, clearance of necrotic stroma, which is a source of collagenase and shields the bare stroma from the tears neutrophil [5].

In this series, the decision for patch graft was made due to many reasons. The author attempted corneal patch graft

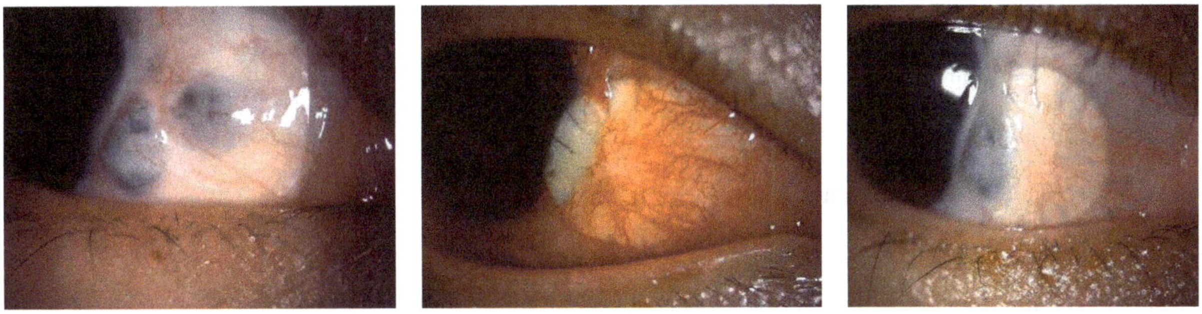

(a) (b) (c)

FIGURE 5: (a) Presence 2 area of scleral thinning at inferonasal quadrant. (b) Immediate post-operative scleral patch graft extending up to inferonasal limbal area. (c) Post-operative 5 months once the scleral melting has stabilized.

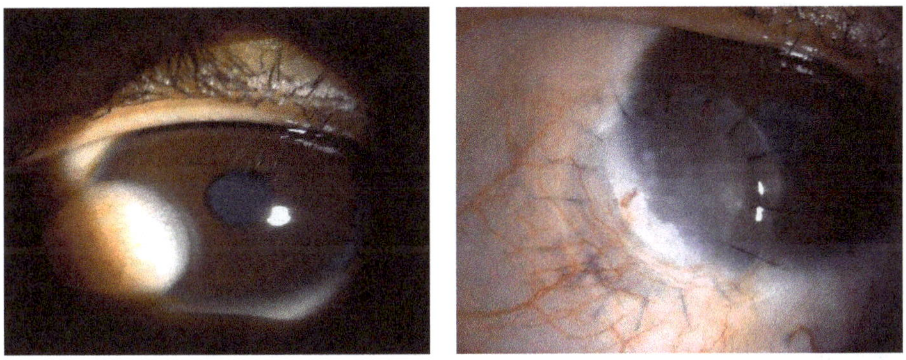

(a) (b)

FIGURE 6: (a) Presence of left eye inferonasal limbal dermoid. (b) Post limbal dermoid removal and corneoscleral graft, 2 weeks post operatively.

as patients were not responding to pharmacological management.

Small cornea perforation as in case 1, was initially managed with cyanoacrylate glue, however, this method was not fruitful in this case. Application of corneal patch graft helped to seal off the perforation and maintained the anterior chamber. Post-operatively this patient had persistent epithelial defect because of uneven surface. This results in unequal distribution of tear film which can result in persistent epithelial defect. The patient underwent graft re-suturing twice before he responded well. A round trephined corneal patch graft was used in this patient had minimal effect on visual axis [5].

Case 2, 3 and 4 involves the usage of corneal patch graft in Mooren's ulcer. Stepwise approach involving; conjunctival resection, amniotic membrane graft and corneal patch graft with concurrent systemic and topical immunosuppressant, manage to control the disease activity. Conjunctival resection is known to remove the presence of complements, immunoglobulins and inflammatory cells [6]. Two patients underwent conjunctival resection together with cornea patch grafting. These helped to halt cornea melting and protect the graft while waiting to buy time for systemic immunosuppressant to work [5]. For instance, in case 3, following corneal patch graft surgery, the patient endured conjunctiva resection for 3 times before the disease activity managed to be controlled.

Scleral thinning has been shown to respond well with corneal patch graft. As in case 5, the usage of corneal patch graft can be cosmetically acceptable as the curvature of cornea was able to cover large area of scleral bed defect [7]. Conjunctiva flap with subsequent graft opacification can limit the visibility of choroid [7]. Post op management is very crucial in any successful surgery. Tapering down oral corticosteroid too soon may impose the risk of graft melting as in this case, but as soon as the corticosteroid was stepped up, the melting has ceased and the graft remains stable.

Corneal patch graft similarly used in post limbal dermoid excision. It has proven to consume less time and labor force [8]. The cosmetic result is comparable with previous study conducted by Wu et al. Their study using similar method has shown no complication such as tissue over riding, wound dehiscence and suture related complications [8].

All patients who underwent this cornea patch graft surgery were treated with topical corticosteroid and topical antibiotic. The author advocate the usage of topical prednisolone acetate 1% and topical levofloxacin 0.5% along with adequate lubricants. Systemic corticosteroid; oral prednisolone was started peri-operatively to control the ocular inflammatory process. Apart from oral corticosteroid, systemic immunosuppressant such as oral azathioprine was given in cases where the patients were treated for Mooren's ulcer.

4. Conclusion

Corneal patch graft has evidence to improve the outcome in treating anterior segment disorders especially involving cornea and sclera. Its advantages have made it possible to produce good post-operative result; be it functionally or cosmetically.

References

[1] O. Spierer, M. Waisbourd, Y. Golan, H. Newman, and R. Rachmiel, "Partial thickness corneal tissue as patch graft material for prevention of glaucoma drainage device exposure," *BMC Opthalmology*, vol. 16, no. 1, 2016.

[2] Y. Yao and V. Jhanji, "Short term observation and management of scleral patch graft used in scleral defects," *Annals of Eye Science*, vol. 2, p. 30, 2017.

[3] T. Raviv, D. S. Greenfield, J. M. Liebmann, P. A. Sidoti, H. Ishikawa, and R. Ritch, "Pericardial patch graft in glaucoma implant surgery," *Journal of Glaucoma*, vol. 7, no. 1, pp. 27–32, 1998.

[4] G. Schaab, C. Clavell, and H. Goyal, "Corneal patch graft: a review of indication, technique and success rates. ARVO annual meeting abstract," *Investigative Ophthalmology & Visual Science*, vol. 53, no. 14, p. 6044, 2012.

[5] H. K. Soong, A. A. Farjo, D. Katz, R. F. Meyer, and A. Sugar, "Lamellar corneal patch graft in the management of cornea melting," *Cornea*, vol. 19, no. 2, pp. 126–134, 2000.

[6] I. Lal, S. B. Shivanagari, M. H. Ali, and J. Vazirani, "Efficacy of conjunctival resection with cyanoacrylate glue application in preventing recurrences of Mooren's ulcer," *British Journal of Ophthalmology*, vol. 100, no. 7, pp. 971–975, 2016.

[7] C. C. de Farias, T. de Sterlenich, L. B. Souza, L. A. Vieira, and J. A. P. Gomes, "Randomized trial comparing multilayer amniotic membrane transplantation with scleral and corneal graft for the treatment of scleral thinning after pterygium surgery associated with beta therapy," *Cornea*, vol. 33, no. 11, pp. 1197–1204, 2014.

[8] K. I. Wu, H. S. Chu, A. S. I. Pai et al., "Surgical management of limbal dermoid using anterior corneal button from descemet stripping automated endothelial keratoplasty donor tissue as patch graft," *Cornea*, vol. 36, no. 1, pp. 64–67, 2017.

28

A Novel Technique for Recurrent Tube Exposure Repair

J. Minjy Kang, Yen Cheng Hsia, and Ying Han

UCSF Department of Ophthalmology, USA

Correspondence should be addressed to Ying Han; ying.han@ucsf.edu

Academic Editor: Cristiano Giusti

Purpose. Tube exposure can lead to vision-threatening consequences and requires prompt surgical attention. Posterior repositioning of the tube to the pars plana has previously been reported as a successful technique. However, this method requires a pars plana vitrectomy (PPV). Here, we describe a novel technique of repositioning the tube into the ciliary sulcus without requiring PPV. *Methods.* This is a retrospective interventional case report of two patients who had undergone prior glaucoma drainage device implantation and prior tube exposure repair and developed recurrent tube exposure. Tube exposure in the subjects was repaired by repositioning the tube in the ciliary sulcus. *Results.* The two eyes remained exposure free postoperatively with 51- and 60-month follow-ups. *Conclusions.* Repositioning the tube to the ciliary sulcus may be an effective technique to avoid reexposure.

1. Introduction

Tube exposure after glaucoma drainage device (GDD) implantation is a postoperative complication that can occur in 1-7% of cases [1, 2]. Possible mechanisms of tube exposure include conjunctival tension over the tube, desiccation from exposure, or mechanical trauma from the eyelid. Younger age, presence of ocular inflammation prior to tube exposure, and inferior placement of the GDD are also potential risk factors [1, 3, 4]. Conflicting evidence exists for other risk factors such as race, diabetes mellitus, history of prior ocular surgery, type of patch graft, and preoperative medications [1, 5, 6]. Tube exposure may lead to endophthalmitis, and therefore, it requires prompt surgical revision [7, 8].

Several surgical techniques for tube revision have been described, most involving the reinforcement of tube coverage with various types of patch grafts (e.g., Tutoplast dura mater (Biodynamics International, Inc., Tampa, FL), sclera, pericardium, and fascia lata) [9, 10]. However, direct coverage with patch grafts may lead to recurrent tube exposure over time [10, 11]. An alternative approach to avoid such recurrence is to reposition the tube posteriorly into the pars plana (PP). This reduces the extraocular portion of the tube where it is subjected to the exposure, desiccation, and mechanical trauma from the eyelid [12–14]. However, PP placement requires concurrent pars plana vitrectomy (PPV) and may subject the patient to additional perioperative risks such as retinal tears, cataract progression, macular edema exacerbation, postoperative hypotony, or retinal detachment [15–17]. Here, we reported two cases with repeated tube exposure repaired by repositioning the tubes into the ciliary sulcus (CS) without requiring PPV with long-term success.

2. Methods

This is a retrospective, noncomparative, interventional case series that adhered to the tenets of the Declaration of Helsinki. All surgeries were performed by one of the authors (YH) at the University of California, San Francisco in 2013, with follow-up until October 2018. Patient charts were reviewed for relevant past medical history, past surgical history, operative notes, and postoperative course.

2.1. Surgical Technique. The patient is dilated in the preoperative area. A limited conjunctival peritomy is made in the area of tube exposure. Tenon's capsule is dissected away from underlying episclera. The anterior chamber (AC) is filled with an ophthalmic viscoelastic device (OVD) via a limbal

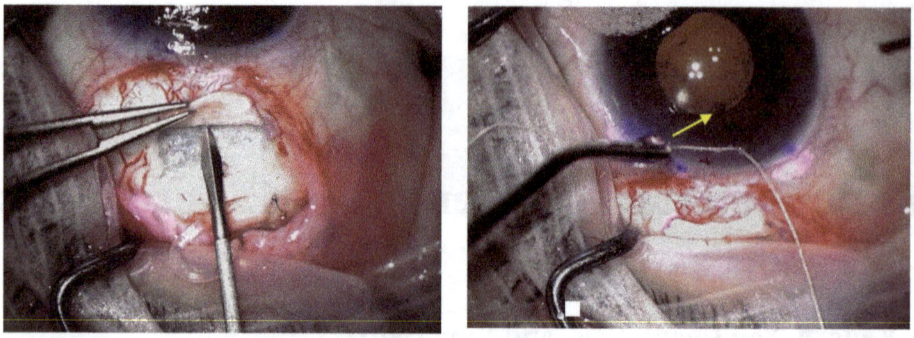

(a) (b)

Figure 1: (a) A bent 20-guage MVR blade is used to enter the sulcus at 4 mm from the limbus in the plane parallel to the iris. (b) The tube (yellow arrow) placement in the CS is confirmed by direct visualization at the pupillary border.

Table 1: Patient characteristics and outcomes.

Case	Glaucoma type	Time to exposure	Prior tube exposure repair	Preop VA	Postop VA	Pre IOP	Post IOP	Pre # drops	Post # drops	Follow-up
1	SI-OAG	39 mo	Conjunctiva oversewn	20/200	HM	15	11	4	2	60 mo
2	NVG	1 mo	K/AMG	HM	LP	17	19	0	1	51 mo

Abbreviations: SI-OAG=steroid-induced open angle glaucoma; NVG=neovascular glaucoma; Time to exposure=time from initial GDD implantation to first exposure of tube; K/AMG=corneal and amniotic membrane patch graft.

paracentesis site, and the tube is removed from the AC. The original sclerotomy site is closed with interrupted nylon sutures. OVD is injected into the CS space via the limbal paracentesis site. A bent 20-gauge MVR blade is then used to enter the CS at 4 mm from the limbus in a plane parallel to the iris (Figure 1(a)). The placement of the blade in the CS is directly visualized through the cornea, ensuring its location posterior to the iris but anterior to the intraocular lens. OVD is injected into the track using a cannula. The tube is then trimmed to a bevel-down configuration and inserted through the track. Tube placement is confirmed with direct visualization (Figure 1(b)). In cases of poor dilation, a pupil retractor can be used. A patch graft or a half-thickness scleral flap of the patient's own sclera is then used to cover the extraocular tube. Conjunctiva, or amniotic membrane in cases with inadequate conjunctiva, is secured over the patch graft.

Standard postoperative care is applied, including topical antibiotic eye drops for one week and topical steroid eye drops, such as prednisolone acetate 1%, starting at QID and tapering over four weeks.

3. Results

Case 1 was performed on a 60-year-old man with steroid-induced open-angle glaucoma (OAG), bilateral Baerveldt glaucoma devices, pseudophakia, and corneal edema, who initially developed tube exposure in the right eye following DSAEK/tube shortening (Table 1). Initial repair was performed by covering the tube with Tutoplast and conjunctiva. However, the tube was reexposed one-year postoperatively. The 2nd repair was performed by repositioning the tube to the CS as described above. At postoperative month 60, in the right eye, the tube remained well covered and intraocular pressure (IOP) was controlled with two drops. The patient developed endothelial graft failure in the right eye over time leading to loss of vision. Case 2 was a 75-year-old woman with Sjogren's syndrome, pseudophakia, neovascular glaucoma secondary to central retinal vein occlusion, and Ahmed glaucoma valve implantation. Tube erosion was initially repaired with a corneal patch graft and amniotic membrane graft. Recurrent tube exposure occurred 10 months later. The second repair was performed by repositioning the tube to the CS. At postoperative month 51 of the 2nd repair, the tube remained well covered and IOP was at goal on one drop. Case 2 maintained relatively stable vision at their last follow-up visit compared to their preoperative visit.

4. Discussion

To our knowledge, this is the first report of addressing recurrent tube exposure by repositioning the AC tube into the CS. While the number of cases is limited, the patients who have undergone tube repositioning to the CS have had excellent results with a nearly 5-year follow-up without recurrent tube exposure. This is promising given a study by Huddleston et al. reporting that 18% of the cases developed recurrent tube exposure after initial tube exposure repair (average follow-up 46.6 weeks, range 3-168 weeks) [11]. In Huddleston et al.'s study, most initial repairs used scleral patch grafts (74%) and none reported repositioning of the tube. Kalenak describes tube exposure repair with dermis graft tissue, resulting in a 13% tube reexposure rate in 30 cases (median follow-up 12 months, range 1-42 months) [10]. These reports suggest that covering the exposed tube with a patch graft may not be adequate for long-term success.

Several reasons may explain why repositioning the tube into CS prevents recurrent tube exposure. First, repositioning the tube posteriorly decreases the extraocular portion of the tube which is subject to exposure, desiccation, and repetitive mechanical trauma from the eyelid. Second, posterior positioning of the tube may help avoid a sharp angle of entry at the limbus, which can increase friction and pressure against the overlying patch graft and/or conjunctiva. Lastly, repositioning the tube posteriorly allows the tube to be covered partially by a ciliary body and by thicker tenon and conjunctiva. The combination of these factors likely contributes to the decreased rate of recurrent erosion.

These factors also likely contribute to the previously reported success in treating recurrent tube exposure by repositioning to the PP in four patients with a follow-up ranging from 2 to 42 months [13]. However, inserting a tube into the PP requires complete PPV to prevent vitreous occlusion of the tube, necessitating the added cost and time for a vitreoretinal surgeon to be present. This also increases the risk of various postoperative complications such as retinal tears or cataract progression associated with a PPV [15–17]. Our approach of inserting the tube into CS space applies a similar concept, but with a simpler approach and avoiding the additional cost and risk of complications.

Insertion of GDD tubes in the CS has been shown to be safe and effective in the past [18–21]. In fact, this technique may not only be used to treat tube exposure but may also be considered during primary implantation to avoid any future tube exposure. In a paper comparing outcomes of Ahmed GDD with tube insertion in the AC versus the CS, tube/plate exposure was reported in 2.9% in the AC group, compared to 0% in the CS group [20]. Although this difference did not reach statistical significance due to a limited sample size, it suggests a trend towards decreased exposure with posterior insertion.

In summary, we present a practical method to repair recurrent tube exposure by repositioning the tube to the CS. This method may be as effective as repositioning it to the PP, but it avoids the additional cost, operating time, and perioperative risks associated with PP tube placement.

Acknowledgments

This work was made possible in part by NIH-NEI EY002162—Core Grant for Vision Research and by the Research to Prevent Blindness Unrestricted Grant.

References

[1] P. Netland, M. Chaku, K. Ishida, and D. Rhee, "Risk factors for tube exposure as a late complication of glaucoma drainage implant surgery," *Clinical Ophthalmology*, vol. 10, pp. 547–553, 2016.

[2] D. L. Budenz, W. J. Feuer, K. Barton et al., "Postoperative complications in the Ahmed Baerveldt comparison study during five years of follow-up," *American Journal of Ophthalmology*, vol. 163, pp. 75–82.e3, 2016.

[3] J. D. Levinson, A. L. Giangiacomo, A. D. Beck et al., "Glaucoma drainage devices: risk of exposure and infection," *American Journal of Ophthalmology*, vol. 160, no. 3, pp. 516–521.e2, 2015.

[4] M. Pakravan, S. Yazdani, C. Shahabi, and M. Yaseri, "Superior versus inferior Ahmed glaucoma valve implantation," *Ophthalmology*, vol. 116, no. 2, pp. 208–213, 2009.

[5] Y. S. Byun, N. Y. Lee, and C. K. Park, "Risk factors of implant exposure outside the conjunctiva after Ahmed glaucoma valve implantation," *Japanese Journal of Ophthalmology*, vol. 53, no. 2, pp. 114–119, 2009.

[6] N. Geffen, Y. M. Buys, M. Smith et al., "Conjunctival complications related to Ahmed glaucoma valve insertion," *Journal of Glaucoma*, vol. 23, no. 2, pp. 109–114, 2014.

[7] A. A. Al-Torbak, S. Al-Shahwan, I. Al-Jadaan, A. Al-Hommadi, and D. P. Edward, "Endophthalmitis associated with the Ahmed glaucoma valve implant," *The British Journal of Ophthalmology*, vol. 89, no. 4, pp. 454–458, 2005.

[8] S. J. Gedde, I. U. Scott, H. Tabandeh et al., "Late endophthalmitis associated with glaucoma drainage implants," *Ophthalmology*, vol. 108, no. 7, pp. 1323–1327, 2001.

[9] S. Oana and J. Vila, "Tube exposure repair," *Journal of Current Glaucoma Practice*, vol. 6, no. 3, pp. 139–142, 2012.

[10] J. W. Kalenak, "Revision for exposed anterior segment tubes," *Journal of Glaucoma*, vol. 19, no. 1, pp. 5–10, 2010.

[11] S. M. Huddleston, R. M. Feldman, D. L. Budenz et al., "Aqueous shunt exposure: a retrospective review of repair outcome," *Journal of Glaucoma*, vol. 22, no. 6, pp. 433–438, 2013.

[12] D. K. Heuer, D. Budenz, and A. Coleman, "Aqueous shunt tube erosion," *Journal of Glaucoma*, vol. 10, no. 6, pp. 493–496, 2001.

[13] K. M. Joos, A. M. Lavina, K. A. Tawansy, and A. Agarwal, "Posterior repositioning of glaucoma implants for anterior segment complications," *Ophthalmology*, vol. 108, no. 2, pp. 279–284, 2001.

[14] T. Puustjarvi, S. Ronkko, and M. Terasvirta, "A novel oculoplastic surgery for exposed glaucoma drainage shunt by using autologous graft," *Graefe"s archive for clinical and experimental ophthalmology = Albrecht von Graefes Archiv fur klinische und experimentelle Ophthalmologie*, vol. 245, no. 6, pp. 907–909, 2007.

[15] O. P. Gupta, E. D. Weichel, C. D. Regillo et al., "Postoperative complications associated with 25-gauge pars plana vitrectomy," *Ophthalmic Surgery, Lasers & Imaging*, vol. 38, no. 4, pp. 270–275, 2007.

[16] O. P. Gupta, A. C. Ho, P. K. Kaiser et al., "Short-term outcomes of 23-gauge pars plana vitrectomy," *American Journal of Ophthalmology*, vol. 146, no. 2, pp. 193–197.e1, 2008.

[17] K. Yoneda, K. Morikawa, Y. Oshima, S. Kinoshita, and C. Sotozono, "Surgical outcomes of 27-gauge vitrectomy for a consecutive series of 163 eyes with various vitreous diseases," *Retina*, vol. 37, no. 11, pp. 2130–2137, 2017.

[18] J. A. Alvarado, D. A. Hollander, R. P. Juster, and L. C. Lee, "Ahmed valve implantation with adjunctive mitomycin C and 5-fluorouracil: long-term outcomes," *American Journal of Ophthalmology*, vol. 146, no. 2, pp. 276–284, 2008.

[19] Y. Eslami, M. Mohammadi, G. Fakhraie, R. Zarei, and S. Moghimi, "Ahmed glaucoma valve implantation with tube

insertion through the ciliary sulcus in pseudophakic/aphakic eyes," *Journal of Glaucoma*, vol. 23, no. 2, pp. 115–118, 2014.

[20] A. Bayer and M. Onol, "Clinical outcomes of Ahmed glaucoma valve in anterior chamber versus ciliary sulcus," *Eye*, vol. 31, no. 4, pp. 608–614, 2017.

[21] T. S. Prata, A. Mehta, C. G. De Moraes, C. Tello, J. Liebmann, and R. Ritch, "Baerveldt glaucoma implant in the ciliary sulcus: midterm follow-up," *Journal of Glaucoma*, vol. 19, no. 1, pp. 15–18, 2010.

Improvements in Optical Characteristics after Excision of an Overhanging Bleb Developed following Trabeculectomy

Yu Mizuno,[1] Atsushi Hirota,[2] Kazuyuki Hirooka,[1] and Yoshiaki Kiuchi[1]

[1]*Department of Ophthalmology and Visual Science, Hiroshima University, 1-2-3 Kasumi Minamiku, Hiroshima 734-8551, Japan*
[2]*Hirota Eye Clinic, 1-25-1 Shinmachi Shyunanshi, Yamaguchi 745-0017, Japan*

Correspondence should be addressed to Yu Mizuno; ymizuno@hiroshima-u.ac.jp

Academic Editor: Tetsuya Kawakita

Introduction. To examine the corneal total higher-order aberrations before and after the excision of an overhanging bleb that developed following trabeculectomy. *Case Presentation.* Two patients who developed overhanging blebs following trabeculectomy with a fornix-based conjunctival flap using mitomycin C (MMC) were assessed. We measured the corneal total higher-order aberrations for a 4 mm pupil diameter using the TOPCON KR-1W wavefront analyzer and the visual acuity before and after bleb excision. The corneal total higher-order aberration (HOA) improved from 0.50 μm to 0.38 μm in case 1 and from 0.59 μm to 0.49 μm in case 2 after bleb excision. The intraocular pressure was identical before and after bleb excision in both cases. No significant changes in the best-corrected visual acuity (BCVA) were noted in case 1; however, BCVA was improved from 20/25 to 20/20 in case 2. Both cases showed improvements in the symptoms of dysesthesia. *Conclusion.* Excision of the overhanging bleb developed following trabeculectomy may have beneficial possibility in some cases where corneal total HOA is affected and reduces the symptoms of dysesthesia.

1. Introduction

Glaucoma is an optic neuropathy characterized by gradual progressive morphological changes in the optic disc that leads to visual field loss [1]. Trabeculectomy is an effective surgery that is performed for lowering the intraocular pressure (IOP) in patients with glaucoma to hinder the progression of visual field loss. However, following this surgery, patients occasionally complain of foreign body sensation, poor cosmetic appearance, and reduction in vision. Several studies have shown that trabeculectomy results in changes in the corneal keratometry, astigmatism, and topography, which lead to change in vision [2, 3]. In such patients, some have overhanging blebs (OHBs), which are defined as oversized filtering blebs that cover part of the cornea. Recently, advances in ocular aberrometry have revealed that ocular surgeries increase ocular and corneal higher-order aberrations (HOAs). Here, we report cases of two patients who developed OHB following trabeculectomy using mitomycin C (MMC). We examined the optical characteristics before and after excision of OHBs by a wavefront analyzer, which can objectively simulate the retinal image of Landolt C using its simulation system for the first time.

2. Higher-Order Aberration Measurement and Surgical Procedures

The corneal total higher-order aberrations for a 4 mm pupil diameter without dilating pupil were measured before and after bleb excision to examine the effects of the excision of the OHB using the TOPCON KR-1W wavefront analyzer (Topcon Corporation, Tokyo, Japan). The wavefront aberrometer was a device for measuring the wavefront aberrations of the eye; the retinal image of Landolt C was objectively simulated using its simulation system. The retinal image resulted from the convolution of the paraxial image and the point-spread function [4]. It could also be calculated by considering only the effect of the anterior cornea. The surgical technique of OHB excision was followed. The overhanging portion of the bleb was removed from the cornea by excising it immediately anterior to the limbus using scissors. Following the dissection, a conjunctival incision was made

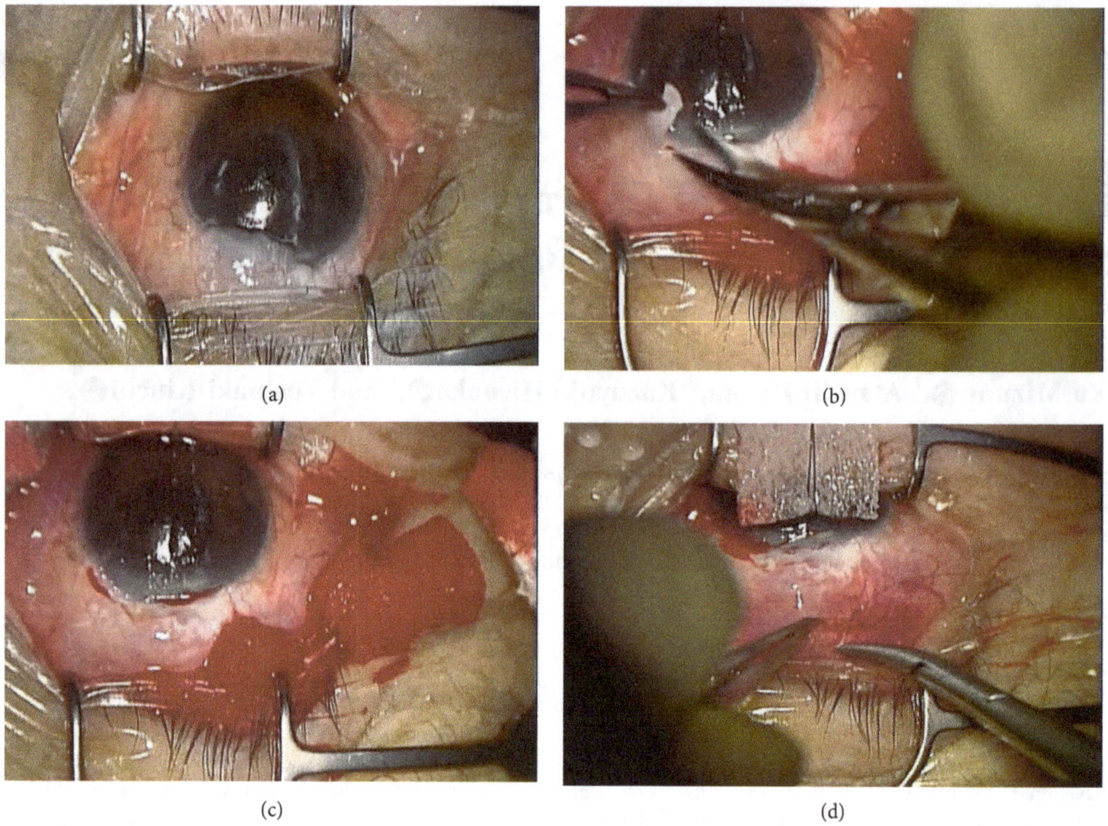

Figure 1: Intraoperative photographs of the excision of the overhanging bleb (OHB). The yellow arrows are the range of the OHB. The OHB is avascular and thin walled (a). A portion of the OHB, which is easy to remove from the cornea, is excised immediately anterior to the limbus using scissors (b). Several sponges soaked in 0.04% MMC solution are applied for 5 min in the scleral surgical site (c). The incision were sutured using a 10-0 nylon suture (d).

7–8 mm posterior to the limbus. An elongated crescent knife was inserted into the conjunctival edge to peel the strong adhesion in order to allow the aqueous humor drain to the fornix side of the eye, preventing the recurrence of OHB. Subsequently, though there was possibility to become avascular bleb, we inserted several sponges soaked in 0.04% MMC solution for 5 min application on the scleral surgical site to prevent strong fibrosis of the conjunctiva and sclera. This area was then washed with 100 ml of balanced salt solution. Thereafter, the incision was sutured with a 10-0 nylon suture (Figure 1).

3. Case Presentation

3.1. Case 1. A 56-year-old man presented with visual disturbances, discomfort, and poor cosmetics in his left eye. He has been undergoing treatment for primary open-angle glaucoma (POAG) when he was 32 years old. Before visiting our hospital, he had undergone trabeculectomy for the first time when he was 45 years old and underwent second surgery of trabeculectomy at age 46 in his left eye using a fornix-based conjunctival flap with MMC. A slit-lamp examination of the left eye revealed a large OHB; the anterior chamber has a normal depth and the lens status was IOL (intraocular lens) (Figure 2(a)). Fundus examination revealed the cup disc ratio of 1.0 in the left eye. The best-corrected visual acuity (BCVA) was 20/125 in the right eye and 20/60 in the left eye. IOP was 11 mmHg in the right eye and 9 mmHg in the left eye without the use of antiglaucoma drugs. We resected the OHB in his left eye. There was a slight leakage around the fornix margin of the excision, but it stopped naturally on postoperative day 5 (Figure 2(c)). At 2 months after the operation, the residual bleb was diffused, there was no leakage, the BCVA was similar to that before the excision, and the IOP of the left eye remained at around 10 mmHg. The corneal total HOAs improved from 0.50 μm to 0.38 μm. Simulated retinal images of Landolt C based on corneal wavefront data had improved clearly with reduced total corneal HOAs. The symptom of constant foreign body sensation was also reduced, and improvement of poor cosmetic was also seen (Figures 2(b) and 2(c)).

3.2. Case 2. A 79-year-old woman presented with discomfort, poor cosmetics, and reduced vision in her right eye. She has been undergoing treatment for POAG since she was 59 years old. She had undergone trabeculectomy using a fornix-based conjunctival flap with 0.04% MMC for the first time when she was 60 years old in the right eye. However, IOP was increased gradually and she underwent second surgery of trabeculectomy at age 61, a third at age 75, and a fourth at age 77.

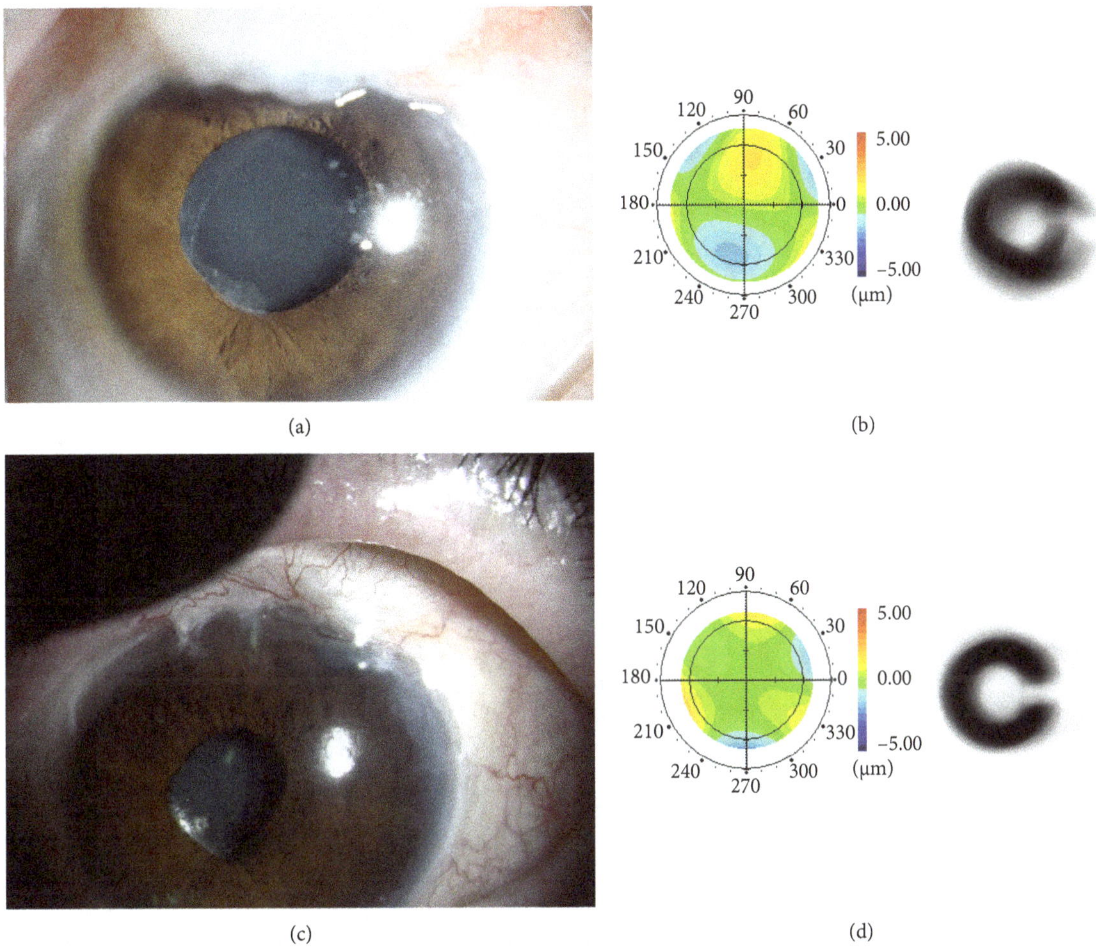

FIGURE 2: Slit-lamp examination of the OHB in case 1 (a). Excision of the OHB (c). Corneal total higher-order aberrations before (b) and after bleb excision (d) with the simulated retinal images of Landolt C from corneal total higher-order aberrations on the right side.

A slit-lamp examination of the right eye revealed an OHB; the anterior chamber has a normal depth and the lens status was IOL (intraocular lens) (Figure 3(a)). Fundus examination revealed the cup disc ratio of 1.0 in the right eye. The BCVA was 20/25 in the right eye, and she could discern the hand motion with her left eye. The IOP, without the use of antiglaucoma drugs, was 12 mmHg and 16 mmHg in the right eye and left eye, respectively. The patient underwent OHB excision in the right eye. No leakage was observed around the margin of the excision following the operation (Figure 3(c)). At 4 months after the operation, the residual bleb was diffused without any leakage and the right eye showed good IOP (10 mmHg). The corneal total HOAs improved from 0.59 μm to 0.49 μm; coma aberrations and spherical aberration also improved from 0.21 μm to 0.12 μm and from 0.19 μm to 0.05 μm, respectively. Simulated retinal images of Landolt C based on corneal wavefront data had clearly improved with reduced total corneal HOAs (Figures 3(b) and 3(d)). The BCVA was improved from 20/25 to 20/20 at 1 year after bleb excision. The symptoms of constant foreign body sensation and poor cosmetics were also reduced. Written informed consent was obtained from both patients to publish these findings and images.

4. Discussion

OHBs are a late complication following glaucoma filtration surgery, and the incidence of these blebs appears to be increasing with the use of antimetabolites [5]. Antimetabolites aid the antiproliferation of fibroblast cells, thereby preventing excessive postoperative scarring and enhancing the growth of the large bleb [6]. The mechanism underlying the formation of OHBs is complex. Several factors, such as the action of gravity on the OHB, the action of the eyelid, scar hyperplasia, and excessive aqueous overfiltration, may together contribute to the formation of OHBs. Following trabeculectomy, patients sometimes complain of a change not only in vision but also of dysesthesia and poor cosmesis. For patients with OHBs, treatment for extensive bleb migration onto the corneal surface requires surgical excision for long-term improvement in vision and symptoms. However, bleb leak that required suture repair may occur for the surgical excision [7]. The mechanism that results in the change of vision has yet not been fully understood. Recent advances in wavefront analysis have shown that ocular surgeries, such as trabeculectomy, corneal transplantation, and pterygium surgery, increase ocular and corneal HOAs, which affect the

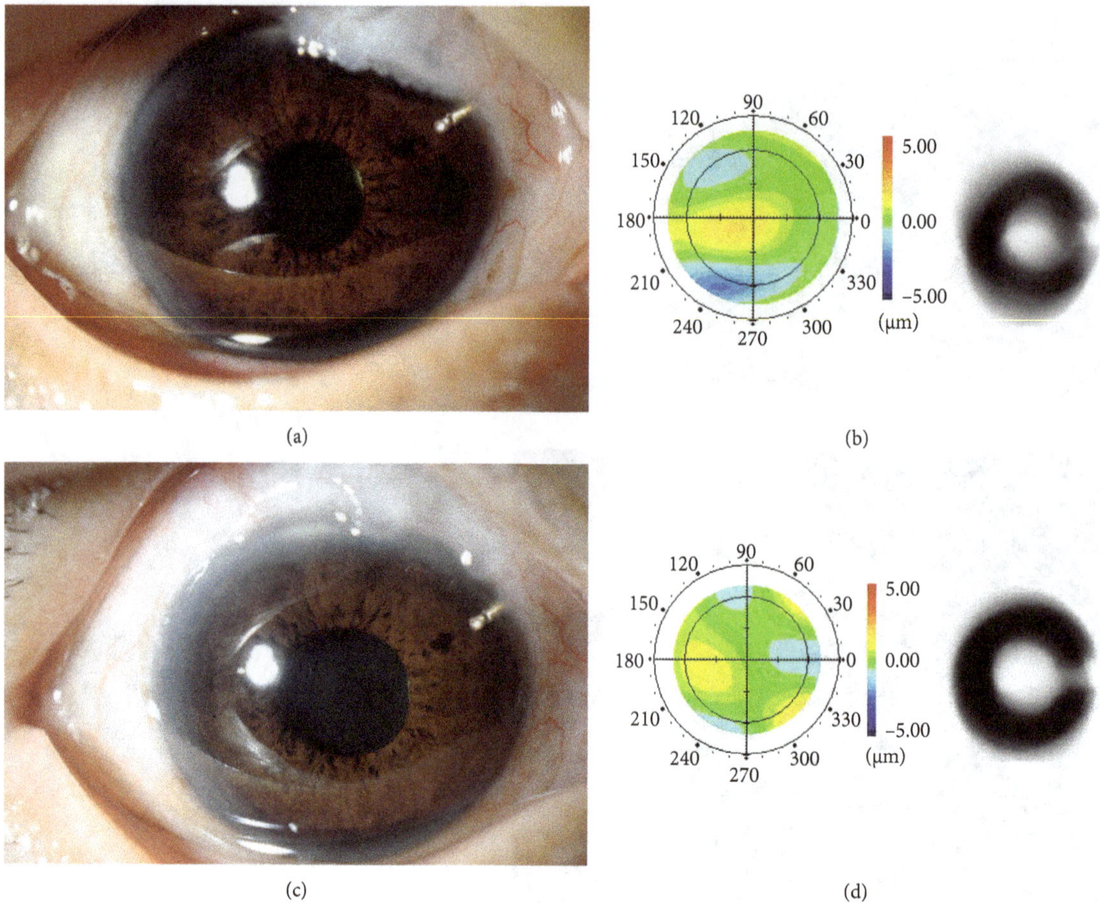

FIGURE 3: Slit-lamp examination of the OHB before (a) and after bleb excision (c) in case 2. Corneal total higher-order aberrations before (b) and after bleb excision (d) with the simulated retinal images of Landolt C from corneal total higher-order aberrations on the right side.

postsurgical visual function [3, 8, 9]. These are the first cases wherein OHB excision objectively improved comfort, poor cosmetics, and visual function by the wavefront aberrations without causing any significant change in IOP. Improvement in the corneal HOAs and the disappearance of the bleb on the cornea supported their subjective symptoms. BCVA did not improve in case 1 following the operation probably because of severe glaucoma and scotoma near the fixation points. Further clinical research by collecting data on OHB removal, wavefront analyzer, and visual outcome is needed to produce a definitive answer in the future. Our results should be compared with the results of data on those without OHB removal, so further research by collecting those data was also needed.

5. Conclusion

In conclusion, OHB excision may have beneficial possibility in some cases where corneal total HOAs are affected. Improvement of corneal total HOAs results in better quality of vision.

Authors' Contributions

All the authors contributed significantly to this report, and all authors agree to be accountable for all aspects of the work. All authors read and approved the final manuscript.

References

[1] H. A. Quigley, E. M. Addicks, W. R. Green, and A. E. Maumenee, "Optic nerve damage in human glaucoma," *Archives of Ophthalmology*, vol. 99, no. 4, pp. 635–649, 1981.

[2] K. G. Claridge, J. K. Galbraith, V. Karmel, and A. K. Bates, "The effect of trabeculectomy on refraction, keratometry and corneal topography," *Eye*, vol. 9, no. 3, pp. 292–298, 1995.

[3] S. Fukuoka, S. Amano, N. Honda, T. Mimura, T. Usui, and M. Araie, "Effect of trabeculectomy on ocular and corneal higher order aberrations," *Japanese Journal of Ophthalmology*, vol. 55, no. 5, pp. 460–466, 2011.

[4] S. Perches, M. V. Collados, and J. Ares, "Retinal image simulation of subjective refraction techniques," *PLoS One*, vol. 11, no. 3, article e0150204, 2016.

[5] H. G. Scheie and J. J. Guehl III, "Surgical management of overhanging blebs after filtering procedures," *Archives of Ophthalmology*, vol. 97, no. 2, pp. 325-326, 1979.

[6] P. B. Ou-Yang, X. Qi, and X. C. Duan, "Histopathology and treatment of a huge overhanging filtering bleb," *BMC Ophthalmology*, vol. 16, p. 175, 2016.

[7] S. Anis, R. Ritch, W. Shihadeh, and J. Liebmann, "Sutureless revision of overhanging filtering blebs," *Archives of Ophthalmology*, vol. 124, no. 9, pp. 1317–1320, 2006.

[8] K. Pesudovs and D. J. Coster, "Penetrating keratoplasty for keratoconus: the nexus between corneal wavefront aberrations and visual performance," *Journal of Refractive Surgery*, vol. 22, no. 9, pp. 926–931, 2006.

[9] K. Pesudovs and F. C. Figueiredo, "Corneal first surface wavefront aberrations before and after pterygium surgery," *Journal of Refractive Surgery*, vol. 22, no. 9, pp. 921–925, 2006.

30

Cyclodialysis Clefts following Microinvasive Glaucoma Surgery with Consecutive Intraocular Pressure Spikes

Ahmed Alshaikhsalama and Niraj Nathan

Department of Ophthalmology, UT Southwestern Medical Center, Dallas, TX, USA

Correspondence should be addressed to Niraj Nathan; niraj.nathan@utsouthwestern.edu

Academic Editor: Hsin Yi Chen

The purpose of this study is to report a case of cyclodialysis clefts associated with microinvasive glaucoma surgery (MIGS) having two distinct consecutive IOP spikes during cleft closure. A 65-year-old female with a history of primary open angle glaucoma was evaluated for right eye blurry vision since cataract surgery 11 months prior. She reported a MIGS procedure that resulted in a cyclodialysis cleft, with resultant hypotony without resolution. On gonioscopy, two clock hours of widened angle were noted nasally, with small clefts (0.5 clock hour) inferonasally and superonasally. Conservative therapy with cycloplegia was unsuccessful. Argon laser photocoagulation was performed for cleft closure. Initially, while there was visible improvement in the cleft size, it did not close completely, and IOP remained low. Additional laser was performed, one week following, she presented with an acute IOP increase to 55 mmHg. On gonioscopy, it was noted that despite the IOP spike indicating inferonasal closure, the superonasal cleft remained small but open. She was started on IOP-lowering therapy. Her IOP normalized shortly thereafter. Two weeks later, she experienced another acute IOP spike to 54 mmHg. On gonioscopy, the residual cleft had closed. Again, her IOP normalized shortly after and has remained normal since. While IOP spikes after cyclodialysis cleft closure have been reported many times, two consecutive IOP spikes of similar magnitude during sequential closure of two concurrent cyclodialysis clefts have not been reported in the literature. This case raises interesting questions about the physiology underlying an acute increase in IOP following cleft closure.

1. Introduction

Cyclodialysis is rare and usually presents after blunt trauma or as a complication from surgery and can cause a decrease in intraocular pressure < 5 mmHg [1]. It can be diagnosed via gonioscopy (gold standard) as well as anterior segment OCT and ultrasound biomicroscopy (UBM) [2]. In many cases, a cyclodialysis cleft (CDC) can resolve spontaneously or with conservative therapy; however, laser and surgical intervention can be performed for cases that fail conservative management [3]. Once the cyclodialysis cleft resolves, a spike in IOP (often as high as 70 mmHg) often occurs [4]. The reasons for this increase in IOP following cleft closure are unclear, but multiple mechanisms have been hypothesized. It could be due to a compensatory upregulation of ciliary body function to counteract the increased uveoscleral outflow caused by the cleft; it could also be due to disrupted drainage function through the trabecular meshwork and Schlemm's canal due to collapse or fibrosis while outflow is preferentially through the cleft [4]. With both mechanisms, the thought is that with sudden closure of the cleft, these compensatory changes take time to normalize, with the result being elevated intraocular pressure until they do. In this case report, we present a patient with two discrete cyclodialysis clefts in one eye that closed at separate times despite simultaneous treatment, resulting in two separate IOP spikes of equal magnitude. This course of two discrete consecutive IOP spikes of similar magnitude has not been previously reported and raises interesting questions about the mechanism of IOP increase after cyclodialysis cleft closure.

2. Material Summary

This case report examines a patient with a cyclodialysis cleft following microinvasive glaucoma surgery that caused a repeated IOP spike. The cyclodialysis cleft was monitored with gonioscopy. Following partial cleft closure, the IOP peaked to 55 mmHg. After a 2-week period of controlled IOP and therapy, an equal IOP elevation was observed, which coincided with complete cleft closure on gonioscopy. Thus, it is hypothesized that the increase in IOP could be a reaction to cleft closure beyond compensatory mechanisms.

3. Case Report/Case Presentation

A 65-year-old female with a history of primary open angle glaucoma was evaluated for right eye blurry vision since cataract surgery 11 months prior. She reported a microinvasive glaucoma procedure (MIGS) was attempted at the time and resulted in a cyclodialysis cleft, with resultant hypotony that had not resolved since. Prior to her procedure, she had a history of primary open angle glaucoma, mild in the right eye, and moderate in the left eye with maximum IOP in the 20s, per her recollection. She was on latanoprost at bedtime and dorzolamide-timolol twice daily in both eyes. Since the procedure in the right eye, her IOP remained in the 4 to 6 mm Hg range, even after the cessation of her IOP lowering drops in that eye. The fellow eye underwent cataract surgery without a MIGS procedure in the interval prior to presentation, complicated by elevated IOP following, so brimonidine twice daily was added to the left eye.

On gonioscopy, two clock hours of widened angle were noted nasally, with small cyclodialysis clefts (approximately 0.5 clock hour) on each side of the widened area, inferonasally and superonasally. On exam, she was noted to have uncorrected visual acuity of 20/50-2 with a manifest refraction of plano $+2.25 \times 090$, suggesting her toric was IOL 90 degrees malrotated, which was eventually confirmed by keratometry. She had an IOP of 4 mmHg in the affected eye and 19 mmHg in the fellow eye. She was noted to have 0.5+ anterior chamber cell. Mild choroidal folds were noted on exam and OCT (shown in Figure 1). Best corrected visual acuity was 20/25 + 2, suggesting that most of her blur was related to her malrotated toric lens, but she noted subjectively that even with the correction it seemed blurry still. Still, it was felt most prudent that the hypotony should be addressed prior to attempting intraocular surgery to rotate her toric IOL.

Given her anterior chamber inflammation, a trial of topical steroids and cycloplegia was performed, first with lotemax four times daily then with prednisolone, given her history of significant steroid response, along with atropine twice daily. After 3 months of attempted conservative therapy, her IOP remained low at 4 mmHg with continued choroidal folds on OCT. The decision was made to attempt argon laser photocoagulation to close the cleft with continuation of cycloplegia. Laser therapy (800-830 milliwatts, 500 millisecond duration, 200-micron spot size, 38 total spots) was performed with laser applied to visible cleft openings and surrounding sclera and iris to close the clefts. Two weeks post laser therapy, on gonioscopy, the clefts appeared smaller but not closed, and IOP remained low at 4 mmHg, so a second session of laser was performed (900 milliwatts, 500 millisecond duration, 200-micron spot size, and 50 total spots).

One week later, the patient began experiencing pain above the right eyebrow; her IOP was 26 mmHg, which was notable since this was the first time her IOP was above 6 mmHg in over a year. She was started on dorzolamide-timolol twice daily. The next day, the patient presented to the ER in the night with increased ocular pain, vomiting, and cloudy vision with an IOP of 55 mmHg. She was advised to add latanoprost at bedtime, brimonidine three times daily, and oral Diamox 500 mg twice daily. She was seen the following day with IOP down to 14 mmHg. On gonioscopy, her clefts were mostly closed but one small portion of the superonasal cleft was still visibly not closed. Diamox was held, but topical therapy with latanoprost, brimonidine, and dorzolamide-timolol was continued to be safe. On follow up a week later, her IOP was 7 mmHg. Only brimonidine was stopped, to reduce the risk of IOP increase, and she continued on latanoprost at bedtime and dorzolamide-timolol twice daily.

Two weeks later, the patient abruptly developed right eye pain, cloudy vision, and nausea with an IOP of 54 mmHg. An anterior chamber paracentesis was performed that reduced the pressure down to 14 mmHg; topical brimonidine and oral Diamox were added again. On gonioscopy, the superonasal cleft was now noted to be completely closed. At subsequent follow up visits, the patient's IOP remained stable around 20 mmHg on latanoprost, dorzolamide-timolol, and brimonidine. The choroidal folds on exam resolved and did not recur. Numerical hypotony did not recur as well. She subsequently underwent rotation of her toric IOL and then YAG capsulotomy, with subsequent improvent in her incorrect visual acuity from 20/60-2 to 20/20-1. She was eventually able to be tapered off brimonidine, with IOP 14-15 mmHg in each eye.

4. Discussion

CDC is a rare consequence of trauma and/or surgery. It involves a separation between the ciliary muscle and the scleral spur enabling aqueous humor to flow into the suprachoroidal space resulting in ocular hypotension. Persistent hypotony can lead to permanent vision loss, and so it is important to be corrected [3, 5]. Once the CDC closes, a spike in IOP is frequently observed [4]. Although transient, an increase in IOP can cause eye pain, retinal vascular occlusion, ischemic ocular neuropathy, and glaucoma progression [6].

Our case presents as an eye with two cyclodialysis clefts as a complication of microinvasive glaucoma surgery. In this case, the clefts closed sequentially, leading to two discrete acute IOP spikes of similar magnitude (55/54 mmHg).

With the prevailing theories of IOP spike after cyclodialysis cleft closure being due to compensation for hypotony/over filtration by the cleft either by increased aqueous production or decreased trabecular outflow, it is reasonable to hypothesize that if these mechanisms had at least partially normalized to the point of normotension after the first spike, albeit on topical medications; then, the second spike should likely have been of less magnitude than the first, given some renormalization of aqueous production and trabecular

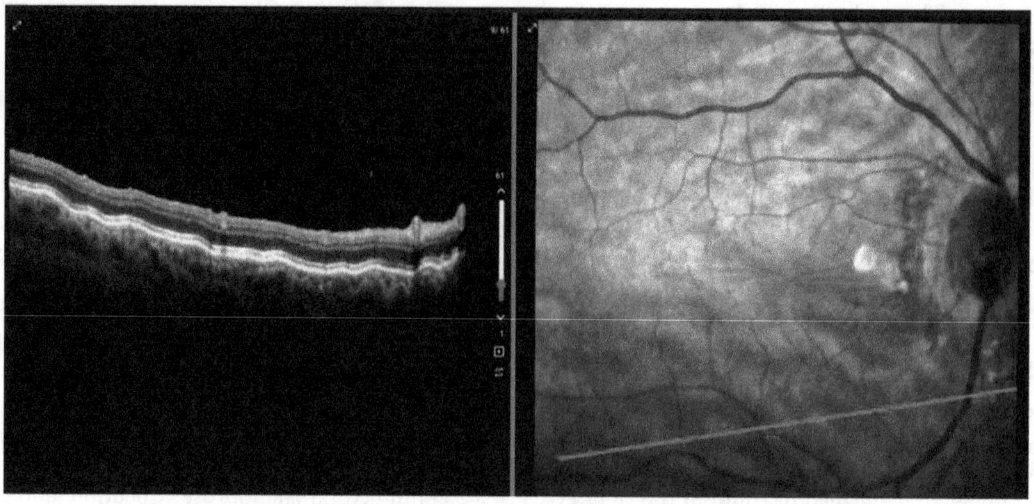

Figure 1: Spectralis OCT of the right macula showing choroidal folds.

outflow, even if partial, if this is indeed the mechanism underlying cleft closure-related IOP spikes.

Two points are important to note to support this hypothesis. First, in this instance, the second IOP spike is very unlikely to be related directly to tapering of medications after the first spike, as the medications were tapered very conservatively (one agent at a time over multiple visits), and the patient presented with an acute (within hours) symptomatic IOP rise two weeks after the tapering of a single drop, while still on three topical IOP-lowering medications. Further, the acute rise coincided with the closure of the residual second cleft on gonioscopy.

Second, it is possible the use topical antihypertensives at the time of the second spike could have masked some ongoing increased aqueous production and/or impaired trabecular function, despite the patient being normotensive; that is, that the traditional aqueous production and trabecular outflow had not fully normalized due to the residual cleft or due to timing. That being said, the prevailing theory is that the eye readjusts these compensatory mechanisms after cleft closure, which accounts for resolution of the IOP spike, typically allowing for cessation of the increased IOP lowering therapy.

If some trabecular outflow had been restored and/or aqueous production reduced more to typical physiologic levels, it would seem to suggest that one would have expected less of an IOP spike the second time, when the eye was no longer hypotonous and had returned at least some trabecular outflow restored after resolution of the initial IOP spike even allowing tapering of medications over multiple visits. It is impossible to say if the patient's preexisiting glaucoma and presumably impaired outflow facility at baseline could have played a role in the phenomenon; it remains a worthy consideration.

In the authors' opinions, this patient's course perhaps suggests that IOP spike may be a direct reaction to cleft closure itself and not just related to compensatory changes in aqueous production and trabecular outflow while the cleft is open. We feel this warrants further investigation as to what physiologic processes mediate this IOP response and resolution.

5. Conclusions

IOP spikes are a frequent consequence of CDC and can be dangerous. Two consecutive IOP spikes of similar magnitude during sequential cleft closure have not been reported in the literature and could be important for understanding the physiology underlying an acute increase in IOP. Understanding these mechanisms and the associated factors may allow better prevention and treatment. Further studies are required to investigate the mechanisms underlying an IOP spike in patients after CDC closure.

Consent

This report does not contain information that would identify the patient. However, written informed consent to publish the case report was obtained through our institutional electronic medical record (EPIC) from the patient including the figure used in this report.

Authors' Contributions

Ahmed Alshaikhsalama did the drafting of manuscript, data acquisition, and manuscript revision. Niraj Nathan did the conception of project along with revision and final approval of published work.

References

[1] B. Mushtaq, M. Y. Chiang, V. Kumar, U. S. Ramanathan, and P. Shah, "Phacoemulsification, persistent hypotony, and cyclodialysis clefts," *Journal of Cataract and Refractive Surgery*, vol. 31, no. 7, pp. 1428–1432, 2005.

[2] A. S. Ioannidis and K. Barton, "Cyclodialysis cleft: causes and repair," *Current Opinion in Ophthalmology*, vol. 21, no. 2, pp. 150–154, 2010.

[3] A. S. Ioannidis, C. Bunce, and K. Barton, "The evaluation and surgical management of cyclodialysis clefts that have failed to respond to conservative management," *The British Journal of Ophthalmology*, vol. 98, no. 4, pp. 544–549, 2014.

[4] L. M. Provencher and M. M. Shah, "Cyclodialysis cleft repair with goniotomy for the control of post-operative ocular hypertension," *American Journal of Ophthalmology Case Reports*, vol. 19, article 100781, 2020.

[5] M. Thomas, T. S. Vajaranant, and A. A. Aref, "Hypotony maculopathy: clinical presentation and therapeutic methods," *Ophthalmology and Therapy*, vol. 4, no. 2, pp. 79–88, 2015.

[6] E. N. Fang and M. A. Kass, "Increased intraocular pressure after cataract surgery," *Seminars in Ophthalmology*, vol. 9, no. 4, pp. 235–242, 1994.

31

The Role of Early Vitrectomy in the Healing of Retinal Lesions in Progressive Outer Retinal Necrosis

Hamid Riazi-Esfahani, Arash Mirzaei, Masoud Mirghorbani, Fariba Ghassemi, Mohammad Zarei, Elias Khalili Pour, and Nazanin Ebrahimiadib

Retina Service, Farabi Eye Hospital, Tehran University of Medical Sciences, Tehran, Iran

Correspondence should be addressed to Elias Khalili Pour; ekhalilipour@gmail.com

Academic Editor: Kamal Kishore

Purpose. To report on the efficacy of early pars plana vitrectomy (PPV), silicone oil (SO) tamponade, and intravitreal ganciclovir injection in the treatment of a case with progressive outer retinal necrosis (PORN). *Case Presentation.* A 33-year-old man with a history of shingles on the chest skin 2.5 months ago presented with progressive vision loss in both eyes over the past 20 days. Fundus examination revealed retinal necrosis with perivascular clearance. Human immunodeficiency virus (HIV) infection was confirmed by western blot analysis. Treatment with intravenous acyclovir and intravitreal ganciclovir injections was unable to stop the progression of retinitis. Along with highly active antiretroviral therapy, the patient underwent PPV with SO tamponade and intravitreal ganciclovir injection in both eyes. A few days after surgery, retinal lesions started to improve. *Conclusion.* Early PPV, SO tamponade, and intravitreal ganciclovir injection may be considered an effective intervention in PORN patients with an unfavorable response to medical treatment.

1. Introduction

Progressive outer retinal necrosis (PORN) syndrome was first identified in 1990 in two patients with acquired immunodeficiency syndrome (AIDS) [1]. It is distinguished from acute retinal necrosis by its rapid progression and vision loss caused by early posterior pole involvement, absence of vitreous reactivity, and relative sparing of the retinal vascular system. Varicella-zoster virus (VZV) infection is the most common cause [2].

This condition is characterised by a poor response to standard antiviral medications, and the visual prognosis remains guarded [2]. Final visual acuity has been reported to be no light perception (NLP) in up to 67 percent of patients with PORN [3]. Due to rapid progression and ominous outcomes, empiric therapy usually begins before a definitive diagnosis.

Herein, we report a case of PORN syndrome with an initial unfavorable response to medical treatment and subsequent successful management with early pars plana vitrectomy (PPV), silicone oil (SO) tamponade, and intravitreal ganciclovir injection.

2. Case Report

A 33-year-old man presented to the retina clinic with progressive vision loss in both eyes over the past 20 days. The best-corrected visual acuity (BCVA) was 20/40 in both eyes. He reported an unintentional weight loss of 17 kg over the past two years. His medical history was notable for a zoster infection involving his chest dermatome as well as oral candidiasis 2.5 months prior to presentation.

Slit-lamp examination of external adnexal and anterior segment revealed unremarkable findings in both eyes. Funduscopy of the right eye showed round white patches distributed across the posterior fundus, becoming denser in the inferonasal quadrant. There were no obvious vascular involvement and vitreous inflammation. (Figure 1(a)). Similar retinal

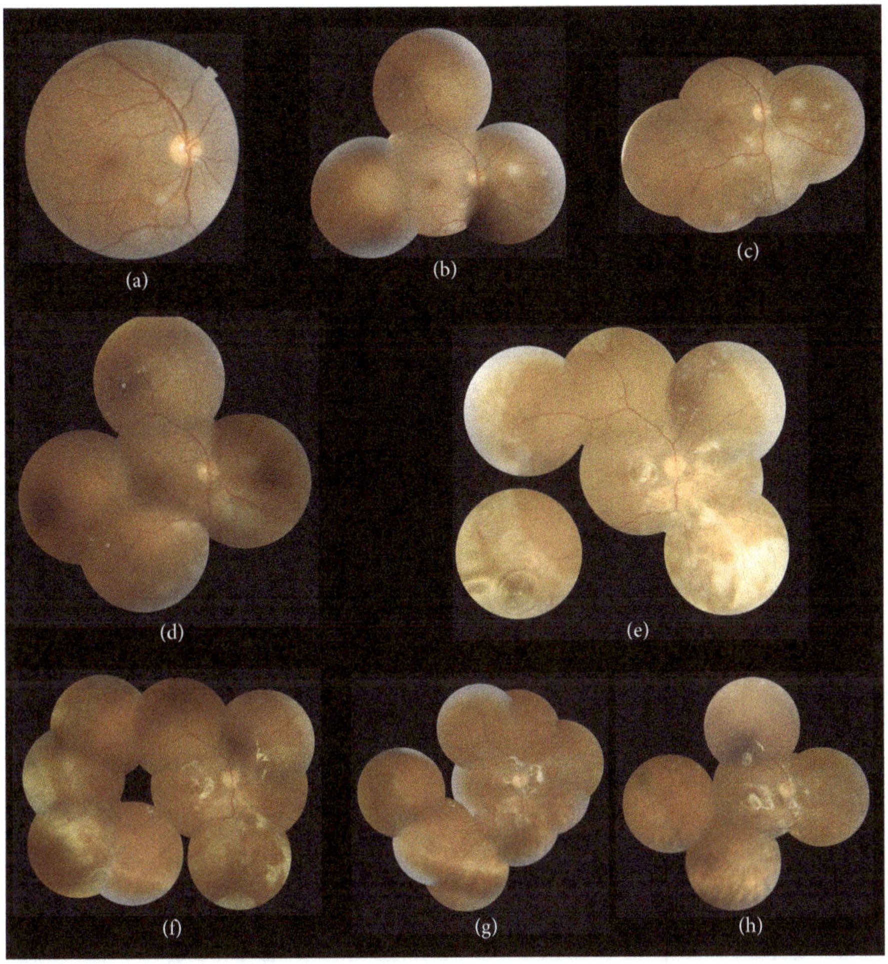

FIGURE 1: (a) Fundus photograph of the right eye (OD) at presentation shows white necrotic patches in the vicinity of the inferior arcade. (b) Montage fundus photograph of OD on day 4: retinal lesions progressed, intravenous acyclovir dosage was increased to 850 mg three times per day, and the second dose of intravitreal ganciclovir (2 mg/0.1 cc) was administered. (c) Three days later, despite medical treatment, the lesions continued to progress. (d) On day 10, lesions coalesced and showed an increase in size. (e) One day after pars plana vitrectomy with silicone oil tamponade and prophylactic endolaser. (f) One week after the right eye surgery (day 20). (g) One month after the right eye vitrectomy, the lesions regressed significantly. (h) Seven months after initial presentation, lesions near completely healed.

lesions with more extensive involvement were observed in the left eye. The patches coalesced in the area posterior to the equator, particularly in the inferior quadrants. Some small dot hemorrhages were noticed, especially along the inferior arcade. No vitreous inflammation was observed. (Figure 2(a)).

On admission, intravenous (IV) acyclovir 700 mg (10 mg/kg), three times per day, and oral aspirin 80 mg daily were commenced. On day 1, the patient underwent intravitreal injection of ganciclovir in both eyes (2 mg/0.1 cc). Polymerase chain reaction (PCR) of the aqueous sample was positive for Varicella zoster virus (VZV) and Human Herpes Virus 6 (HHV6). Additionally, positive serum human immunodeficiency virus (HIV) antibodies were detected using an initial enzyme-linked immunosorbent assay (ELISA) method and validated using a western blot test. At the time of admission, the CD4 count was 42 cells/mm3.

On day 4, retinal lesions continued to progress in both eyes. The intravenous acyclovir dose was increased to 850 mg three times per day, and both eyes received a second dose of intravitreal ganciclovir (2 mg/0.1 cc) (Figures 1(b) and 2(b)). The patient first attempted to deny HIV diagnosis and resisted the initiation of highly active antiretroviral therapy (HAART), but after a few days, he participated for treatment with the help of psychiatric counselling. Finally on day 7, the patient was started on HAART.

Three days later, despite medical treatment, the lesions expanded with sparing of perivascular areas and the BCVA of the left eye dropped to the counting fingers (CF) at 1 meter (Figures 1(c) and 2(c)). On day 10, the patient underwent 23-gauge PPV and SO tamponade along with intravitreal ganciclovir (2 mg/0.1 cc) injection in the left eye (Figure 2-D). Three days following surgery (day 13), the lesions in the left eye began to heal, while the lesions in the right eye continued to enlarge, lowering the BCVA to 20/200 (Figures 2(e) and 1(d). The same surgical procedure was scheduled for the right eye (Figure 1(e)). Barrier endolaser photocoagulation along the posterior border of the retinal lesions was performed in the right eye in contrast to the left eye (Figures 1(e) and 2(e)). Due to the proximity of the necrosis to the macula, posterior vitreous detachment

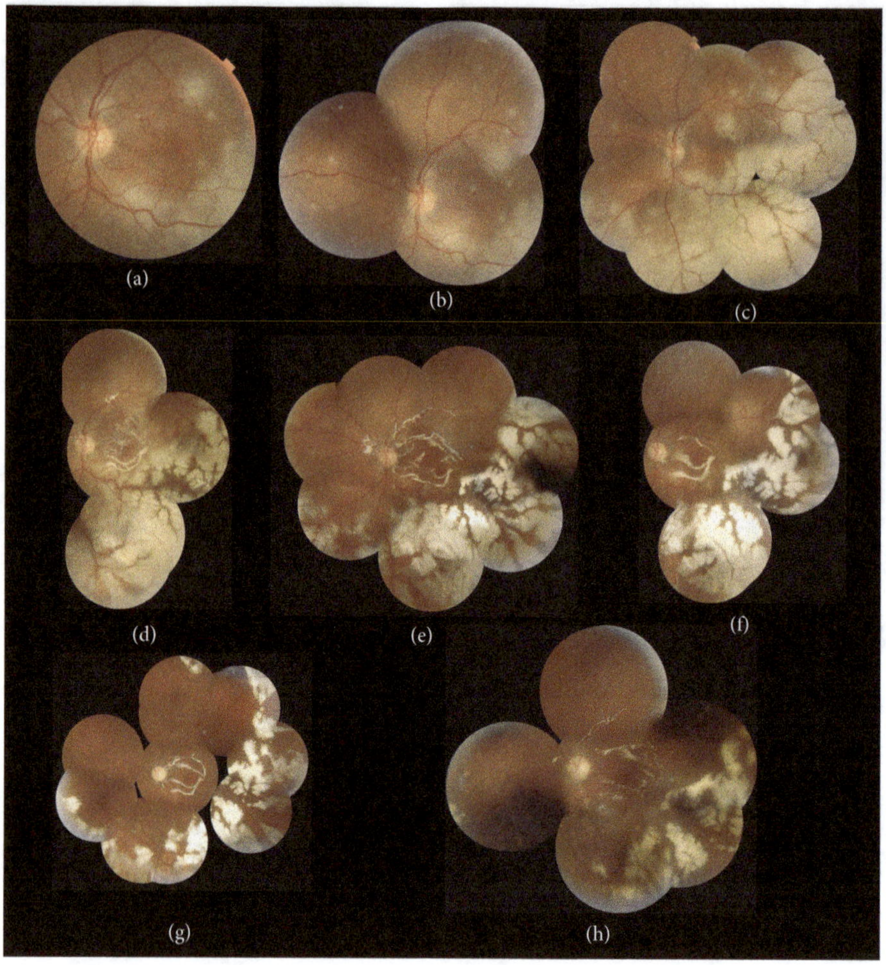

FIGURE 2: (a) Fundus photograph of the left eye (OS) at presentation shows white necrotic retinitis patches encroaching the macula from the inferior and temporal area. Scattered hemorrhages are evident along the inferior arcade. There is no significant vitritis. (b) Montage fundus photograph of OS on day 4: retinal lesions progressed, the intravenous acyclovir dosage was increased to 850 mg three times per day, and the second dose of intravitreal ganciclovir (2 mg/0.1 cc) was administered. (c) Three days later, despite medical treatment, the lesions coalesced and showed an increase in size. Perivascular sparing can be appreciated. (d) One day after pars plana vitrectomy with silicone oil tamponade and intravitreal ganciclovir injection. (e) On day three postoperatively, lesions regressed, especially from the macular area. (f) One week after the left eye surgery (day 20). (g) One month after vitrectomy, the lesions resolved obviously and got sharper borders. (h) Seven months after initial presentation, the lesions regressed significantly.

(PVD) was not induced during the vitrectomy of the left eye, and the vitreous was shaved over the necrotic regions and towards the vitreous base using a very low aspiration mode. The posterior hyaloid was separated from the optic disc up to the equator using triamcinolone for better visualization of vitreous during the vitrectomy of the right eye, and the remaining vitreous was meticulously shaved using the shaving mode of the vitrectomy instrument.

After two weeks of IV acyclovir, the patient was switched to oral valacyclovir 1 g three times daily. On day 20, the BCVA improved to 20/60 in the right eye (OD) and 20/200 in the left eye (OS) (Figures 1(f) and 2(f)).

One month after PPV, the lesions of both eyes improved dramatically. The BCVA was stabilized at 20/60 OD and 20/200 OS (Figures 1(g) and 2(g)). After the posterior lesions in the left eye were resolved, prophylactic barrier laser photocoagulation was performed on the areas away from the fovea. On day 60, the CD4 count had increased to 124 cells/mm^3.

Seven months after presentation, all lesions significantly regressed and the BCVA was 20/60 OD and 20/100 OS (Figures 1(h) and 2(h)). As the patient's CD4 count remained subnormal at 147 cells/mm3, valacyclovir 1 g three times daily was continued in addition to HAART.

3. Discussion

PORN is a potentially blinding disease that often responds poorly to currently available antiviral therapies. This condition is most frequently found in immunocompromised patients with a shingles history [1–3]. Due to the disease's rarity, there has been no prospective, randomised clinical trial; hence, management recommendations are based on case reports/series.

The patient did not respond to the initial intravenous acyclovir treatment or the subsequent intravitreal ganciclovir injection in this report. We had limited access to more potent antivirals such as Foscarnet, as a result, we used PPV in conjunction with SO tamponade and intravitreal ganciclovir injection. Within two days of surgery, this approach resulted in a dramatic improvement of the lesions, which lasted for seven months.

Mehrotra et al. recently described a case of PORN in a 43-year-old male who was originally treated with intravenous acyclovir and intravitreal ganciclovir, followed by oral valacyclovir. One month later, the patient had retinal detachment. After one month, PPV with SO tamponade and intravitreal and intravenous ganciclovir injection resulted in retinal reattachment and an improvement in visual acuity to 20/200 [4].

To the best of our knowledge, this is the first report of an early vitrectomy for a PORN syndrome patient. We propose two possible explanations for the effectiveness of simultaneous SO tamponade and intravitreal ganciclovir injection. The first possibility is that the injected ganciclovir concentration is greater in the "subsilicone space," which is in close proximity to the retinal lesions. The other possibility is that SO has an antiviral effect, as demonstrated in an in vitro investigation against HSV-1 [5]. However, there is no data of SO antiviral effect against VZV or CMV in the literature.

Although the findings of a recent meta-analysis in patients with acute retinal necrosis support early vitrectomy in lowering the rate of retinal detachment as a potentially devastating complication, more research is needed to determine the efficacy of early vitrectomy in individuals with PORN syndrome in terms of controlling retinal inflammation and preventing retinal detachment [6].

While the patient has a promising BCVA with attached retina in both eyes seven months after PPV and SO tamponade, the patient's final outcome, particularly after SO removal, requires long-term follow-ups.

Finally, our limited experience, in this case, illustrates that for progressive PORN patients despite conventional antiviral regimens or in situations with limited access to more potent antivirals, early vitrectomy and silicone oil tamponade with concomitant intravitreal ganciclovir injection can show short-term efficacy.

References

[1] D. J. Forster, P. U. Dugel, G. T. Frangieh, P. E. Liggett, and N. A. Rao, "Rapidly progressive outer retinal necrosis in the acquired immunodeficiency syndrome," *American Journal of Ophthalmology*, vol. 110, no. 4, pp. 341–348, 1990.

[2] R. B. Austin, "Progressive outer retinal necrosis syndrome: a comprehensive review of its clinical presentation, relationship to immune system status, and management," *Clinical eye and vision care.*, vol. 12, no. 3-4, pp. 119–129, 2000.

[3] A. Takeda, M. Arima, K. Ishikawa, E. Hasegawa, Y. Murakami, and K.-H. Sonoda, "Acute Retinal Necrosis and Progressive Outer Retinal Necrosis," in *Inflammatory and Infectious Ocular Disorders*, pp. 215–220, Springer, 2020.

[4] N. Mehrotra, J. Khandelwal, and M. Nagpal, "Surgical management of complications in a case of progressive outer retinal necrosis," *Taiwan Journal of Ophthalmology*, vol. 10, no. 4, pp. 312–314, 2020.

[5] H. Yan and J. Li, "Experimental study on antiviral activity of silicone oil in vitro," *Graefe's archive for clinical and experimental ophthalmology = Albrecht von Graefes Archiv fur klinische und experimentelle Ophthalmologie*, vol. 246, no. 9, pp. 1285–1289, 2008.

[6] S. Fan, D. Lin, and Y. Wang, "Role of prophylactic vitrectomy in acute retinal necrosis in preventing rhegmatogenous retinal detachment: systematic review and meta-analysis," *Systematic Review and Meta-analysis. Ocular immunology and inflammation.*, pp. 1–5, 2020.

32

Button Battery-Induced Necrotizing Keratoconjunctivitis: Case Report

Nima Koosha, Leila Babaei, and Mohsen Pourazizi

Isfahan Eye Research Center, Department of Ophthalmology, Isfahan University of Medical Sciences, Isfahan, Iran

Correspondence should be addressed to Mohsen Pourazizi; m.pourazizi@yahoo.com

Academic Editor: Kamal Kishore

We report a case of a 2-year-old girl who presented to the ocular emergency department with a button battery retained in the inferior fornix of the left eye for more than 48 hours. The child developed necrotizing keratoconjunctivitis, which was treated with antibiotics, amniotic membrane graft, prompt removal of button battery, and other supportive measures.

1. Introduction

The usage of button batteries (BBs) has become more common in recent years to power electronic equipment and toys. On one hand, BBs are increasingly used in devices including electronic games, watches, and new electronic toys. On the other hand, the advent in size reduction and also the smooth and shiny appearance of BB make them quite attractive and interesting to young children, and the number of serious injuries or deaths as a result of small BBs has increased in the last decade [1, 2].

BBs can be extremely dangerous for children due to electrochemical mechanism of injury [1, 3, 4]. If BBs are swallowed or placed in the any orifice of the body, they can cause significant damage to the mucosa and potentially cause long-term complications [1–3]. The clinical course of a child with a BB depends on several factors including the location, duration of exposure, battery size, power of BB, remaining voltage in the battery, and chemical composition of the battery [1, 2].

Locations for BBs injury in children include aerodigestive tract, nose, vagina, and ear [2, 5]. Embedded BB in the eye is very rare, and there is limited report of ocular surface damage from BBs [6–9]. The purposes of this report are to present our experience in the diagnosis and management of a new case of BB foreign body in a young child and review the related literature.

2. Case Presentation

A 2-year-old girl was brought to emergency department of the referral eye center of Feiz Hospital affiliated to Isfahan University of Medical Sciences, Isfahan, Iran, by her mother with complaints of redness, tearing, and pain. The patient also had bloody stained discharge in her left eye. The interval between initiation of ocular symptoms and first visit was about 48 hours. The patient was otherwise healthy with no significant medical or ophthalmic history. Prior to injury, she had been left playing alone. There was no history of ocular trauma.

In the emergency room, physical exam revealed stable vital signs and swollen left upper and lower eyelids (Figure 1).

Slit-lamp examination in the emergency room showed a disc foreign body in the inferior fornix. The pupil was reactive with normal size. The extraocular movements were normal. The foreign body was an alkaline 1.5 volt, 6 millimeter BB obtained from a musical toy. The button battery was removed in the emergency room, and a chemical ocular injury in the left eye was suspected (Figure 2).

Due to poor cooperation of child in the emergency room, the pH of the ocular surface tear film in the affected eye was not evaluated. The eyes were irrigated with balanced salt solution. Fluorescein solution was applied over the ocular surface to identify the extent of injury. Multiple scattered epithelial defects (ED) and an area of epithelial necrosis in

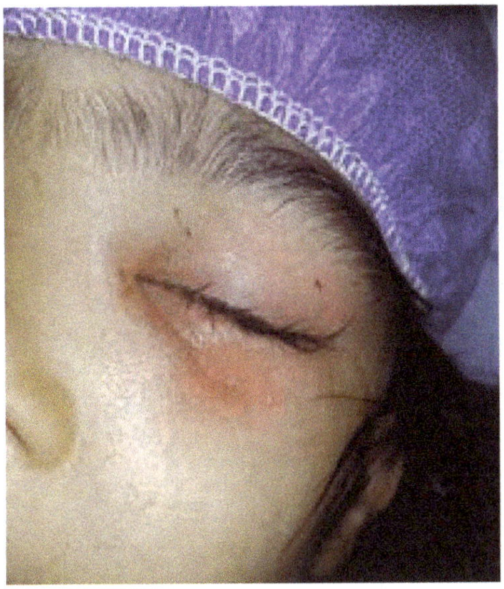

Figure 1: Edema of left upper and lower eyelids.

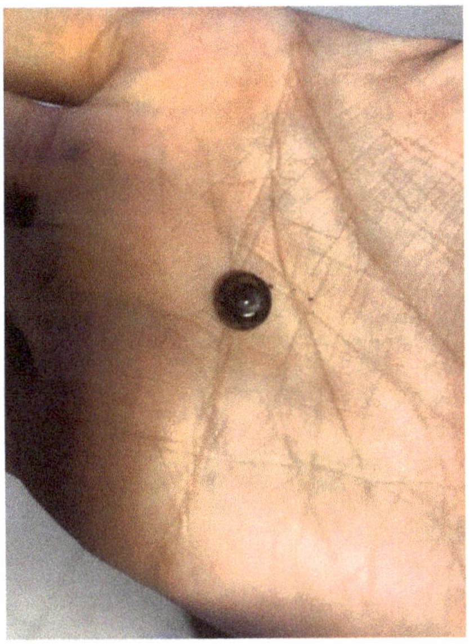

Figure 2: Removed alkaline button battery from left inferior fornix in a child.

inferior fornix were discovered. Apart from the corneal ED, the inferior limbus from 4 to 8 o'clock was ischemic and conjunctiva also had evidence of chemical toxicity and necrosis inferiorly (Figure 3).

The anterior chamber was quiet, and the sclera was intact. The rest of the anterior segment examination was unremarkable in the left eye, and the posterior segment was within normal limits. To rule out the rare possibility of any intraorbital foreign body, an axial and coronal CT were also done, which revealed air in the inferior orbital space-like necrotic tissue. A complete ophthalmic exam was performed under general anesthesia in the operating room. Intraocular pressure was in a normal range.

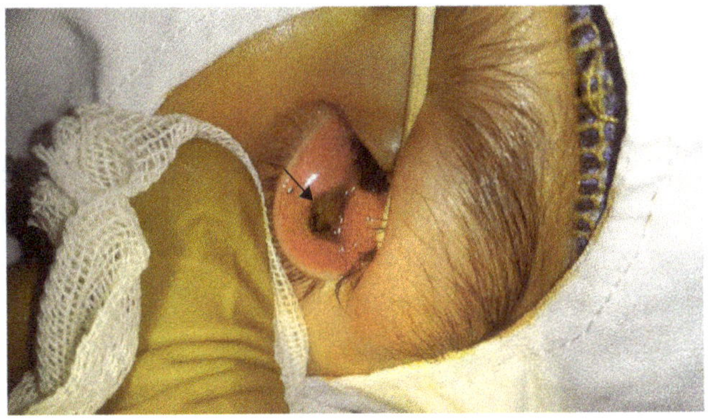

Figure 3: Necrosis in the inferior fornix of the left eye due to button battery exposure (black arrow).

During exploration of the conjunctiva, severe tissue destruction was noted in the lower palpebral conjunctiva caused by the alkaline BB. In the operation room, irrigation was continued until normal surface pH unit.

All necrotic tissue of cornea and conjunctiva was debrided. A commercial amniotic membrane was applied to cover the raw surface as a biological bandage and to promote epithelialization. The amniotic membrane is secured with multiple 8-O Vicryl™ absorbable sutures. The patient was given systemic intravenous antimicrobial treatment (cefazolin; 1 mg/kg body weight) postoperatively for 72 hours.

The eye treated with topical ciprofloxacin every 4 hours, topical betamethasone every 6 hours, and a preservative-free artificial tear frequently. The patient's condition continuously improved, and the epithelial defect had completely healed. Both the cornea and conjunctiva gradually became normal without fluorescein staining after 2 weeks. All medications tapered off within 4 weeks. On 6-month follow-up, there was no sign of limbal deficiency, and the clarity of the cornea was preserved (Figure 4).

3. Discussion

We report a case of ocular BB foreign body leading to necrotizing keratoconjunctivitis. The importance of this report lay on (1) the organ-threatening consequence of a delay in removing the BB and (2) the importance of applying AMT when there is a significant tissue loss for repair. Evidence of BB exposure was apparent by the ocular surface necrotizing injury, with confirmation upon discovery of a small BB in the inferior fornix of the left eye.

A toxic keratoconjunctivitis has been reported to be caused by a wide range of toxic foreign body including chemical powder, caustic agents, remnants of shampoo and cosmetic lotions, and chlorinated pool water. Although foreign bodies are usually removed from the ocular surface by the protective mechanisms, embedded foreign bodies can potentially be serious toxic ocular foreign bodies and cause tissue destruction [10].

If the battery is damaged or shows any leakage, the possible mechanism is chemical injury; and if the battery is intact with considerable charge for example in new toys,

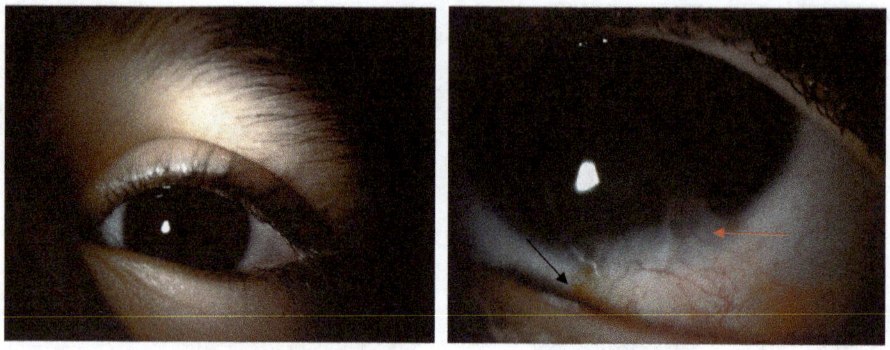

Figure 4: After 6-month follow-up. Sectoral superficial pannus formation in the inferior temporal quadrant with distinct borders, pannus formation (red arrow), and an adhesion band formation (black arrow).

Table 1: Ocular injury after exposure to a BB in the literature.

Case no.	Author(s)/ years	Patient age/sex	Latency until examination	Ocular manifestations	Management	Prognosis
1	Ogasawara et al./2011 [6]	3/F	8 hours	(i) Hard and polished white opacity on the cornea (ii) Conjunctival injection	(1) Removal button battery (2) Ocular surface irrigation	Improvement of the opacity gradually secondary pterygium formation
2	Mazer-Amirshahi et at./2013 [7]	18/F	90 min	(i) Conjunctival ulceration (ii) Subconjunctival hemorrhage (iii) Vitreous opacification (iv) Partially dilated pupil	(1) Removal button battery in the operating room (2) Ocular surface irrigation (3) Topical antibiotics (4) Topical steroids (5) Daily rodding procedure using glass rod to separate the bulbar and tarsal conjunctiva	Healing over the subsequent 6 months, normal visual acuity
3	Ratnarajan et al./2013 [8]	2/F	18 hours	(i) Lower eyelid edema and erythema (ii) Severe eye pain	(1) Removal button battery (2) Daily rodding procedure for 3 days (3) Betamethasone 1% ointment four times a day (gradually tapered over 3 months)	Symblepharon between the bulbar and tarsal conjunctiva without eye movements restriction
4	Khan et al./2014 [9]	2/F	3 hours	(i) Eye lid erythema and swelling with a pseudoptosis	(1) Removal button battery	Symblepharon formation
5	Our case/2021	2/F	48 hours	(i) Upper and lower eyelid edema and erythema (ii) Tearing (iii) Severe pain (iv) Bloody discharge	(1) Removal button battery (2) Ocular surface irrigation (3) Topical betamethasone (4) Topical ciprofloxacin (5) Systemic antibiotic	Improvement with no sign of limbal deficiency on 6-month follow up

the possible mechanisms like electrical burns or generation of hydroxide can be considered [1, 3–5].

In our case, the suspected mechanism of injury was likely chemical as the removed BB was not intact.

Exudation of tissue fluids caused by a burn injury creates a moist environment. In vitro studies have shown that spontaneous leakage of electrolyte solution occurs when alkaline batteries are exposed to moisture. The leaked alkaline electrolyte solution can penetrate deeply into tissues producing a liquefying necrosis. This results in dissolution of protein and collagen, saponification of lipids, dehydration of tissue cells, and consequential extensive tissue damage [1, 4].

BBs ocular injury is a rarely reported condition in the literature. Some reports revealed ocular toxicity or injury after exposure to a BB [6–9] (Table 1). Given the unusual site of BBs as a foreign body in eye, occurrences of ocular toxicity due to BBs are rare; therefore, some ophthalmologists may never have encountered ocular BBs injury and would not recognize the clinical and ocular characteristics of retained BBs in the eye.

In 2011, in an experimental study, a button battery was placed on an eyeball of a pig. The result of the study demonstrated corneal opacity development in five minutes [6]. Ogasawara et al. report a case of button battery-induced ocular injury in a 3-year-old girl that presented with corneal opacity and conjunctival injection. Over several months, scar tissue was replaced by secondary pterygium [6]. In a similar report, Mazer-Amirshahi et al. report an 18-year-old girl with severe conjunctival ulceration, subconjunctival hemorrhage, vitreous opacification, and a partially dilated pupil associated BB injury. The patient was treated with topical antibiotics, steroids, and a daily rodding procedure using glass rod to separate the bulbar and tarsal conjunctiva to prevent the tarsal conjunctival scar and finally healed over the subsequent 6 months [7]. In another case, Ratnarajan et al. report severe ocular injury from a BB with a delayed presentation after about 18 hours exposure to the BB [8]. Khan et al. report a rapid onset case of severe ocular injury after exposure to a BB. Their case presented with swelling and redness of the eye within 3 hours after exposure. Due to severe ocular injury, symblepharon formation occurred [9].

Since only few hours may be needed to result in major complications, the most important issue in management of BB foreign bodies is rapid diagnosis and prompt removal of any BB contacting any mucosal membranes [1, 4]. In our patient, the BB remain for more than 48 hours and induced severe necrotizing injury. The toxic reaction in our patient was more severe possibly due to the long-lasting retained BB within the lower eyelid and continuous release of toxic electrolytes in an alkaline condition, which could contribute to additional ocular surface damage.

A previous study reported successful treatment of BB ocular burn using steroid. Steroid plays a major role in controlling inflammation, especially in the acute stage and subsequently prevent of development of symblepharon and deformation of the ocular surface. We also used amniotic membrane to promote the healing process that had a favorable result in our patient.

Transplantation of amniotic membrane has been shown to promote epithelialization and reduce inflammation, scarring, and neovascularization [11]. Our report is also not without limitations. The study was a single case report; and therefore, generalisation of this report is cautioned by the authors. Another limitation of current report included absences of more follow-up period.

4. Conclusion

Our report provides new insight in clinical presentation and the significance of early removal, copious irrigation, medical treatment, and the unique treatment of amniotic membrane as an adjunct to the BB injuries in the eye. Due to the common use of these batteries, physicians should be more aware of the serious risks associated with BBs. Since there is no standard of protocol for treatment of BB-induced ocular injury, it seems prevention is the best approach for to be safe from BB-induced ocular injury.

Consent

No written consent has been obtained from the patients as there is no patient identifiable data included in this case.

Acknowledgments

The study was supported by Vice Chancellery for Research and Technology, Isfahan University of Medical Sciences, Isfahan, Iran. Funding organization participated in ethical and scientific approval before the study began.

References

[1] A. Mubarak, M. A. Benninga, I. Broekaert et al., "Diagnosis, management, and prevention of button battery ingestion in childhood: a European Society for Paediatric Gastroenterology Hepatology and Nutrition position paper," *Journal of pediatric gastroenterology and nutrition.*, vol. 73, no. 1, pp. 129–136, 2021.

[2] L. C. Oyama, "Foreign bodies of the ear, nose and throat," *Emergency medicine clinics of North America.*, vol. 37, no. 1, pp. 121–130, 2019.

[3] T. Litovitz, N. Whitaker, and L. Clark, "Preventing battery ingestions: an analysis of 8648 cases," *Pediatrics*, vol. 125, no. 6, pp. 1178–1183, 2010.

[4] S. Jayachandra and G. D. Eslick, "A systematic review of paediatric foreign body ingestion: presentation, complications, and management," *International Journal of Pediatric Otorhinolaryngology*, vol. 77, no. 3, pp. 311–317, 2013.

[5] J. A. Kurowski and M. Kay, "Caustic ingestions and foreign bodies ingestions in pediatric patients," *Pediatric clinics of North America.*, vol. 64, no. 3, pp. 507–524, 2017.

[6] M. Ogasawara, S. Goto, T. Shiba et al., "A case of button battery-induced corneal and conjunctive burn injury and experimental findings of local damage," *Nippon Ganka Gakkai Zasshi*, vol. 115, no. 8, pp. 711–717, 2011.

[7] M. Mazer-Amirshahi, N. Whitaker, L. Kayewilson, and T. Litovitz, "Severe ocular injury after button battery exposure," *The Journal of Emergency Medicine*, vol. 44, no. 2, pp. e187–e189, 2013.

[8] G. Ratnarajan, D. Calladine, K. J. Bird, and S. L. Watson, "Delayed presentation of severe ocular injury from a button battery," *Case Reports*, vol. 2013, no. may02 1, article bcr2013009094, 2013.

[9] Y. Khan, S. Maqsood, S. Marpuri, S. Bhermi, and V. Geh, "Rapid onset of severe ocular injury after exposure to a button battery," *Journal of AAPOS*, vol. 18, no. 6, pp. 600-601, 2014.

[10] A. Malik and C. Claoué, "Transport and interaction of cosmetic product material within the ocular surface: beauty and

the beastly symptoms of toxic tears," *Contact Lens and Anterior Eye.*, vol. 35, no. 6, pp. 247–259, 2012.

[11] A. Kheirkhah, D. A. Johnson, D. R. Paranjpe, V. K. Raju, V. Casas, and S. C. Tseng, "Temporary sutureless amniotic membrane patch for acute alkaline burns," *Archives of Ophthalmology*, vol. 126, no. 8, pp. 1059–1066, 2008.

33

Endogenous Endophthalmitis Associated with Liver Abscess Successfully Treated with Vitrectomy and Intravitreal Empirical Antibiotics Injections

Sung Woong Lim, Youngje Sung, Hee Jung Kwon, and Won Kyung Song

Department of Ophthalmology, CHA Bundang Medical Center, CHA University College of Medicine, Seoul, Republic of Korea

Correspondence should be addressed to Won Kyung Song; songwkmd@daum.net

Academic Editor: Kevin J. Blinder

Purpose. Klebsiella pneumoniae is the most common pathogen of endogenous endophthalmitis accompanying liver abscess in East Asia. The treatment may be different for the patients with endogenous endophthalmitis from the postoperative endophthalmitis. Prompt administration of both intraocular (vancomycin and ceftazidime) and systemic (ceftriaxone, aminoglycoside, and/or metronidazole) antibiotics have been a mainstay of treatment. However, ceftriaxone has been proven to more effectively kill K. pneumoniae than ceftazidime in in vitro studies, and the safety of intravitreal ceftriaxone has been confirmed in animal studies. *Methods.* Two diabetic female patients with liver abscess presented with decreased visual acuity of the unilateral eyes. Fundus photography, ocular ultrasonography, and abdominal computed tomography were performed. *Results.* A 50-year-old diabetic female patient with liver abscess presented decreased visual acuity of the left eye. In fundus examinations, a yellowish necrotic lesion was noted throughout the eye. The results of culture of the blood culture was positive for K. pneumoniae. She was successfully treated with intravitreal ceftazidime injections, and the remaining vitreous opacity was treated with vitrectomy. A 62-year-old female with liver abscess presented a visual symptom of floaters in the right eye. The fundus had a hazy appearance through the vitreous opacity. A yellowish-white subretinal abscess was noted at the temporal macula. Cultures of blood were negative. She underwent intravitreal injections of empirical antibiotics. However, she did not respond to intravitreal vancomycin and ceftazidime. Thus, we changed the intravitreal antibiotics from ceftazidime to ceftriaxone and performed vitrectomy. Her ocular status significantly improved after this change. *Conclusion.* Our results indicate that for cases with EE, prompt initial treatment with broad spectrum antibiotics, followed by rapid use of antibiotics selected according to culture results, and empirical use of antibiotics in cases of a negative culture may be an effective treatment. Vitrectomy also can be an effective treatment option for vitreous opacity refractory to the treatment.

1. Case Report

The prognosis of patients who develop endogenous endophthalmitis (EE) is devastating despite aggressive therapy, with many cases resulting in irreversible vision loss [1]. We report EE cases in which intravitreal antibiotic treatment saved the patients from visual losses.

A 50-year-old female was referred under suspicion of hepatitis because of vomiting and jaundice symptoms for 2 weeks. Her only medical history was uncontrolled diabetes mellitus. A computed tomography scan of the abdomen showed a 16 cm gas-forming abscess in the right lobe and left medial segment of the liver (Figure 1(c)). Intravenous administration of antibiotics (ceftriaxone, metronidazole, and amikacin) was started, and emergent percutaneous drainage was performed for the liver abscess. On the fourth day of admission, the patient was referred to the ophthalmology clinic because of decreased visual acuity in the left eye. The best-corrected visual acuity (BCVA) was hand motion in the left eye. In slit lamp examinations, many cells and a 3 mm high hypopyon were observed in the anterior chamber of the left eye. In fundus examinations, the optic disc was not visualized, and a yellowish necrotic lesion was noted throughout the eye (Figure 1).

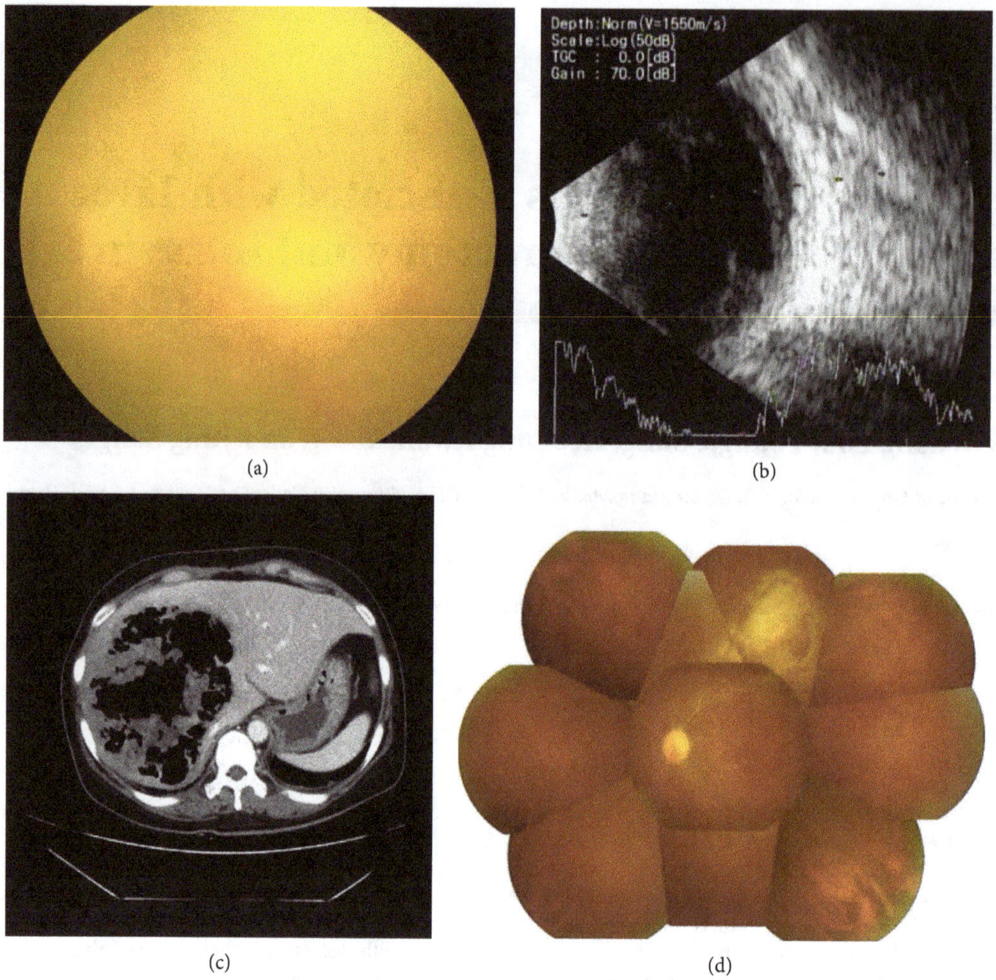

FIGURE 1: (a) Funduscopy shows a large necrotic lesion in the macular and superotemporal area with vitreous opacity of the left eye. (b) Ultrasound shows opacity and a diffuse abscess formation. (c) Abdominal computed tomography shows a gas-forming pyogenic liver abscess of the right lobe. (d) Fundus after 1 month of surgery, showing an atrophic lesion in the superotemporal area, and retinal hemorrhage around the macula.

She underwent intravitreal vancomycin (1 mg/0.1 mL) and ceftazidime (2.5 mg/0.1 mL) injections on the fourth day of admission. She was also prescribed topical antibiotics (fortified cefazolin, fortified tobramycin, and moxifloxacin), as well as treatment with corticosteroids and anticholinergics. The results of culture of the intra-abdominal abscess cavity and blood culture were positive for *Klebsiella pneumoniae* (negative for extended spectrum beta-lactamase (ESBL)) on the third day of admission. This strain was resistant to ampicillin only but was susceptible to all other antibiotics. Intravitreal injections of ceftazidime without vancomycin were given nine times, and dexamethasone was given four times every 3–4 days. Despite several intravitreal injections, vitreous opacity remained. Pars plana vitrectomy (PPV) and an intravitreal ceftazidime (2.5 mg/0.1 mL) injection were performed in the left eye 30 days after admission. An intraoperative superotemporal subretinal abscess was noted. On postoperative day 39, a fundus examination showed a resolved abscess and a decreased whitish lesion. On the last follow-up at 18 months, stable atrophy at the location of the retinal abscess area was noted and best-corrected visual acuity was 0.08 (Figure 1(d)).

A 62-year-old female presented with a 3-day history of chilling, diarrhea, and a visual symptom of floaters in the right eye. The initial BCVA was counting fingers in the right eye, 0.63 in the left eye, and a normal intraocular pressure. Slit lamp examination revealed ciliary injection as well as subconjunctival hemorrhage and many cells with flare in the anterior chamber of the right eye. The fundus had a hazy appearance through the vitreous opacity. A yellowish-white, round, elevated lesion three times the diameter of the optic disc was noted at the temporal macula (Figure 2(a)). Ultrasonography revealed multiple vitreous opacities and an elevated lesion with a height of 5 mm at the posterior pole, consistent with a subretinal abscess (Figure 2(b)). In a computed tomography scan of the abdomen, a pyogenic liver abscess was detected in segments VII/VIII (Figure 2(c)).

She was initially treated with empirical antibiotics (systemic moxifloxacin). She also underwent intravitreal injections of antibiotics (1 mg/0.1 mL vancomycin, 2.5 mg/0.1 mL

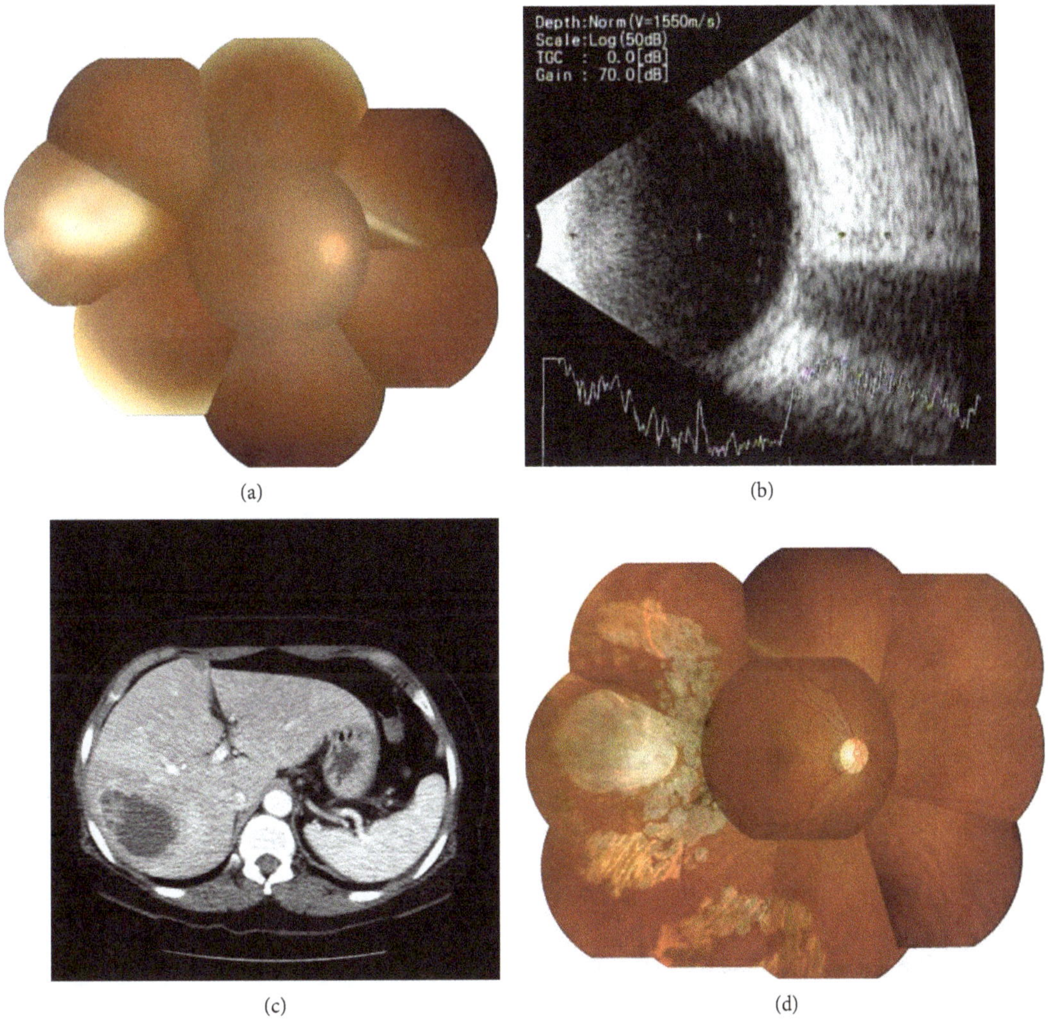

FIGURE 2: (a) Funduscopy shows a large necrotic lesion in the superotemporal area with vitreous opacity of the right eye. (b) Ultrasound shows abscess formation with a height of 5 mm at the temporal macula (c) Abdominal computed tomography shows a pyogenic liver abscess of the right lobe. (d) Fundus, 18 months after admission showing a resolved abscess and atrophic retina at the original abscess site.

ceftazidime, and 400 μg/0.1 mL dexamethasone) on the initial visit day. She was admitted to the internal medicine department, and the liver abscess was drained with pigtail catheterization. Systemic antibiotics were changed to ceftriaxone, amikacin, and metronidazole according to the recommendation of a gastroenterology specialist. The results of cultures of blood and drained fluid on the initial day of admission were negative. The results of vitreous and anterior chamber cultures on the initial day were negative on the fourth day after admission. Cultures of blood and the liver abscess were also negative. On the third day, the visual acuity of the right eye worsened to hand motions and the vitreous turbidity became denser. She underwent PPV and intravitreal injection. The antibiotics were changed to 2 mg/0.1 mL ceftriaxone from ceftazidime and vancomycin to treat Gram-negative bacteria, the most common pathogens of metastatic endophthalmitis from a liver abscess. Although the vitreous opacity was alleviated dramatically after the vitrectomy, subretinal abscess was remained. She underwent intravitreal ceftriaxone and dexamethasone injection again on the fourth day after the vitrectomy. Vitreous opacity and anterior chamber reactions improved after 1 day, and the size of subretinal abscess was dramatically improved 2 days after the second intravitreal injection. Fourteen days after the second intravitreal injection, the subretinal abscess was completely resolved and the BCVA had improved to 0.2. She was discharged. At the 40-month follow-up, the BCVA of the right eye was 0.5 and a stable atrophic lesion was noted at the previous retinal abscess area (Figure 2(d)).

Klebsiella pneumoniae, the most common pathogen of EE accompanying liver abscess in east Asia, is associated with poor visual outcomes [2, 3]. It is very destructive, with a rapid progression, so prompt use of empirical antibiotics is the most effective treatment. In contrast to postoperative endophthalmitis, there are presently no clear guidelines on the management of EE, in particular, on the selection of systemic antibiotics and the role of vitrectomy in its management [4]. Ceftazidime and amikacin were usually selected as the initial antibiotics according to the Endophthalmitis Vitrectomy Study (EVS) protocol. However, the treatment may be different for the patients with EE because EVS protocol was established for the patients with postoperative endophthalmitis. Lee et al. [4] recommended ceftriaxone for EE complicated with liver abscess as initial antibiotics in Korea, considering the regional variations in the causative pathogens in East Asia. They also reported that early vitrectomy (within 10 days after the presentation) may be helpful in patients with a visual acuity better than hand motion. In *in vitro* studies, ceftriaxone has been proven to more effectively kill *K. pneumoniae* than ceftazidime [5–8], and the safety of intravitreal ceftriaxone has been confirmed in animal studies [9]. The second patient did not respond to intravitreal vancomycin and ceftazidime, suggesting resistance to the antibiotics. Thus, we performed vitrectomy and changed the intravitreal antibiotics from ceftazidime to ceftriaxone. Her ocular status was dramatically improved after this change.

Taken together, our results indicate that for cases with EE, rapid use of antibiotics was selected according to culture results, and empirical use of antibiotics in cases of a negative culture may be an effective treatment. Vitrectomy also can be an effective treatment option for vitreous opacity refractory to the treatment.

Authors' Contributions

Sung Woong Lim and Youngje Sung contributed equally.

References

[1] C.-T. Fang, S.-Y. Lai, W.-C. Yi, P.-R. Hsueh, K.-L. Liu, and S.-C. Chang, "Klebsiella pneumoniae genotype K1: an emerging pathogen that causes septic ocular or central nervous system complications from pyogenic liver abscess," *Clinical Infectious Diseases*, vol. 45, no. 3, pp. 284–293, 2007.

[2] P. P. Connell, E. C. O'Neill, D. Fabinyi et al., "Endogenous endophthalmitis: 10-year experience at a tertiary referral centre," *Eye*, vol. 25, no. 1, pp. 66–72, 2011.

[3] C. S. Yang, H. Y. Tsai, C. S. Sung, K. H. Lin, F. L. Lee, and W. M. Hsu, "Endogenous Klebsiella endophthalmitis associated with pyogenic liver abscess," *Ophthalmology*, vol. 114, no. 5, pp. 876–880.e2, 2007.

[4] S. Lee, T. Um, S. G. Joe et al., "Changes in the clinical features and prognostic factors of endogenous endophthalmitis: fifteen years of clinical experience in Korea," *Retina*, vol. 32, no. 5, pp. 977–984, 2012.

[5] M. E. Levison and J. H. Levison, "Pharmacokinetics and pharmacodynamics of antibacterial agents," *Infectious Disease Clinics of North America*, vol. 23, no. 4, pp. 791–815, 2009, vii.

[6] S. M. Palmer, S. L. Kang, D. M. Cappelletty, and M. J. Rybak, "Bactericidal killing activities of cefepime, ceftazidime, cefotaxime, and ceftriaxone against Staphylococcus aureus and beta-lactamase-producing strains of Enterobacter aerogenes and Klebsiella pneumoniae in an in vitro infection model," *Antimicrobial Agents and Chemotherapy*, vol. 39, no. 8, pp. 1764–1771, 1995.

[7] T. Fekete, H. Tumah, J. Woodwell, V. Satishchandran, A. Truant, and P. Axelrod, "Comparative susceptibilities of Klebsieila species, Enterobacter species, and Pseudomonas aeruginosa to 11 antimicrobial agents in a tertiary-care university hospital," *American Journal of Medicine*, vol. 100, no. 6, pp. 20S–25S, 1996.

[8] S. I. Suh, W. K. Baek, and M. H. Suh, "Antimicrobial drug susceptibility and multidrug resistance of Klebsiella pneumoniae," *Keimyung Med J*, vol. 31, 2012.

[9] W. M. Jay, M. Z. Aziz, J. P. Rissing, and R. K. Shockley, "Pharmacokinetic analysis of intravitreal ceftriaxone in monkeys," *Archives of Ophthalmology*, vol. 103, no. 1, pp. 121–123, 1985.

Accidental Intralenticular Injection of Ozurdex® for Branch Retinal Vein Occlusion: Intact Posterior Capsule and Resolution of Macular Edema

Ali Kurt,[1] **Ali Hakan Durukan**,[2] **and Murat Küçükevcilioğlu**[3]

[1]*Ahi Evran University Faculty of Medicine, Department of Ophthalmology, Turkey*
[2]*Health Sciences University Faculty of Medicine, Department of Ophthalmology, Turkey*
[3]*Gülhane Education and Research Hospital, Department of Ophthalmology, Turkey*

Correspondence should be addressed to Ali Kurt; dralikurt@gmail.com

Academic Editor: Stephen G. Schwartz

Purpose. We present a case of accidental intralenticular injection of Ozurdex implant in a patient with macular edema secondary to branch retinal vein occlusion. *Method*. A case report. *Results*. Intravitreal dexamethasone implant injection had been performed for macular edema due to left superior temporal vein branch occlusion to the left eye of a 78-year-old male patient. The slit-lamp examination 85 days later revealed that the dexamethasone implant was intralenticular. The best-corrected visual acuity (BCVA) was 0.16 on the Snellen chart. Cataract surgery was decided on for the cataract as there was no anterior chamber inflammation, the intraocular pressure (IOP) was normal, and the macular edema had resolved. Uneventful phacoemulsification within the bag intraocular lens placement was performed. *Conclusions*. Accidental intralenticular Ozurdex injection is an extremely rare complication. The surgeon must decide whether to continue to observe or intervene immediately when such a complication is encountered. Cataract surgery can be planned if the macular edema has resolved and a cataract has developed. It is important to evaluate the posterior capsule with ultrasound biomicroscopy and Scheimpflug imaging before the cataract surgery to ensure a safe surgical procedure.

1. Introduction

Retinal vein occlusion (RVO) is only surpassed by diabetic retinal disease as a retinal vascular disorder. The two main types are branch retinal vein occlusion (BRVO) and central retinal vein occlusion (CRVO). The main cause of decreased visual acuity with BRVO is the cystoid macular edema (CME) that develops in 30% of the cases [1]. Dexamethasone intravitreal implant (Ozurdex®; Allergan, Inc., Irvine, Calif., USA) has been approved by the Food and Drug Administration in the USA to treat the macular edema seen with RVO, in addition to central diabetic macular edema and noninfectious posterior uveitis [2].

Increased intraocular pressure (IOP) and the onset or progression of cataracts are the most common adverse ocular reactions with Ozurdex use [3]. However, there have also been increasing reports of accidental injection of Ozurdex into the crystalline lens [3–13]. Some authors feel expectant waiting is better [3, 4, 7, 10, 11] while others suggest immediate phacoemulsification (PE) for the cataract [5, 6, 13].

We present a case of accidental intralenticular Ozurdex implant injection where the macular edema recovered and was followed by uneventful PE.

1.1. Case Presentation. A hypertensive and diabetic 78-year-old male presented with decreased left visual acuity. There was a history of intravitreal Ozurdex implantation approximately 85 days ago for upper temporal RVO and CME. The best-corrected visual acuity (BCVA) was 0.16 on the Snellen chart and the IOP was 16 mmHg. Slit lamp examination revealed a Grade II nuclear cataract without anterior chamber inflammation and there was an intralenticular dexamethasone implant in the upper part of the lens (Figure 1(a)). Fundus examination revealed findings

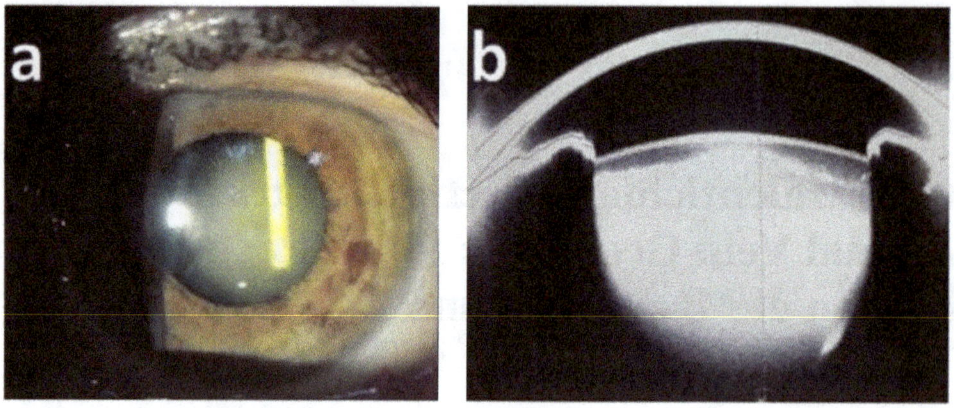

(a) (b)

FIGURE 1: (a) Slit lamp photograph showing the intralenticular Ozurdex implant. (b) Scheimpflug image showing the intralenticular Ozurdex implant together with the intact posterior capsule.

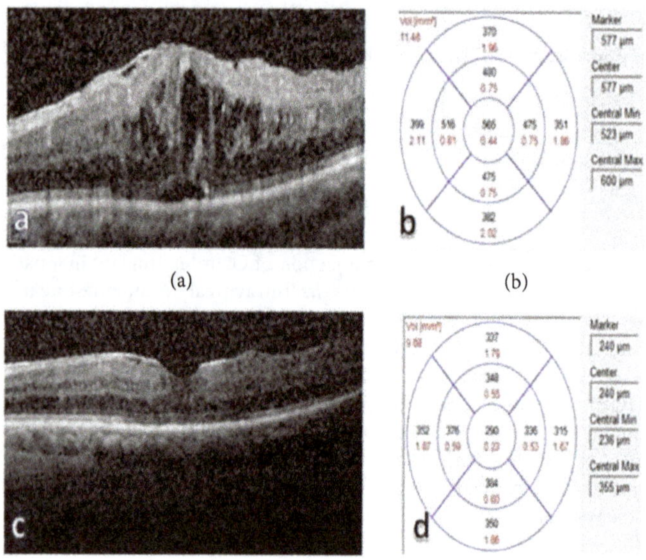

(a) (b)

(c) (d)

FIGURE 2: (a)-(b) Optical Coherence Tomography image showing the macular edema before Ozurdex injection (CMT: 565 μm). (c)-(d) Optical Coherence Tomography images 85 days after the following Ozurdex administration showing resolution of the macular edema (CMT: 290 μm).

secondary to upper temporal RVO. Scheimpflug photograph of the left eye showed the intralenticular Ozurdex implant with an intact posterior capsule (Figure 1(b)). Comparison of OCT images of the macular edema prior to Ozurdex injection (central macular thickness (CMT): 565 μm) (Figures 2(a) and 2(b)) and 85 days afterwards (CMT: 290 μm) demonstrated resolution of the edema (Figures 2(c) and 2(d)).

1.2. Surgical Procedure Outline. Anterior continuous curvilinear capsulorrhexis was performed using viscoelastic material protection (Figure 3(a)). The nucleus was rotated following gentle hydrodelineation and hydrodissection. The intralenticular Ozurdex implant rotated together with the nucleus (Figure 3(b)). After a groove was created with the phaco probe (Figure 3(c)), the nucleus, and Ozurdex implant were easily removed. The cortical remnants (Figure 3(d)) were removed with irrigation-aspiration. We observed that the posterior capsule was intact (Figure 3(e)). A hydrophopic acrylic three-piece IOL (Sensar AR40e; Abbott Medical Optics, Santa Ana, California, USA) was then placed inside the capsule using 1% sodium hyaluronate (Figure 3(f)).

2. Discussion

Ozurdex (Allergan Inc., Irvine, CA, USA) is a rod-shaped biodegradable dexamethasone (0.7 mg) implant that is 6 mm in length and 0.46 mm in diameter. It is injected into the vitreous cavity through a 22-gauge needle. The implant is

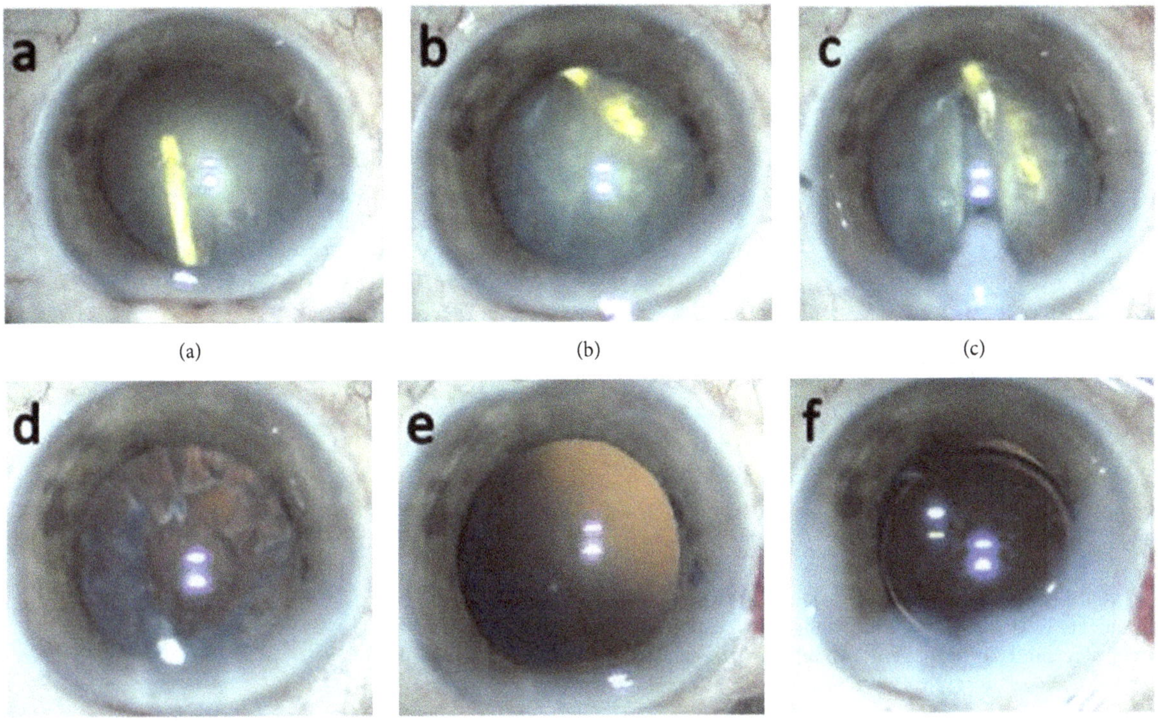

(a) (b) (c)

(d) (e) (f)

FIGURE 3: (a) Completed anterior continuous curvilinear capsulorrhexis, (b) image of intralenticular Ozurdex rotated with nucleus, (c) creating a groove with phaco probe, (d) cortical remnants, (e) image of intact posterior capsule, and (f) intraocular lens implantation.

injected into the mid-vitreous, 3.5 mm to 4 mm posterior to the limbus. The muzzle velocity has been calculated as 0.8 m/s [14]. There have been many case reports of accidental Ozurdex injection in the crystalline lens in recent years [3–13]. The contributing factors are thought to be lack of experience or inappropriate technique on the surgeon's part and uncontrolled head movement during the procedure by the patient [3].

Accelerated cataract development has been reported in some intralenticular Ozurdex implant administration cases [4–6], while other cases had increased IOP [8] or both these complications together [9, 10]. Poornachandra et al. [11] and Clemente-Tomás et al. [3] have reported no acceleration of cataract progression. Many authors [3, 4, 7, 10, 11] have found a gradual resolution of the macular edema with an intralenticular implant but Baskan et al. [12] found decreasing vision and no edema improvement. Coca-Robinot et al. [9] have observed very little effect of the intralenticular implant on the macular edema.

An intralenticular implant can be monitored in several different ways. The wait-and-see approach and later cataract surgery are used by most authors [3, 4, 7, 10, 11]. In contrast, some authors [5, 6, 13] suggest early removal of the implanted Ozurdex device with phacoemulsification, followed by repositioning within the vitreous, but this approach can have several disadvantages. First of all, the potential for fibrosis development at the posterior capsule tear is eliminated. It is also possible for the increased posterior capsule stress during phacoemulsification to enlarge the tear. The implant repositioning in the vitreus cavity can be difficult because of vitreus resistance. The implant can also become fragmented during repositioning in the vitreus cavity with altered drug absorption and increased glaucoma risk [15]. Another risk of this approach is the migration of the reinserted implant to the anterior chamber through the posterior capsule defect, resulting in corneal decompensation [2].

We presented a case of intralenticular Ozurdex implantation where the macular edema had resolved and a cataract had accelerated developed 85 days later without an increase in IOP, necessitating phacoemulsification. We believe the resolution of the macular edema in our case was due to the release of the drug in small amounts from the part of the implant that contacted the vitreus outside the capsule and attributed the uncomplicated phacoemulsification surgery and in the bag IOL implantation success to the closure of the posterior capsule with fibrosis at the implant entry point.

In conclusion, accidental intralenticular injection of Ozurdex is an extremely rare complication. However, the surgeon must decide on whether to wait and see or intervene immediately when confronted with such a case. The various factors that need to be taken into account are decreased visual acuity (due to cataract progression or the implant obstructing the visual axis), increased intraocular pressure, and the state of the macula. Cataract surgery may be necessary when the macular edema is resolved and a cataract has developed. We believe using ultrasound biomicroscopy and Scheimpflug imaging to evaluate the posterior capsule before cataract surgery if possible will make it easier to foresee the potential complications that may develop during phacoemulsification.

Consent

Informed consent was obtained from individual participant included in the case.

Disclosure

The authors alone are responsible for the content and writing of the paper.

References

[1] J. Li, Y. M. Paulus, Y. Shuai, W. Fang I, Q. Liu, and S. Yuan, "New developments in the classification, pathogenesis, risk factors, natural history, and treatment of branch retinal vein occlusion," *Journal of Ophthalmology*, vol. 2017, Article ID 4936924, 18 pages, 2017.

[2] R. N. Khurana, S. N. Appa, C. A. McCannel et al., "Dexamethasone implant anterior chamber migration: Risk factors, complications, and management strategies," *Ophthalmology*, vol. 121, no. 1, pp. 67–71, 2014.

[3] R. Clemente-Tomás, D. Hernández-Pérez, P. Neira-Ibáñez et al., "Intracrystalline Ozurdex®: therapeutic effect maintained for 18 months," *International Ophthalmology*, pp. 1-5, 2017.

[4] K. A. Regan, C. R. Blake, Z. L. Lukowski, and S. S. R. Iyer, "Intralenticular ozurdex® - One year later," *Case Reports in Ophthalmology*, vol. 8, no. 3, pp. 590–594, 2017.

[5] F. Fasce, M. Battaglia Parodi, K. A. Knutsson et al., "Accidental injection of dexamethasone intravitreal implant in the crystalline lens," *Acta Ophthalmologica*, vol. 92, no. 4, pp. e330–e331, 2014.

[6] K. Chalioulias and M. M. K. Muqit, "Vitreoretinal surgery for inadvertent intralenticular Ozurdex implant," *Eye (Basingstoke)*, vol. 28, no. 12, pp. 1523-1524, 2014.

[7] M. A. Sekeroglu, M. A. Anayol, F. Koc, H. Tirhis, S. S. Ozkan, and P. Yilmazbas, "Intralenticular sustained-release dexamethasone implant: Is it still effective on macular edema," *Case Reports in Ophthalmology*, vol. 7, no. 1, pp. 85–89, 2016.

[8] K. Lee, A. Park, S. Jang, and Y.-R. Chung, "Elevation of intraocular pressure after inadvertent dexamethasone implant injection into the lens," *Canadian Journal of Ophthalmology*, vol. 51, no. 3, pp. e103–e105, 2016.

[9] J. Coca-Robinot, B. Casco-Silva, F. Armadá-Maresca, and J. García-Martínez, "Accidental injections of dexamethasone intravitreal implant (Ozurdex®) into the crystalline lens," *European Journal of Ophthalmology*, vol. 24, no. 4, pp. 633–636, 2014.

[10] R. Chhabra, K. Kopsidas, and S. Mahmood, "Accidental insertion of dexamethasone implant into the crystalline lens - 12 months follow-up," *Eye (Basingstoke)*, vol. 28, no. 5, pp. 624-625, 2014.

[11] B. Poornachandra, V. M. B. Kumar, C. Jayadev, S. H. Dorelli, N. K. Yadav, and R. Shetty, "Immortal Ozurdex: A 10-month follow-up of an intralenticular implant," *Indian Journal of Ophthalmology*, vol. 65, no. 3, pp. 255–257, 2017.

[12] B. Baskan, A. Cıcek, A. Gulhan, M. Gundogan, and S. Goktas, "Ozurdex completely located inside a crystallized lens - Results of 14 months," *American Journal of Ophthalmology Case Reports*, vol. 4, pp. 38–40, 2016.

[13] M. Munteanu and C. Rosca, "Repositioning and follow-up of intralenticular dexamethasone implant," *Journal of Cataract & Refractive Surgery*, vol. 39, no. 8, pp. 1271–1274, 2013.

[14] C. H. Meyer, A. Klein, F. Alten et al., "Release and velocity of micronized dexamethasone implants with an intravitreal drug delivery system: kinematic analysis with a high-speed camera," *Retina*, vol. 32, no. 10, pp. 2133–2140, 2012.

[15] R. Roy and S. Hegde, "Split Ozurdex implant: A caution," *Canadian Journal of Ophthalmology*, vol. 48, no. 1, pp. e15–e16, 2013.

35

Successful Technique for Closure of Macular Hole Retinal Detachment using Autologous Retinal Transplant

Juan Abel Ramirez-Estudillo[1] **Geovanni Rios-Nequis**[1] **Martin Jimenez-Rodríguez**[1] **Hugo Valdez-Flores**[1] **and Ximena Ramirez-Galicia**[2]

[1]*Retina Department, Fundacion Hospital Nuestra Señora De La Luz IAP, Mexico*
[2]*Research Department, Faculty of Medicine, Universidad La Salle, Mexico*

Correspondence should be addressed to Martin Jimenez-Rodríguez; martinretina@icloud.com

Academic Editor: Claudio Campa

Macular hole retinal detachment (MHRD) for the most part develops in highly myopic eyes. Several surgical methods have been introduced to treat MHRD. We describe our experience with the autologous retinal transplant in patient with MHRD. A 49-year-old female presented with a 2-week history of a sudden decrease in the central vision in the right eye (RE). A 3-port, 25-gauge pars plana vitrectomy was performed with the ILM dye staining and peeling. Endodiathermy was applied around a 1.5-disc diameter neurosensory donor site in the supertemporal retina. The graft was cut with standard 25-gauge curved scissors. Perfluoro-n-octane (PFO) was instilled. The free graft was gently handled until its packing into the macular hole. Two months following the initial PPV, the macular hole was closed, and vision improved from 0.05 to 0.25 logMAR.

1. Introduction

Macular hole retinal detachment (MHRD) mostly develops in highly myopic eyes. Since Gonvers and Machemer reported using pars plana vitrectomy (PPV) and gas tamponade in 1982 [1], several surgical methods have been introduced to treat MHRD, such as macular buckling, vitrectomy, and gas or silicon oil tamponade fluid with internal limiting membrane (ILM), inverted ILM flap technique, and scleral imbrication [1–6]. In recent years, the autologous neurosensory retinal transplant has been considered like a surgical technique in the treatment for closure of the refractory macular hole. We describe our case with the autologous retinal transplant in patient with MHRD.

2. Case Presentation

A 49-year-old female presented with a 2-week history of a sudden decrease in the central vision in the right eye (RE). The patient had no significant history of systemic disease. At her initial visit, the best corrected visual acuity (BCVA) was 0.05 logMAR in her RE and 1.00 logMAR in her left eye. The slit-lamp examination of the anterior segment and intraocular pressure were normal, and the lens status was phakic of both eyes. A fundus examination revealed macular hole retinal detachment in her RE, lattice degeneration, and atrophic holes were found.

The surgery was performed under general anaesthesia, and we elected to use no. 41 circumferential scleral buckle owing to the fact that another predisposal lesions were found

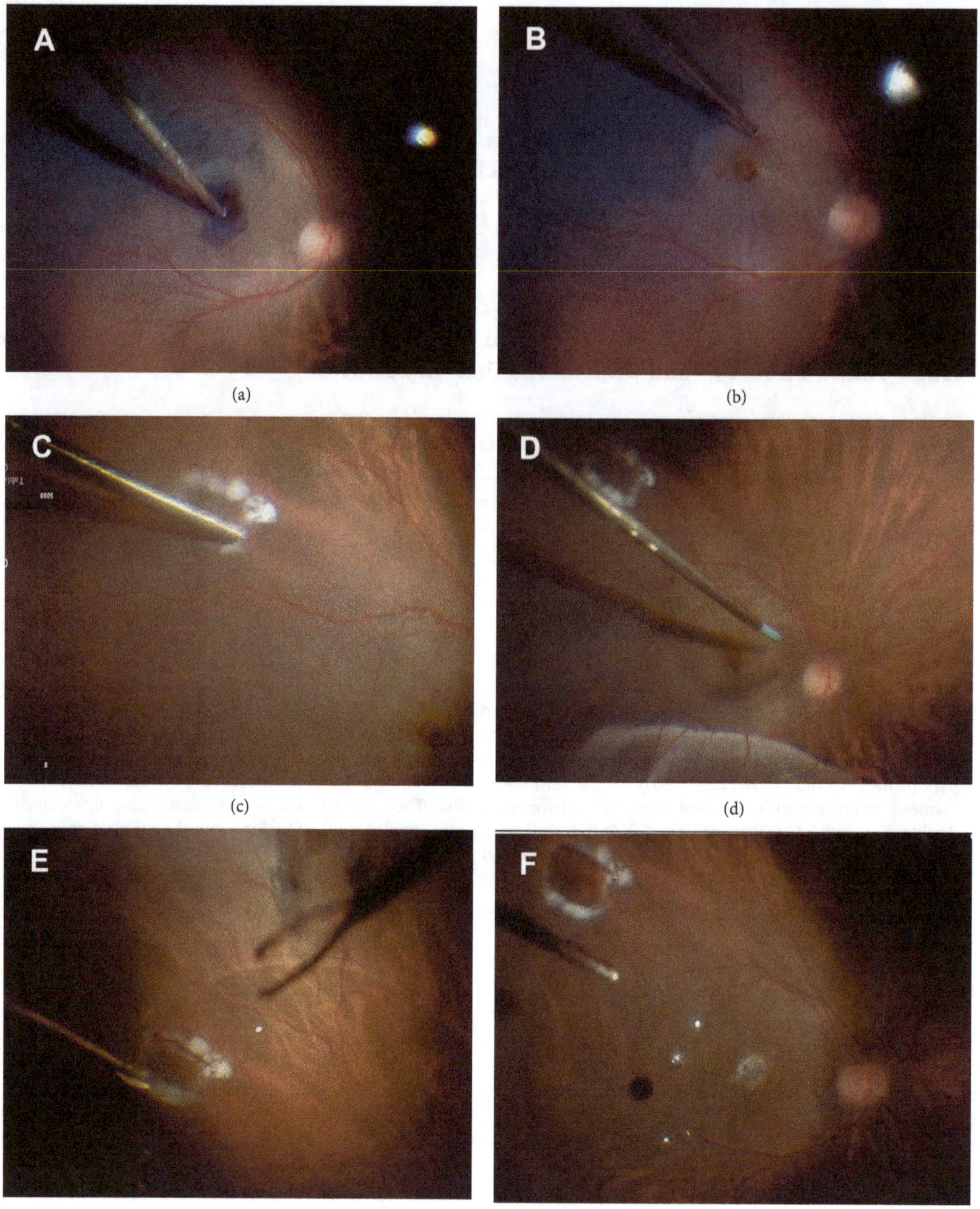

(a) (b) (c) (d) (e) (f)

Figure 1: Continued.

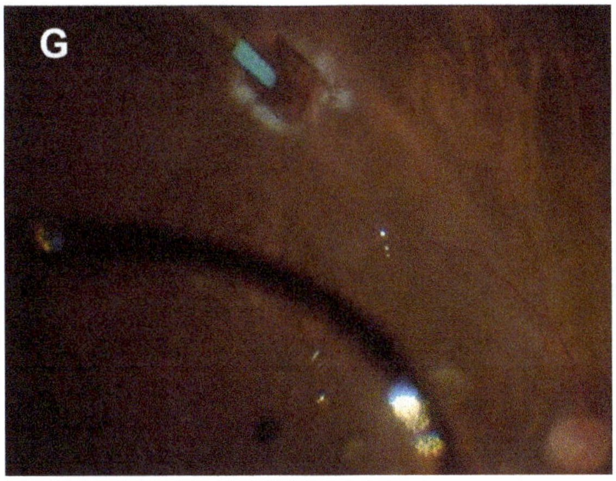

(g)

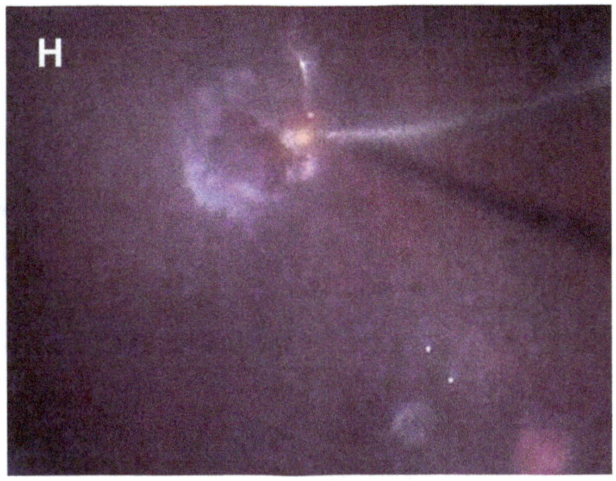

(h)

FIGURE 1: (a) Intraoperative digital photography showing subretinal migration of brilliant blue during dye staining. (b) The internal limiting membrane has been removed and is grasped with the vitreous forceps. Notice the absence of blue coloration at the macular area at the region of internal limiting membrane ablation. (c) Endodiathermy was applied around a 1.5-disc diameter neurosensory retina. (d) Injection of the perfluoro-n-octane in the retinal interface. (e) The graft cuts were linear, being a square graft. (f) Image showing free graft packing inside the macular hole. (g) A fluid air exchange was performed, and subretinal fluid was extracted through the area where the graft was taken. (h) Laser around the area where the graft was taken.

in the inferior retina. A standard vitrectomy equipment (Constellation, Alcon Surgical, Ft. Worth, TX), Lumera 700 microscope (Carl Zeiss Germany) and NGENUITY 3D visualization system (Alcon Surgical, Ft. Worth, TX) were used. A 3-port, 25-gauge PPV was performed; after posterior hyaloid detachment, the ILM was dyed (TissueBlue, DORC). The ILM peeling was performed on the detached retina in a circular fashion, pulling off approximately 1.0 disk diameters of ILM centered on the foveal defect. We should mention that subretinal migration of brilliant blue was detected; opportunely, when the dye was aspirated, part of the subretinal fluid came out at the same time with the dye (Figure 1). Peripheral vitrectomy with indentation was done before taking the graft.

Endodiathermy was applied around a 1.5-disc diameter neurosensory donor site. The harvest location was selected in the more bullous zone of the retina (superior and temporal) in order to avoid touching the choroid. The graft was cut with standard 25-gauge curved scissors to approximately 90% of its final size to keep the tissue stable.

Perfluoro-n-octane (PFO) was instilled to completely cover the donor site, the free graft was teared and manipulated into the correct position using end grasping forceps, and the tissue was gently handled until packing it into the macular hole.

A fluid air exchange was performed, and subretinal fluid was extracted through the area where the graft was taken. Laser endophotocoagulation was applied as retinopexy in the donor site and the predisposal lesions, and 5000 centistoke silicone oil was used as tamponade to the finish the surgery.

One day after the surgery, the retinal was completely attached, and the free graft stayed inside in the macular hole. Two months following the initial PPV, the macular hole was closed, and the optical coherent tomography (OCT) showed integration of the retinal flap and partial restoration of the internal plexiform layer (Figure 2). Best corrected visual acuity improved to 0.25 logMAR at 2 months of the surgery.

3. Discussion

The coexistent macular hole was described in approximately 1% to 4% of cases of rhegmatogenous retinal detachment. According to the pathological mechanisms, several surgical methods have been introduced to the treatment and the retinal reattachment rate ranged from 40% to 90% [7–10], but the macular hole closure rate was lower, approximately 40% (range 35%-70%) [10]. In 2015, the technique involving the use of an autologous neurosensory retinal free flap for closure of the refractory myopic macular hole was described (MH) [11]; since then, several series have been published that mentions the complete anatomical closure of MH by OCT can reach up to 87.8%.

In this case, single surgery achieved the retina reattachment and MH closure. Although this type or surgery has been referred [12], the technique with detached retina has not described formerly. The presence of retinal detachment was not a problem for the management of free graft of the neurosensory retina; in fact, in our opinion, the subretinal fluid due to retinal detachment facilitated the harvest by maintaining the neurosensory retina separate from the retinal pigment epithelium and helps avoiding touching the choroid instead of developing an hydraulic retinal detachment with the aid of a 38 or 41G syringe that can cause subretinal hemorrhage under the graft or subretinal blood migration

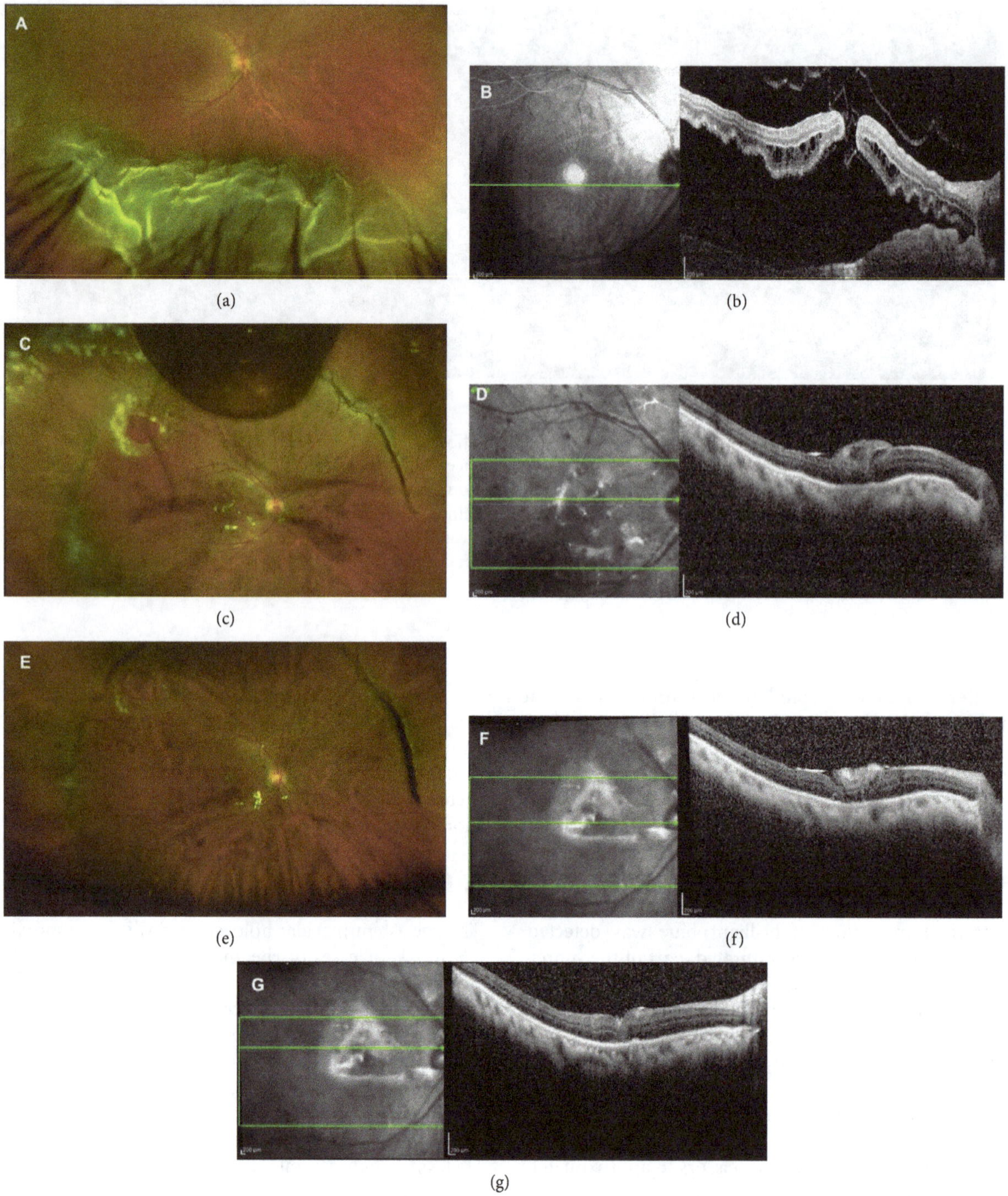

Figure 2: (a) Fundus photo RE shows macular hole retinal detachment. (b) Preoperative optical coherence tomography (OCT) demonstrates macular detachment with full-thickness macular hole. (c) One day after surgery, the foveal contour had improved by the free graft. (d) OCT postop 1 day and the hyperreflective retinal flap are visualized in place over the MH. (e) Color photograph of the fundus of the right eye two months after the autologous retina transplant shows retina reattachment. (f) One month postoperatively, there was significant integration of the retinal flap with improved architecture of the inner retinal layers, and some hyperreflective lines show the graft.(g) At 2 months postoperatively, there was significant integration of the retinal flap.

causing toxicity. 5000 centistoke silicon oil was used because the patient was not able to stay in the city; aside, it allowed us to keep up the graft by OCT image with better quality than SF6 bubble.

4. Conclusions

According to the evolution of this case, we believe it is possible to initiate a series of patients with this technique in order to consider autologous retinal transplant as a first therapeutic possibility in the retinal detachment associated with a macular hole.

Disclosure

The research did not receive any specific funding, although the Hospital Nuestra Señora de la Luz allowed its facilities for exploration, surgery, and patient monitoring.

References

[1] M. Gonvers and R. Machemer, "A new approach to treating retinal detachment with macular hole," *American Journal of Ophthalmology*, vol. 94, no. 4, pp. 468–472, 1982.

[2] F. Ando, "Use of a special macular explant in surgery for retinal detachment with macular hole," *Japanese Journal of Ophthalmology*, vol. 24, pp. 29–34, 1980.

[3] E. H. Ryan, C. T. Bramante, R. A. Mittra et al., "Management of rhegmatogenous retinal detachment with coexistent macular hole in the era of internal limiting membrane peeling," *American Journal of Ophthalmology*, vol. 152, no. 5, pp. 815–819.e1, 2011.

[4] Z. Michalewska, J. Michalewski, R. A. Adelman, and J. Nawrocki, "Inverted internal limiting membrane flap technique for large macular holes," *Ophthalmology*, vol. 117, no. 10, pp. 2018–2025, 2010.

[5] E. Ortisi, T. Avitabile, and V. Bonfiglio, "Surgical management of retinal detachment because of macular hole in highly myopic eyes," *Retina*, vol. 32, no. 9, pp. 1704–1718, 2012.

[6] Z. Hu, X. Gu, H. Qian et al., "Perfluorocarbon liquid-assisted inverted limiting membrane flap technique combined with subretinal fluid drainage for macular hole retinal detachment in highly myopic eyes," *Retina*, vol. 10, no. 2, pp. 140–144, 2016.

[7] C.-C. Lai, Y.-P. Chen, N.-K. Wang et al., "Vitrectomy with internal limiting membrane repositioning and autologous blood for macular hole retinal detachment in highly myopic eyes," *Ophthalmology*, vol. 122, no. 9, pp. 1889–1898, 2015.

[8] X. Li, W. Wang, S. Tang, and J. Zhao, "Gas injection versus vitrectomy with gas for treating retinal detachment owing to macular hole in high myopes," *Ophthalmology*, vol. 116, no. 6, pp. 1182–1187.e1, 2009.

[9] L. S. Lim, A. Tsai, D. Wong et al., "Prognostic factor analysis of vitrectomy for retinal detachment associated with myopic macular holes," *Ophthalmology*, vol. 121, no. 1, pp. 305–310, 2014.

[10] F. U. M. I. T. A. K. A. ANDO, N. O. R. I. O. OHBA, K. O. U. TOUURA, and H. I. R. O. S. H. I. HIROSE, "ANATOMICAL AND VISUAL OUTCOMES AFTER EPISCLERAL MACULAR BUCKLING COMPARED WITH THOSE AFTER PARS PLANA VITRECTOMY FOR RETINAL DETACHMENT CAUSED BY MACULAR HOLE IN HIGHLY MYOPIC EYES," *Retina*, vol. 27, no. 1, pp. 37–44, 2007.

[11] D. S. Grewal and T. H. Mahmoud, "Autologous Neurosensory Retinal Free Flap for Closure of Refractory Myopic Macular Holes," *JAMA Ophthalmology*, vol. 134, no. 2, pp. 229-230, 2016.

[12] D. S. Grewal, S. Charles, B. Parolini, K. Kadonosono, and T. H. Mahmoud, "Autologous retinal transplant for refractory macular holes: multicenter international collaborative study group," *Ophthalmology*, vol. 126, no. 10, pp. 1399–1408, 2019.

36

Surgical Outcomes in Macular Telangiectasia Type 2-Related Macular Holes: A Report on Four Patients

Kinza T. Ahmad, Joseph Chacko, Ahmed B. Sallam, David B. Warner, and Sami H. Uwaydat

Jones Eye Institute, University of Arkansas for Medical Sciences, 4301 W. Markham St. Little Rock, AR 72205, USA

Correspondence should be addressed to Sami H. Uwaydat; shuwaydat@uams.edu

Academic Editor: Stephen G. Schwartz

Introduction. The few published studies that exist on the surgical outcomes of full-thickness macular hole (FTMH) repair in Macular Telangiectasia (MacTel) Type 2 report poor rates of hole closure of around 30%. This study is the largest case series of patients with FTMH in MacTel Type 2 and describes an 80% hole closure rate. *Purpose/Aim.* To describe the outcomes of four patients who underwent surgery for FTMH associated with MacTel Type 2. *Methods.* A retrospective review of clinical, surgical, and imaging data of five eyes in four patients with MacTel Type 2 FTMH who underwent pars plana vitrectomy (PPV) with internal limiting membrane (ILM) peeling and 30% SF_6 or 15% C_3F_8 gas tamponade within 3-9 months of initial vision decline. *Results.* Visual acuity (VA) at the time of surgery ranged from 20/50 to 20/200. Successful hole closure was achieved in four out of five eyes, and final VA ranged from 20/20 to 20/40 at follow-up visits greater than 20 months postoperatively. The single eye that did not achieve hole closure had a final VA of 20/60. *Conclusion.* Our case series describes higher hole closure rates and better final VA than previously published reports for macular hole surgery in patients with MacTel Type 2 FTMH.

1. Introduction

Macular Telangiectasia (MacTel) Type 2 is an idiopathic bilateral foveal degeneration characterized by neurosensory atrophy and changes in the macular capillary network [1]. Clinical findings include angiographic perifoveal vascular leakage, telangiectatic vessels more prominent in the temporal macula, and cystic foveal changes. Full-thickness macular holes (FTMH) in MacTel Type 2 are rare and can be seen at any stage [2]. Given the rarity of FTMH in MacTel Type 2, few published studies exist on the surgical outcomes of these patients. Existing studies have reported that pars plana vitrectomy (PPV) in this setting has a guarded prognosis with a closure rate of about 25-30% [2–7]. In this series, we report successful surgical outcomes of PPV for FTMH in 5 eyes (4 patients) with angiographically confirmed MacTel Type 2. We also report on the postoperative angiographic findings that show persistent vascular leakage following hole closure.

2. Methods

We conducted a retrospective review of the clinical, surgical, and imaging data of 5 eyes in 4 patients who underwent surgery for FTMH associated with MacTel Type 2 at the University of Arkansas for Medical Sciences Hospital in Little Rock, AR. Each eye underwent PPV with indocyanine green- (ICG-) assisted internal limiting membrane (ILM) peeling, gas tamponade, and one week of strict prone positioning. All vitrectomies were performed by one surgeon (SHU). Eyes were evaluated at various time points with fundus photographs, fluorescein angiography (FA), optical coherence tomography (OCT), and OCT-angiography (OCT-A) imaging.

TABLE 1: Summary table of patient characteristics, surgical methods, and outcomes of patients with FTMH associated with MacTel Type 2.

	Case 1 OD	Case 1 OS	Case 2 OD	Case 3 OS	Case 4 OD
Age (years)	62	62	71	65	57
Gender	Female	Female	Male	Female	Female
Preoperative BCVA	20/80	20/80	20/50	20/200	20/60
Time from symptom onset to surgery	1 month	3 months	4 months	9 months	Unknown
Macular hole size (μm)					
Diameter	410	246	225	184	493
Maximum height	426	424	340	403	309
Posterior vitreous detachment	Yes	Yes	No	No	No
Surgical procedure	PPV, ICG-assisted ILM peeling, cataract surgery done at the time of PPV	PPV, ICG-assisted ILM peeling, cataract surgery done at the time of PPV	PPV, ICG-assisted ILM peeling	PPV, ICG-assisted ILM peeling	PPV, ICG-assisted ILM peeling, cataract surgery done 1 month prior to PPV
Tamponading agent	30% SF_6	30% SF_6	30% SF_6	30% SF_6	15% C_3F_8
Positioning, duration	Prone, 1 week	Prone, 1 week	Prone, 1 week	Prone, 1 week	Prone, 1 week
Anatomical hole closure	Closed hole	Closed hole	Closed hole	Closed hole	Not closed
EZ and ELM integrity on most recent OCT	Yes	Yes	Yes	Yes	No
BCVA at last follow-up	20/25	20/20	20/20-1	20/40-1	20/60
Length of follow-up	26 months	37 months	21 months	35 months	22 months

PPV: pars plana vitrectomy; ILM: internal limiting membrane; ICG: indocyanine green; EZ: ellipsoid zone; ELM: external limiting membrane; BCVA: best corrected visual acuity; SF_6: sulfur hexafluoride; C_3F_8: perfluoropropane.

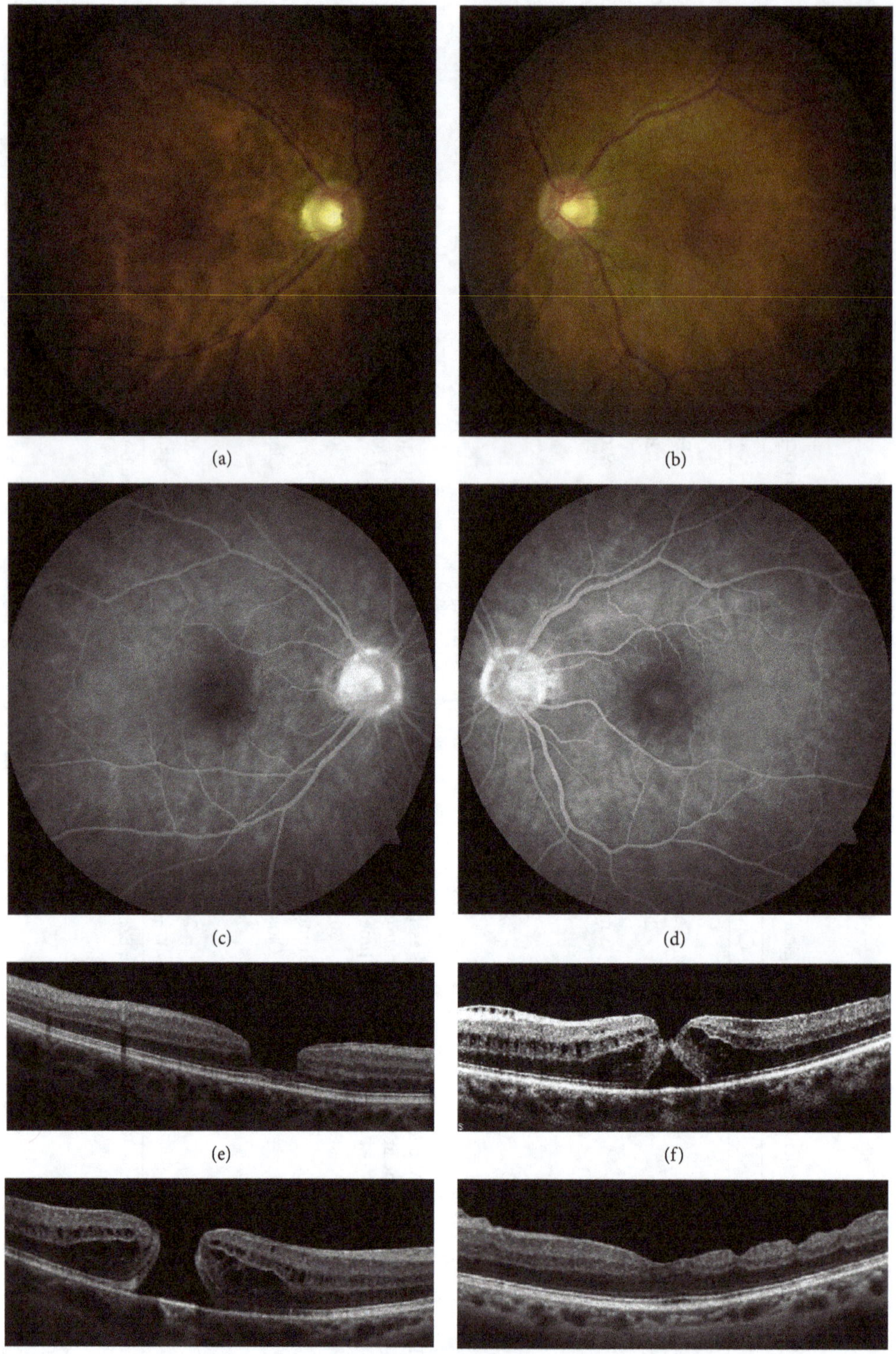

(a) (b)

(c) (d)

(e) (f)

(g) (h)

Figure 1: Continued.

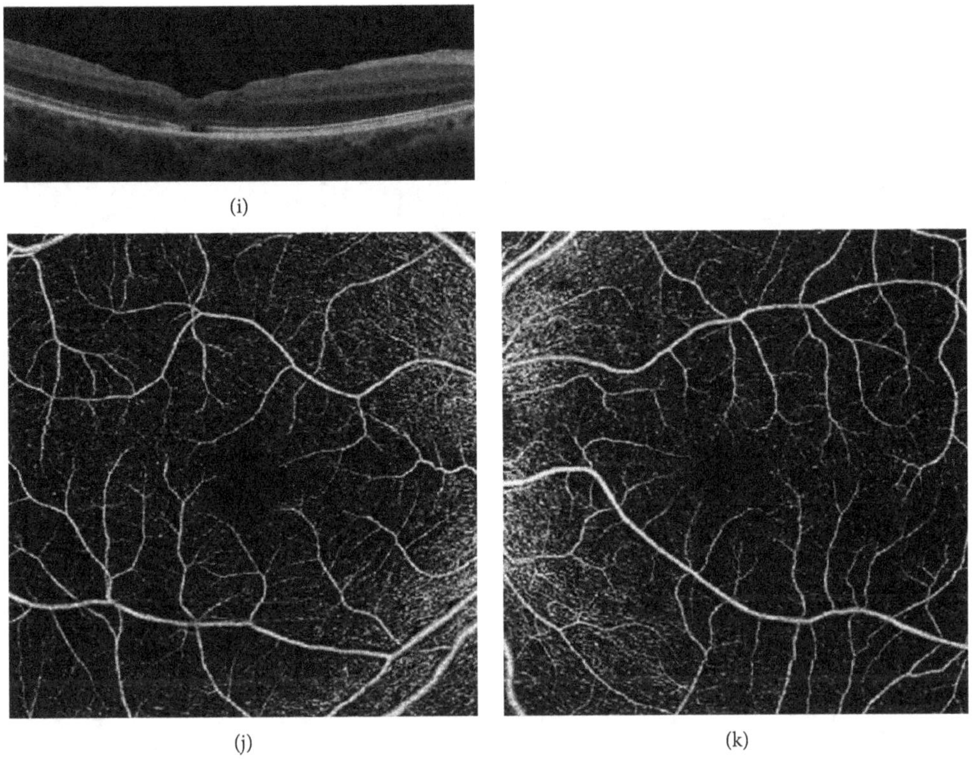

FIGURE 1: Case 1. Fundus image (a, b) and FA (c, d) show features consistent with MacTel Type 2 in both eyes. Preoperative OCT at initial presentation shows foveal thinning with outer neurosensory atrophy OD (e) and a full-thickness macular hole (FTMH) OS (f). The right eye developed a FTMH at a later visit (g). Later, postoperative OCT of each eye shows complete hole closure in each eye (h, i). Postop OCT-A photos in the right eye show areas of capillary dropout in the superficial bed (j) and in the left eye show telangiectasias in the superficial capillary bed temporal to the fovea with areas of capillary dropout (k).

3. Case Presentations

The characteristics, surgical methods, and outcomes of the cases are summarized in Table 1.

3.1. Case 1. A 62-year-old woman presented with a three-month history of blurry vision in her left eye. On examination, her best corrected visual acuity (BCVA) was 20/30 in the right eye and 20/80 in the left eye. Anterior segment evaluation revealed a 2+ nuclear sclerotic cataract (NSC) in both eyes. On fundus examination, there was a loss of the foveal reflex in the right eye and a FTMH in the left eye (Figures 1(a) and 1(b)). OCT showed significant foveal thinning with outer neurosensory atrophy in the right eye (Figure 1(e)) and a FTMH with an associated epiretinal membrane (ERM) in the left eye (Figure 1(f)). Fluorescein angiography was significant for mild leakage temporal to the fovea in both eyes with a window defect corresponding to the macular hole in the left eye (Figure 1(d)). The OCT and FA findings were consistent with the diagnosis of MacTel Type 2. The patient underwent a 23-gauge PPV with ERM/ILM peeling and injection of 30% SF_6, combined with phacoemulsification and intraocular lens (IOL) implantation. Strict prone positioning was maintained for 5 days postoperatively. At the 2-week postoperative visit, closure of the macular hole was confirmed by OCT (Figure 1(h)). The hole remained closed at her most recent visit 37 months postop with a BCVA of 20/20.

The patient presented 10 months following surgery on her left eye with a 2-week history of vision loss in the right eye. The vision had dropped to 20/80, and OCT confirmed the presence of a FTMH (Figure 1(g)). She again underwent phacoemulsification with IOL implantation and PPV with ILM peeling and 30% SF_6 gas tamponade in the right eye approximately 4 weeks after presentation. Postoperative closure of the macular hole was confirmed by OCT 4 days after surgery. The hole remained closed on her most recent follow-up visit 26 months after surgery with the BCVA stable at 20/25 (Figure 1(i)). A postoperative OCT-A photo of the right eye shows areas of capillary dropout in the superficial bed (Figure 1(j)) and in the left eye shows telangiectasias in the superficial capillary bed temporal to the fovea with areas of capillary dropout (Figure 1(k)); these are persistent vascular anomalies associated with MacTel Type 2 that have been described in the literature [8].

3.2. Case 2. A 71-year-old man presented with a few months history of decreased vision in the right eye. BCVA was 20/50 OD and 20/40 OS. Anterior segment examination was significant for 2+ NSC in both eyes. Fundus examination revealed a macular hole in the right eye with pigment clumps temporal to the hole and a lamellar hole in the left macula with intraretinal crystals (Figures 2(a) and 2(b)). OCT confirmed the presence of a full-thickness macular hole in the right eye and a lamellar hole in the left (Figures 2(e) and 2(f)). FA showed leakage temporal to the fovea in both eyes with

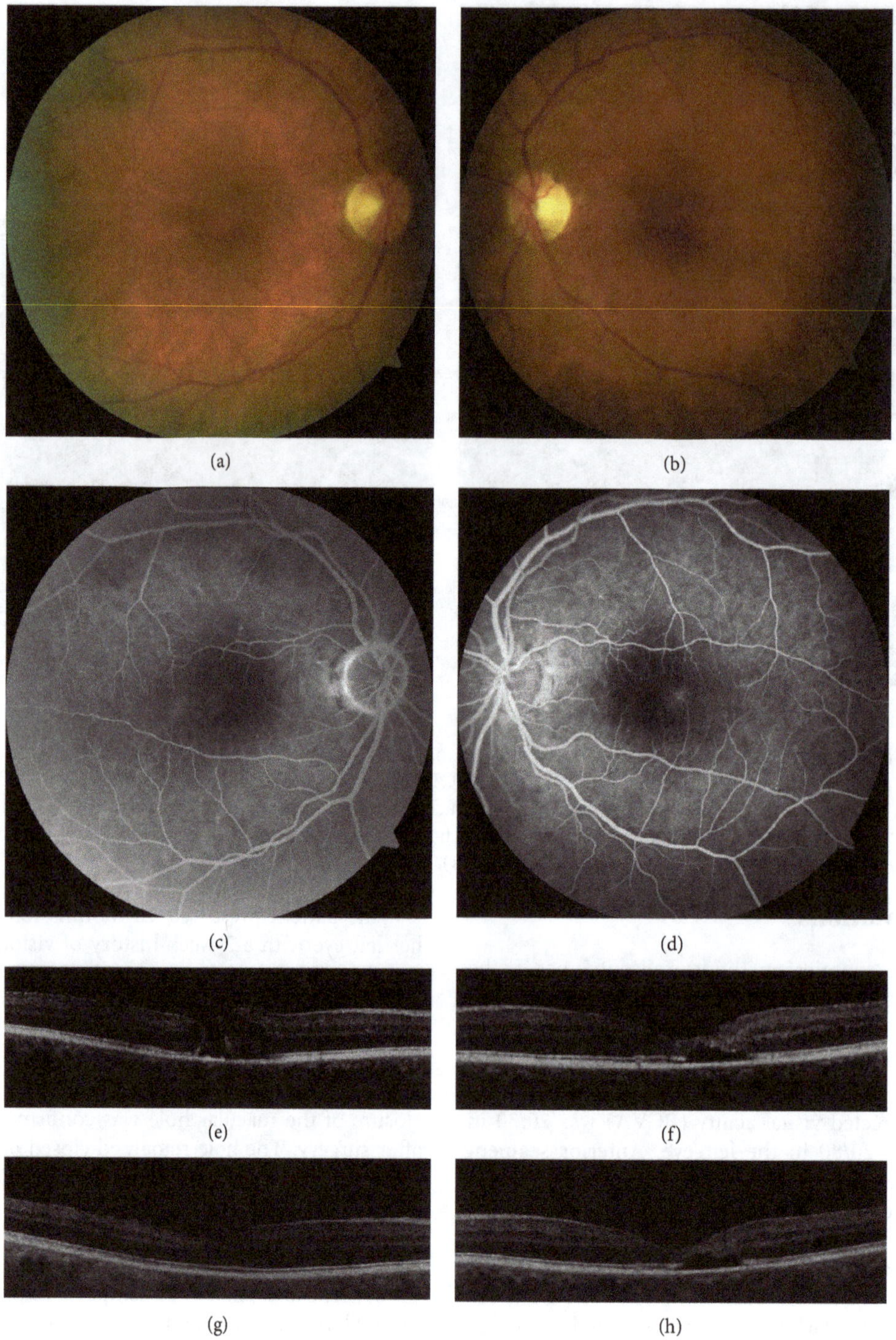

Figure 2: Continued.

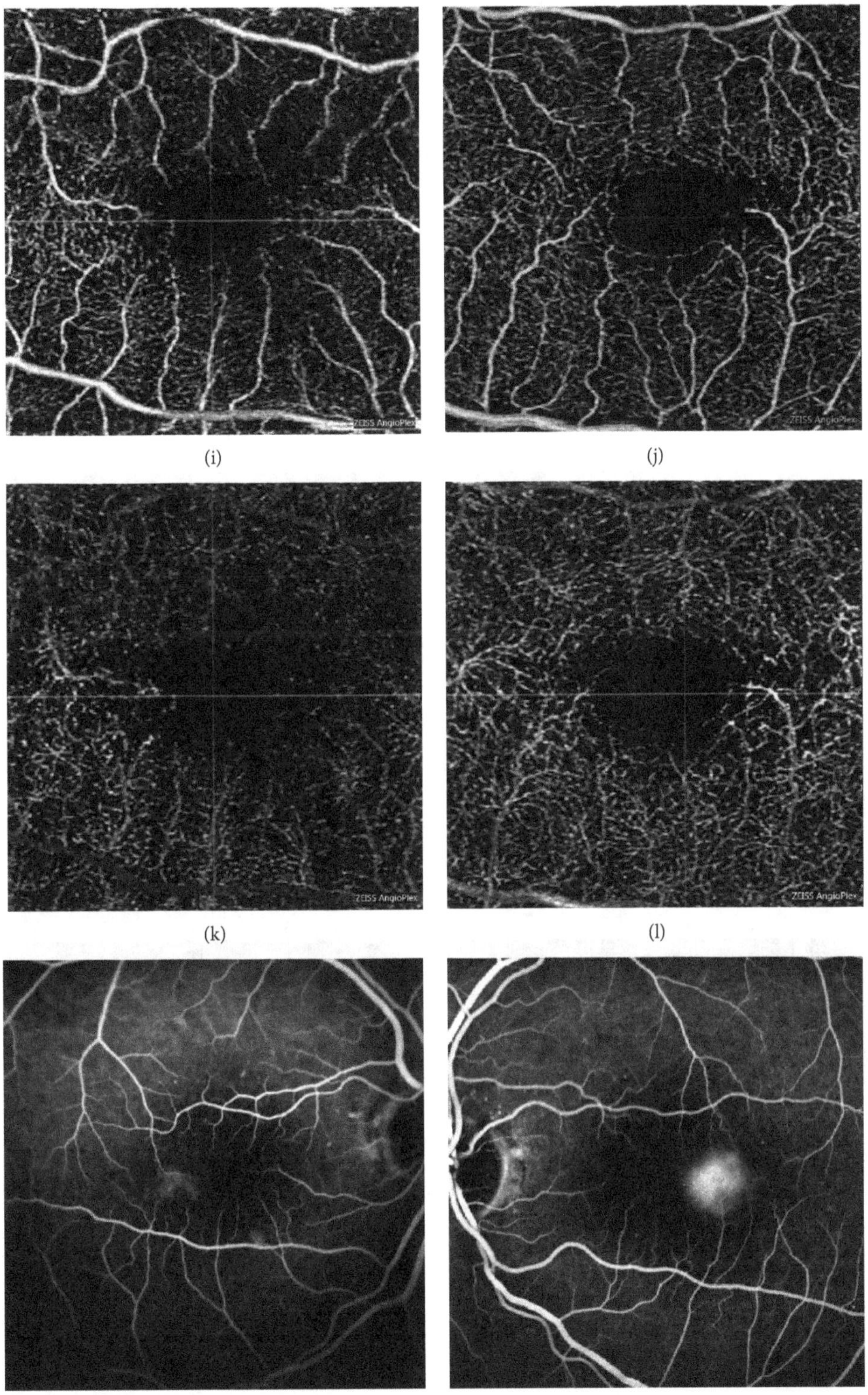

FIGURE 2: Case 2. Fundus image (a, b) and FA (c, d) show loss of the foveal reflex with hyperfluorescence temporal to the fovea in both eyes. On presentation, OCT shows a FTMH in the right eye with intraretinal cysts and loss of the outer foveal layers in the left eye (e, f). Postoperative OCT of the right eye shows a closed macular hole (g). OCT of the left eye demonstrates a stable lamellar hole (f, h). Postop OCT-A shows right-angled venules and FAZ irregularity as well as significant telangiectasias of the deep vascular network with reduced vascular density (i–l). Postoperative FA shows persistent hyperfluorescence temporal to the fovea (m, n).

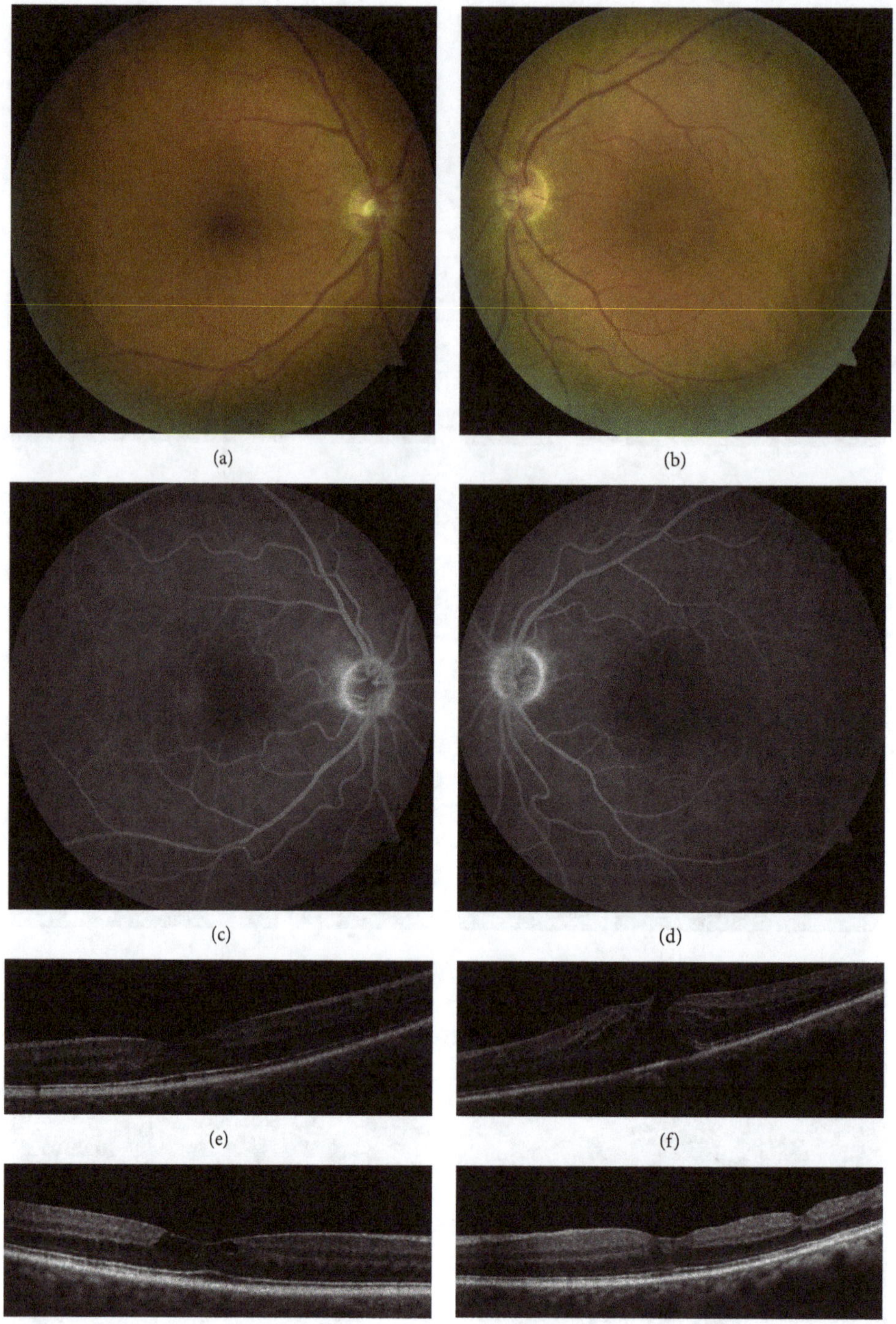

FIGURE 3: Continued.

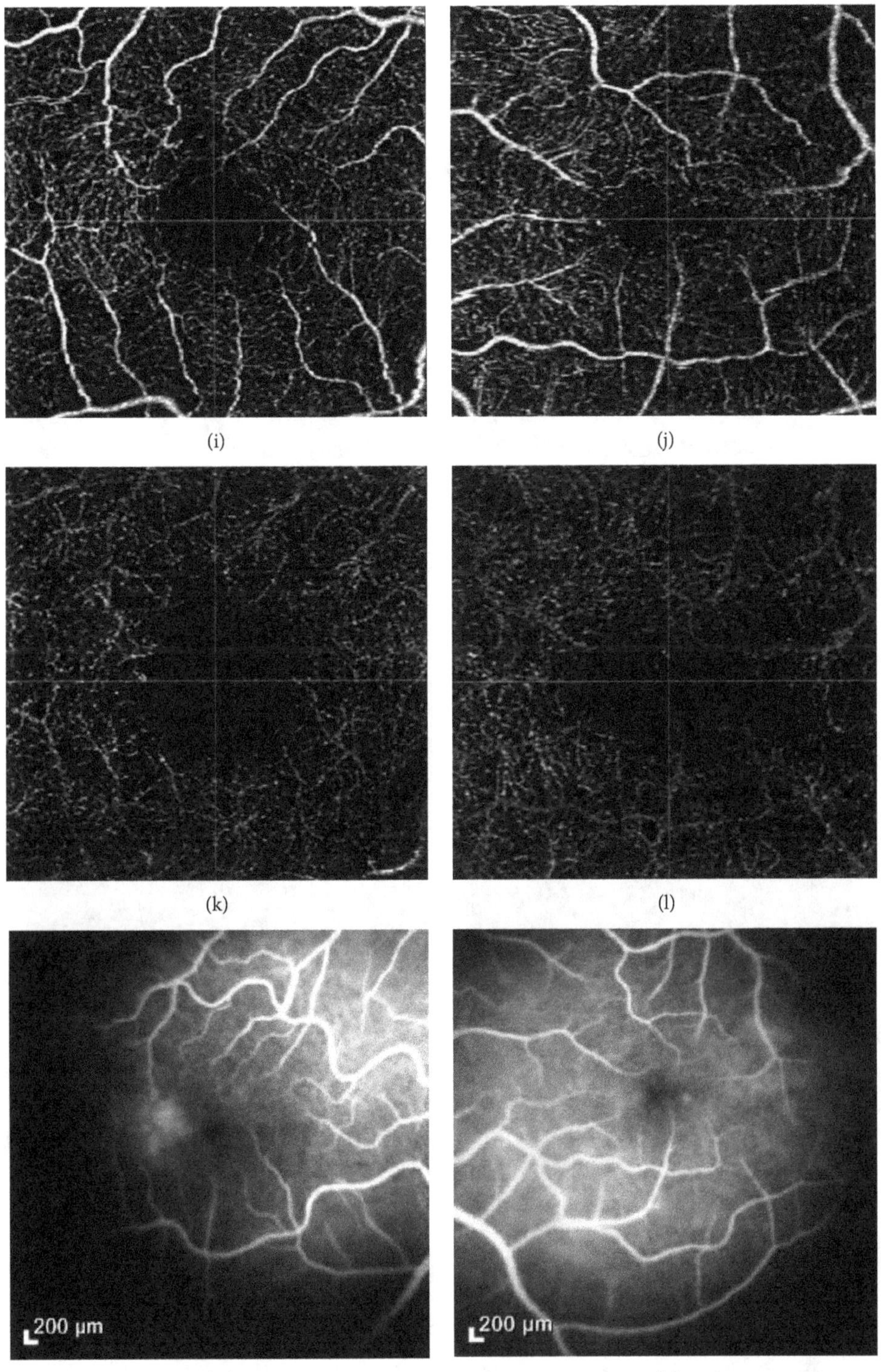

FIGURE 3: Case 3. Fundus image (a, b) and FA (c, d) show features typical of MacTel Type 2 with leakage temporal to the fovea in both eyes. On presentation, OCT (e, f) shows a FTMH in the left eye and some intraretinal cysts in the right eye. Postoperatively, OCT of the left eye (h) shows a closed macular hole. OCT-A of both eyes (i–l) demonstrates telangiectatic vessels, right-angled venules, and enlarged FAZ, with capillary bed closure temporal to the fovea. Postoperative FA of both eyes shows persistent leakage temporally (m, n).

a window defect in the fovea of the right eye (Figures 2(c) and 2(d)). The diagnosis of MacTel Type 2 was made in both eyes. Four weeks after presentation, a 23-gauge PPV with ILM peeling and fluid-gas exchange with 30% SF_6 was performed and prone positioning was maintained for 5 days. On the fifth postoperative day, OCT confirmed the closure of the macular hole. Cataract extraction was performed 7 months after PPV at another facility. Twenty-one months after PPV, the macular hole in the right eye remained closed (Figure 2(g)) and BCVA was 20/20-1. In the left eye, the lamellar hole remained stable.

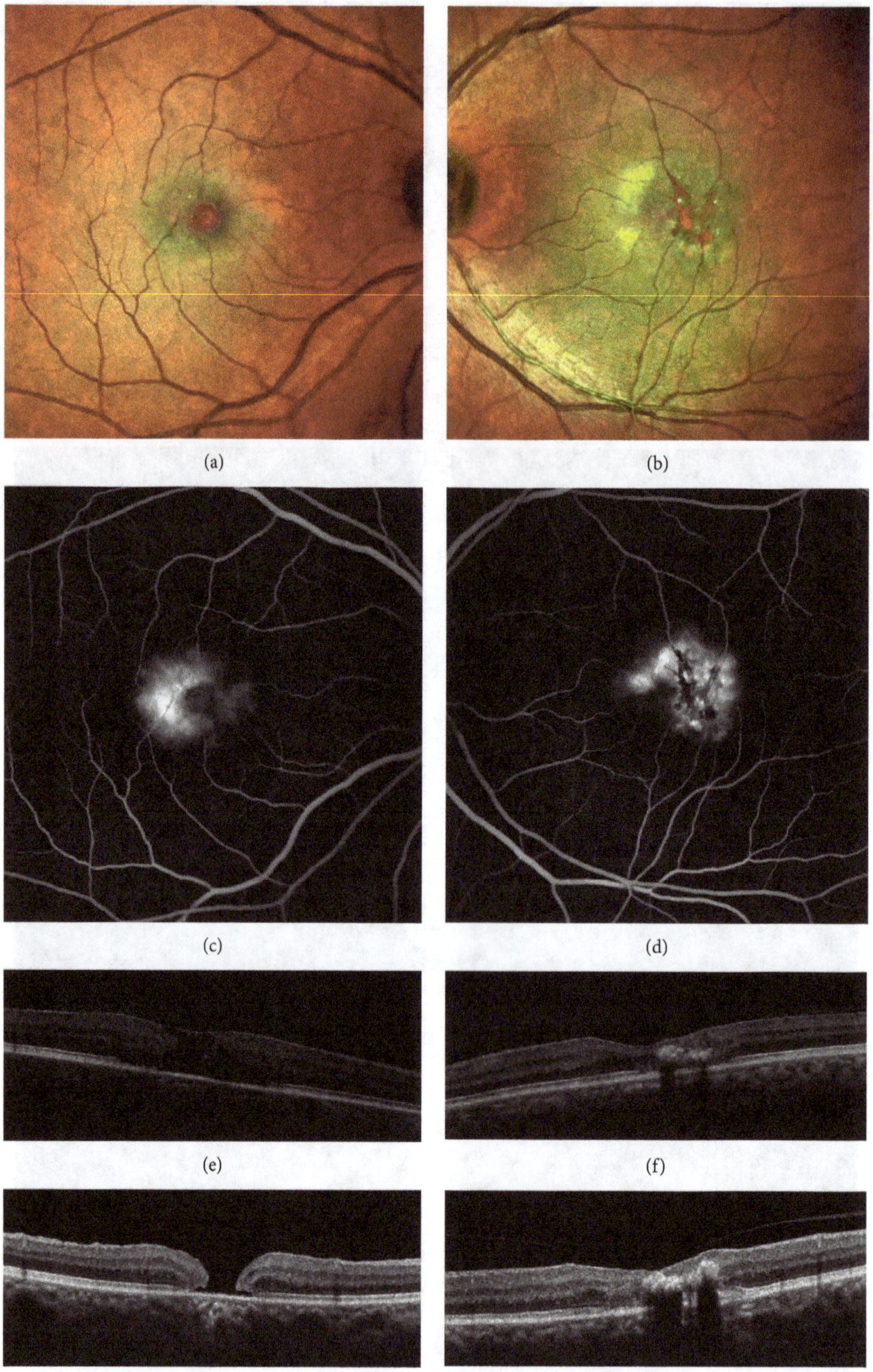

(a) (b)

(c) (d)

(e) (f)

(g) (h)

FIGURE 4: Continued.

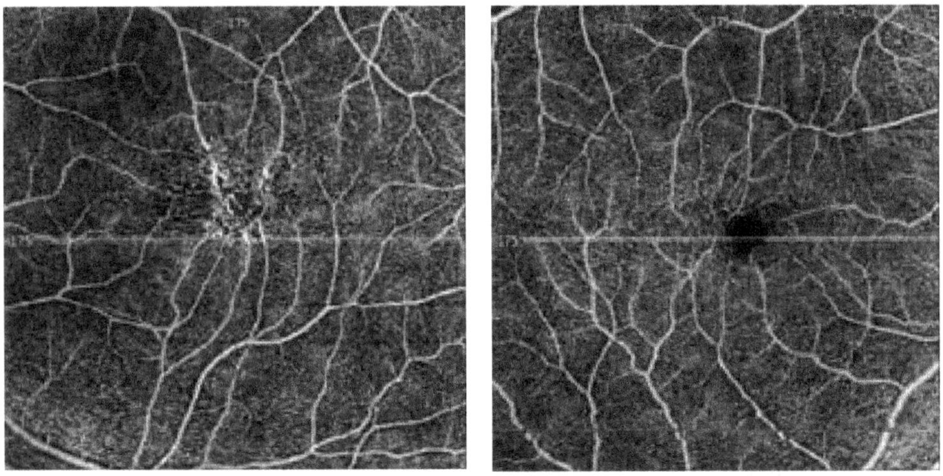

(i) (j)

FIGURE 4: Case 4. Fundus image (a, b) and FA (c, d) show findings consistent with MacTel Type 2. On presentation, OCT confirms a FTMH in the right eye (e). Postoperative OCT (g) shows the hole still being present. OCT-A (i, j) of the superficial layer shows telangiectatic vessels and vascular invasion of the FAZ, especially in the right eye (i).

TABLE 2: Table of anatomical results from published cases of patients with idiopathic Macular Telangiectasia Type 2 and FTMH undergoing surgery [2–7, 9].

Year	Author	Number of eyes	Hole closed	Hole reopened	Hole not closed
2008	Rishi and Kothari	1	0	0	1
2009	Issa et al.	2	0	0	2
2010	Gregori and Flynn	2	1	1	0
2011	Shukla	1	1	0	0
2014	Karth et al.	4	1	1	2
2015	Patel et al.	2	0	0	2
2019	Lee et al.	4	3	1	0
	Subtotal	16	6 (37.5%)	3 (18.75%)	7 (43.75%)
Our study		5	4 (80%)	0 (0%)	1 (20%)
	Total	21	10 (47.6%)	3 (14.2%)	8 (38.1%)

Repeat FA revealed significant dye leakage temporal to the fovea in both eyes. Postoperative OCT-A demonstrated remodeling of the deep capillary plexus characteristic of MacTel Type 2 (Figures 2(k) and 2(l)).

3.3. *Case 3.* A 65-year-old lady with a past medical history of hypertension presented with 8 months of decreased vision in the left eye. BCVA was 20/25 in the right eye and 20/200 in the left. Fundus examination revealed a blunted foveal reflex in the right eye and a FTMH in the left eye (Figures 3(a) and 3(b)). FA revealed faint leakage temporal to the fovea in each eye, consistent with the diagnosis of MacTel Type 2 (Figures 3(c) and 3(d)). She underwent 23-gauge PPV with ILM peeling and 30% SF_6 gas tamponade 7 weeks after presentation. On the 5th postoperative day, the hole was sealed by OCT (Figure 3(g)). The patient underwent cataract extraction in the left eye at another facility. On follow-up, the macular hole in the left eye has remained closed on examination through postoperative month 35 with a BCVA of 20/40. In the right eye, an intraretinal cyst remained stable and vision was maintained at 20/30. Postoperative OCT-A showed persistent features typical of MacTel Type 2 (Figures 3(i)–3(l)). Repeat FA showed significant leakage temporal to the fovea in the right eye and minimal leakage in the left eye (Figure 3(m)).

3.4. *Case 4.* A 57-year-old diabetic female presented with unknown duration of vision loss in her right eye. BCVA in her right eye at presentation was 20/400 and in the left eye 20/50. On anterior segment examination, she had 2+ NSC in both eyes. Fundus examination of the right eye revealed a blunted foveal reflex while the left eye showed pigmentary changes centrally and temporal scarring of the retinal pigment epithelium, without any evidence of diabetic retinopathy (Figures 4(a) and 4(b)). FA revealed bilateral foveal leakage characteristic of MacTel Type 2 (Figures 4(c) and 4(d)). In the right eye, OCT confirmed the clinically apparent FTMH (Figure 4(e)). In the left eye, OCT demonstrated hyperreflective deposits consistent with the macular scarring that was apparent on fundus examination (Figure 4(f)). Three weeks after presentation, she underwent phacoemulsification with IOL implantation in the right eye. Seventeen days after cataract surgery, her BCVA improved to 20/60 in the right eye. Four weeks after cataract surgery, she had a 23-gauge PPV with ILM peeling and 15% C_3F_8 gas tamponade. The hole failed to close as shown on the postoperative OCT (Figure 4(g)), and her BCVA at the 22-month visit was stable at 20/60 in the right eye.

4. Discussion

Surgery for FTMH in the setting of MacTel Type 2 has a guarded prognosis. To date, there are only 16 reported cases that have undergone surgical intervention [2–7, 9]. In these 16 cases, 6 achieved successful hole closure, 3 initially closed but then reopened, and 7 failed to close at all (Table 2). Of the 6 that achieved successful anatomical closure, only 5 had improvement in visual acuity.

The difference in pathophysiology of hole formation is one proposed reason for the much lower success rate of macular hole surgery in MacTel Type 2 as compared to idiopathic macular holes. Idiopathic macular holes are thought to develop from retinal cavitation due to vitreomacular traction [10]. By contrast, in MacTel Type 2, macular holes are postulated to occur from retinal cavitation due to Müller cell degeneration [11]. Histologic analysis also supports this theory as patients with MacTel Type 2 have had reduced expression of Müller cell markers in corresponding areas of the macula [12]. It is thought that the tissue defect from Müller cell atrophy in MacTel Type 2 causes foveal structural instability and leaves an insufficient amount of tissue for the hole to seal. This may account for the historically poor surgical outcomes in MacTel Type 2 FTMH repair. This pathologic process is thought to be independent of the vascular abnormalities in MacTel Type 2. In his initial paper, Gass had proposed a primary role for abnormal retinal vasculature leading to retinal atrophy [13]. However, he later revised this theory to suggest a primary role of parfoveolar Müller cell abnormality since telangiectatic vessels often did not develop till later in the disease [14].

Rishi and Kothari first reported on the surgical management of patients with FTMH in MacTel Type 2. In their series of 2 patients, one achieved successful hole closure and improvement in vision from 20/100 to 20/63, while the other case exhibited initial closure followed by reopening at 4 months and no functional vision improvement [4]. Several case series have followed since then, all with overall poor closure rates. Issa et al. described 2 patients with MacTel Type 2 in whom the FTMH did not close [2]. In 2010, Gregori and Flynn reported on 2 patients both of whom had initial hole closure with reopening of the hole in one of the patients after 4 months [3]. In the patient with successful hole closure, VA improved from 20/50 to 20/30. In 2011, Shukla described successful hole closure in 1 patient with VA improvement from 20/80 to about 20/30 at the 11-month postoperative visit [5]. This was followed by Karth et al. who described FTMH in 4 patients with stage 3 and 4 MacTel Type 2 [6]. The holes successfully closed in one patient, reopened in one, and failed to close in two. In the single patient with successful closure, VA improved from 20/200 to 20/30. This study was followed by Patel and Flaxel who reported on 2 patients in whom the hole did not close following attempted surgical repair [7]. Most recently, a group from Korea published the first case series on Asian patients [9]. They reported on 4 patients with MacTel Type 2 and FTMH with an average thickness of 345 μm. Three of the 4 patients had successful hole closure, and the fourth patient had initial closure with recurrence after 1 month. Among the 3 patients with successful closure, 2 had improved vision—from 20/125 to 20/32 at postop month 43 in one patient and from 20/200 to 20/32 at postop month 6 in the second patient. The third patient with successful closure had worsening of vision from 20/200 to 20/400 at 10 months postoperatively. The results of all these described studies are summarized in Table 2. Before the addition of our cases, the successful hole closure rate was 37.75% with the inclusion of all the most recent cases. By contrast, the rate of hole closure in our cases alone was 80%. The inclusion of our 5 cases to the previously existing data increased the hole closure rate to 47.6%.

Our series of surgical outcomes in 5 eyes with FTMH in MacTel Type 2 is the largest to date and has the highest success rate of hole closure among currently published studies. As described above, we had successful hole closure in 4 out of 5 eyes with final visual acuities ranging from 20/20 to 20/40 at the follow-up visits at least 21 months out from surgery in each patient. There are several possibilities to explain the higher success in our series compared to previously reported cases. We performed ILM peeling in all eyes from major vascular arcade to arcade. Only one of the previously published studies detailed the extent of ILM peeling, and this was the one by Lee et al. Interestingly, similar to us, this group performed ILM peeling of the major vascular arcades as well and three out of four holes remained closed in their series. Given the higher success rate in patients that undergo a larger extent of ILM peeling, it may be that this is what leads to better results in FTMH repair in MacTel Type 2. ILM peeling may activate Müller cells, stimulating the secretion of collagen, basement membrane components, and inflammatory factors which may subsequently activate glial cell-mediated closure of macular holes as suggested in histological studies [15]. Despite the depletion of Müller cells, the foveal structure may be reinforced by the remaining Müller cells, contributing to the hole closure. Another possibility that may have contributed to our successful surgical outcomes was our reinforcement of strict head positioning for 5 days postoperatively. It may also have helped that our patients underwent surgery at an earlier stage of MacTel, as most of our patients did not have the foveal intraretinal pigment changes observed in the later stages of MacTel Type 2. Of note, FA and OCT-A in three of our patients with successful hole closure revealed persistence of foveal vascular anomalies after surgery, evidenced by fluorescein leakage on FA and the presence of abnormal capillary beds on OCT-A. This supports the hypothesis that vascular incompetence is unlikely to have contributed to macular hole formation [14] as 4 of the 5 macular holes remained closed more than 21 months after surgery.

Our study is limited by the small number of cases; however, this is expected given the rarity of the disease. Additionally, there is a possibility that the visual improvement seen in our first patient may have been from the phacoemulsification component of the surgery. However, although this patient had combined cataract and retinal surgery, anatomic closure of the hole was still achieved and it is likely that both surgeries contributed to the final improvement in VA. Additionally, the second and third patients did not have concomitant cataract surgery and these patients also had improvements in VA in addition to anatomical closure. Strengths of our case series include including OCT-A imaging in all five eyes and long-term follow-up of greater than 20 months. Additionally, given that the same vitreoretinal surgeon performed all surgeries, the surgical technique employed was uniform among all five eyes.

5. Conclusion

In conclusion, our case series suggests that a higher rate of success may be achievable in surgical repair of FTMH in MacTel Type 2. Specifically, characteristics that may have contributed to a greater chance of success include operating at an earlier stage of MacTel, operating promptly after initial symptom onset, a more thorough ILM peeling, and strict prone positioning postoperatively. Our data may help inform the preoperative discussion surgeons have with their patients. Finally, our findings of persistent leakage on angiography and lack of vascular remodeling on OCT-A despite successful hole closure suggest that vascular leakage in MacTel Type 2 is unlikely to contribute to the pathophysiology of hole formation or closure.

Abbreviations

FTMH: Full-thickness macular hole
MacTel: Macular Telangiectasia
PPV: Pars plana vitrectomy
ILM: Internal limiting membrane
SF_6: Sulfur hexafluoride
C_3F_8: Octafluoropropane
VA: Visual acuity
ICG: Indocyanine green
FA: Fluorescein angiography
OCT: Optical coherence tomography
OCT-A: Optical coherence tomography-angiography
BCVA: Best corrected visual acuity
NSC: Nuclear sclerotic cataract
ERM: Epiretinal membrane
IOL: Intraocular lens.

Disclosure

The abstract for this manuscript was presented as a poster at the virtual American Society of Retina Specialists Meeting, Seattle, WA, July 2020 (<400-word abstract).

Authors' Contributions

KTA and SHU wrote and edited the manuscript. SHU is the attending physician for all four patients and performed all vitreoretinal surgeries reported. JC performed cataract surgery on one patient and edited the manuscript. DBW performed cataract surgery on one patient and edited the manuscript. ABS edited the manuscript. All authors read and approved the final manuscript.

Acknowledgments

We acknowledge Jones Eye Institute, University of Arkansas for Medical Sciences College of Medicine. This work was supported by Research to Prevent Blindness and the Martha Wood Bentley Chair in Ophthalmology.

References

[1] W. R. Green, H. A. Quigley, Z. de la Cruz, and B. Cohen, "Parafoveal retinal telangiectasis. Light and electron microscopy studies," *Transactions of the Ophthalmological Societies of the United Kingdom*, vol. 100, no. 1, pp. 162–170, 1980.

[2] P. Charbel Issa, H. P. N. Scholl, A. Gaudric et al., "Macular full-thickness and lamellar holes in association with type 2 idiopathic macular telangiectasia," *Eye*, vol. 23, no. 2, pp. 435–441, 2009.

[3] N. Gregori and H. W. Flynn, "Surgery for full-thickness macular hole in patients with idiopathic macular telangiectasia type 2," *Ophthalmic surgery, lasers and imaging retina.*, 2010.

[4] P. Rishi and A. R. Kothari, "Parafoveal telangiectasia (PFT) has been associated with changes in macular architecture and macular holes (lamellar and full thickness)," *Retina*, vol. 28, no. 1, pp. 184-185, 2008.

[5] D. Shukla, "Evolution and management of macular hole secondary to type 2 idiopathic macular telangiectasia," *Eye*, vol. 25, no. 4, pp. 532-533, 2011.

[6] P. A. Karth, S. C. Raja, D. M. Brown, and J. E. Kim, "Outcomes of macular hole surgeries for macular telangiectasia type 2," *Retina*, vol. 34, no. 5, pp. 907–915, 2014.

[7] P. Patel and C. Flaxel, "Visual and anatomic outcomes in eyes with idiopathic juxtafoveal macular telangiectasia (MacTel) and full thickness macular holes undergoing surgical repair," *Enliven: Clin Ophthalmol Res*, vol. 1, no. 1, p. 005, 2015.

[8] H. Nalcı, F. Şermet, S. Demirel, and E. Özmert, "Optic coherence angiography findings in type-2 macular telangiectasia," *Turkish journal of ophthalmology*, vol. 47, no. 5, pp. 279–284, 2017.

[9] S. C. Lee, D. J. Hwang, K. M. Lee, Y. S. Park, and J. H. Sohn, "Surgical outcomes of macular telangiectasia type 2 associated with macular hole," *Journal of Retina*, vol. 4, no. 2, pp. 48–54, 2019.

[10] R. F. Spaide, "Closure of an outer lamellar macular hole by vitrectomy: hypothesis for one mechanism of macular hole formation," *Retina*, vol. 20, no. 6, pp. 587–590, 2000.

[11] H. Koizumi, J. S. Slakter, and R. F. Spaide, "Full-thickness macular hole formation in idiopathic parafoveal telangiectasis," *Retina*, vol. 27, no. 4, pp. 473–476, 2007.

[12] M. B. Powner, M. C. Gillies, M. Zhu, K. Vevis, A. P. Hunyor, and M. Fruttiger, "Loss of Müller's cells and photoreceptors in macular telangiectasia type 2," *Ophthalmology*, vol. 120, no. 11, pp. 2344–2352, 2013.

[13] J. D. Gass and R. T. Oyakawa, "Idiopathic juxtafoveolar retinal telangiectasis," *Archives of Ophthalmology*, vol. 100, no. 5, pp. 769–780, 1982.

[14] J. D. M. Gass, "Histopathologic study of presumed parafoveal telangiectasis," *Retina*, vol. 20, no. 2, pp. 226-227, 2000.

[15] T. Hisatomi, T. Tachibana, S. Notomi et al., "Incomplete repair of retinal structure after vitrectomy with internal limiting membrane peeling," *Retina*, vol. 37, no. 8, pp. 1523–1528, 2017.

37

Tube Length Adjustment and Tube Trimming Technique in Refractory Glaucoma

Iwan Soebijantoro and Nina Asrini Noor

JEC Eye Hospital Kedoya, Jakarta, Indonesia

Correspondence should be addressed to Nina Asrini Noor; nina.asrini.noor@gmail.com

Academic Editor: Huban Atilla

Secondary glaucoma may develop after vitreoretinal surgery as it is a known risk factor for its development. When the risk factors are more than one, for instance along with neovascular glaucoma (NVG), the secondary glaucoma may become recalcitrant and very difficult to manage. Surgical intervention is often warranted to control intraocular pressure (IOP) and prevent progressive glaucomatous damage in patients with refractory glaucoma, and glaucoma drainage implant may be preferred as the primary choice. We describe a patient who develop secondary glaucoma after vitrectomy and silicone oil (SO) injection due to unresolved vitreous hemorrhage in proliferative diabetic retinopathy (PDR) and subsequent NVG. Baerveldt glaucoma implant (BGI) was carried out and placed in the superotemporal quadrant with longer anterior chamber tube placement to prevent escape of SO through the tube. Qualified success was achieved with additional one fixed-drug combination (FDC). However, 3 years later, the tube was blocked by the iris tissue at the inferior edge of the pupil. Tube trimming was performed efficiently using a simple technique. The distal end of the tube was pulled out of the anterior chamber through a paracentesis just next to the tube entrance and trimmed to the appropriate length. More than a year after the surgery, IOP was still well controlled with the same FDC. Unfortunately, the visual acuity could not be recovered due to advanced PDR.

1. Introduction

Refractory glaucoma after vitreoretinal surgery is not rare occurrence. It has been reported in up to 30% of patients 2 years after vitrectomy with silicone oil (SO) injection [1]. It develops due to surgery and tamponade agents, is usually transient, and is generally managed with antiglaucoma therapy [2]. However, when it arises in conjunction with other form of secondary glaucoma, such as neovascular glaucoma (NVG), it may become very difficult to treat. Several factors were thought to play a role in the development of intraocular pressure (IOP) increase after vitreoretinal surgery, although they are not fully understood. Oxidative damage to the trabecular meshwork, secondary scarring, and SO complications were some of the possible mechanisms [3–9].

Glaucoma implants have become very useful for refractory glaucoma in the eyes with previous vitreoretinal surgery and NVG. Both nonvalved and valved implants have been used for the management of refractory glaucoma [7, 8]. Complications in tube shunt surgery are not uncommon, and one of them is tube occlusion which may require tube revision or trimming [9, 10]. However, in certain cases, tube trimming may be considered as major intervention with risk of further complications.

Here, we report the case of a patient who developed secondary glaucoma after vitrectomy surgery and SO injection for unresolved vitreous hemorrhage in proliferative diabetic retinopathy (PDR). The patient also developed NVG subsequently. Baerveldt glaucoma implant (BGI) was performed, and the tube was left longer in the anterior chamber near the inferior pupillary margin to avoid SO passing through the tube as SO removal was deemed not yet possible at that time. Despite being successful in reducing IOP along with one additional fixed-drug combination (FDC), the tube became occluded by the iris tissue three years later. This case briefly explains how we performed tube trimming with an

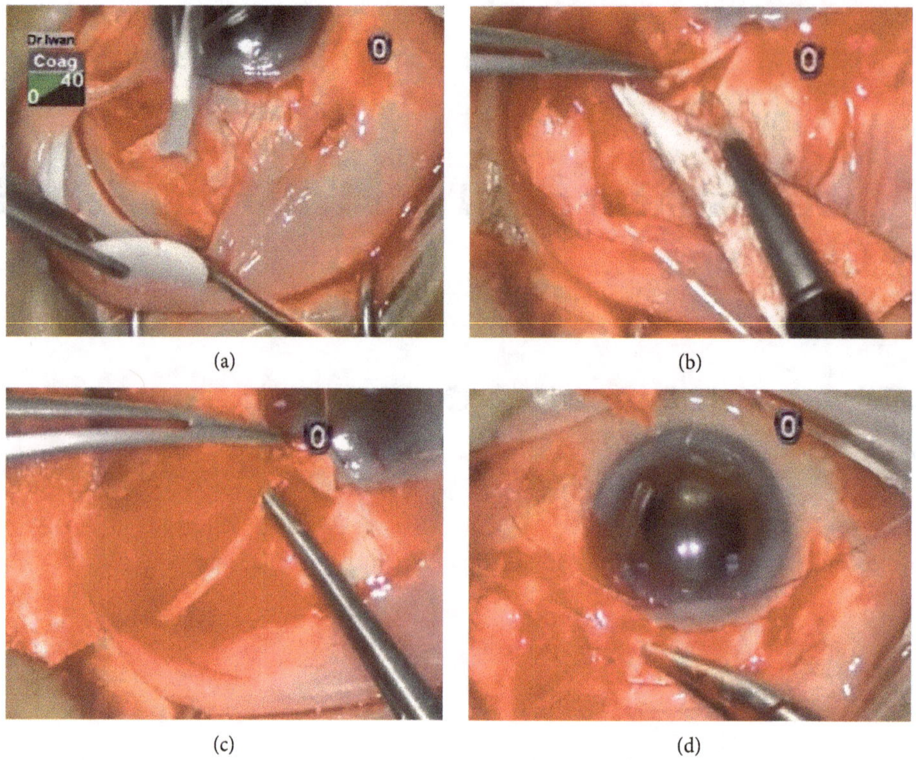

Figure 1: Summary of the Baerveldt glaucoma implant (BGI) surgery. (a) The implant was slipped between the sclera and Tenon's capsule 10 mm posterior to the limbus and then positioned and securely sutured at superotemporal quadrant. (b) A scleral flap was made for the insertion of the tube, and then, the tube was cut and beveled anteriorly. (c) An opening was made underneath the scleral flap, and the tube was inserted into the anterior chamber. (d) The final position of the tube in the anterior chamber was checked, and scleral flap was sutured, followed by closure of Tenon's capsule and conjunctiva.

effective and efficient approach. More than a year after the tube trimming, the IOP is under control while maintaining the same FDC.

2. Case Presentation

A 61-year-old male was referred to the glaucoma service of JEC Eye Hospital in September 2014. In the last one year, he was taken care by the retina service for PDR and diabetic macular edema (DME) from uncontrolled type II diabetes which he already had for 15 years. The patient had undergone multiple panretinal photocoagulation (PRP), intravitreal ranibizumab injections, cataract surgery with IOL implantation of both eyes, and subsequently vitrectomy and SO in August 2014 due to unresolved vitreous hemorrhage of the left eye.

The patient was referred to glaucoma service one month after vitrectomy and SO surgery due to uncontrolled IOP of the left eye despite medication with brimonidine tartrate 0.2% ophthalmic solution (Alphagan®, Allergan Inc., United States) and dorzolamide hydrochloride 2% eye drops (Trusopt®, MSD, United Kingdom) combined with oral extended release acetazolamide 500 mg capsule (Diamox® Sequels, Wyeth Pharmaceuticals Inc., Canada).

He presented with visual acuity 1-meter finger counting and IOP 37 mmHg. Iris neovascularization was markedly observed, and he was diagnosed with NVG as a secondary mechanism contributing to the IOP increase besides postvitrectomy and the presence of SO. The patient was immediately planned to undergo glaucoma implant surgery which took place a couple of days after his initial visit to glaucoma service.

The patient underwent an uncomplicated Baerveldt implant (model BG-101-350, Abbott Medical Optics, Santa Ana, California, United States) surgery (Figure 1). A 350 mm^2 Baerveldt implant was placed in the superotemporal quadrant. A limbus-based conjunctival flap was dissected, and the implant was sutured securely to the sclera. Due to the presence of SO, the tube was left longer and lower in the anterior chamber below the inferior edge of the pupil (Figure 2). This approach was taken to avoid the escape of SO through the tube if it was left shorter.

One week after the surgery, IOP was markedly decreased to 6 mmHg. Since then, he was routinely followed up in glaucoma service every month together under the care of retina service. The patient underwent SO removal of the left eye in January 2015 and several more intravitreal ranibizumab injections of both eyes. During three years of follow-up, the IOP was maintained in the low teens for three years with additional topical FDC of brinzolamide 10 mg/ml and timolol 5 mg/ml ophthalmic suspension (Azarga®, Alcon Laboratories Inc., United States).

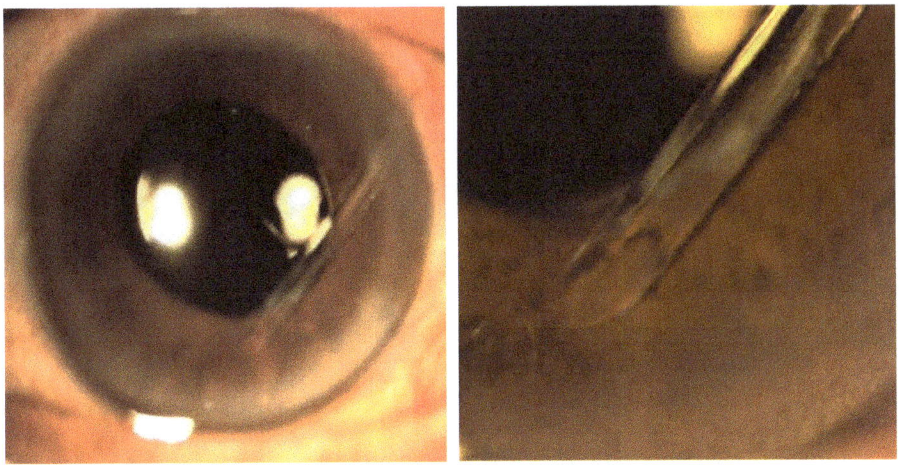

FIGURE 2: The final tube position after the initial BGI surgery. The tube was left longer in the anterior chamber just below the inferior pupillary margin.

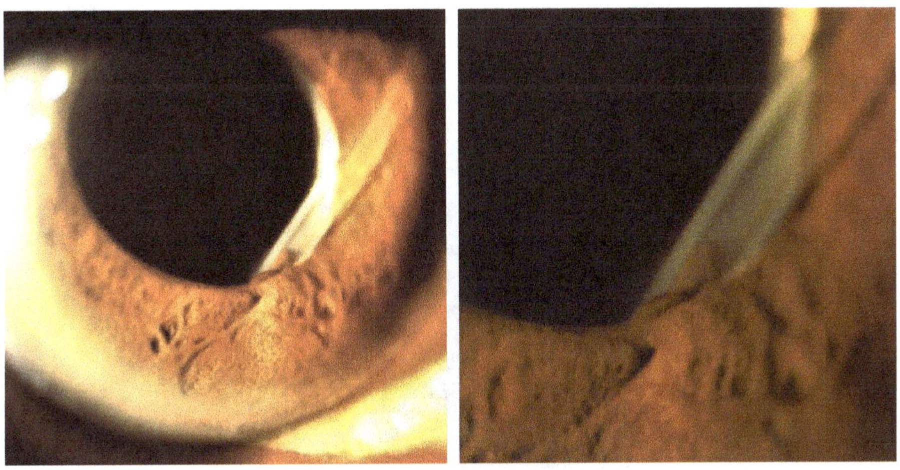

FIGURE 3: The tube was blocked by the iris tissue at the pupillary margin.

In February 2018, the IOP was suddenly elevated to 46 mmHg. From slit lamp examination, the cornea remained clear and there was no tube-corneal touch, but unfortunately, the tube was blocked by the iris tissue (Figure 3). Tube trimming was immediately performed efficiently with a relatively easy technique (Figure 4). A single paracentesis was made next to the tube insertion, followed by injection of viscoelastic to release the iris tissue which was blocking the tube tip. The distal end of the tube was then pulled out from the anterior chamber through the paracentesis using forceps. Next, the tube tip was transected with scissors for the desired length, beveled anteriorly, and subsequently inserted back into the anterior chamber.

One day after the surgery, IOP decreased to 11 mmHg and the tube was well-positioned near the superior pupillary edge. Thereafter, the patient was followed up every 2 months and maintained his previous FDC. Until his last visit in December 2019, the IOP was well-controlled in the low teens. However, the visual acuity was very poor and only hand movement due to the course of advanced PDR.

3. Discussion

Factors that play a role in the development of an IOP elevation after vitreoretinal surgery are not well understood. An increase in oxygen tension in the vitreous cavity after a vitrectomy, which is hypothesized to yield oxidative damage to the trabecular meshwork, is considered to play a role in the pathogenesis [3–6]. SO complications may also be responsible for IOP elevation after vitrectomy [11, 12]. Several mechanisms associated with SO-induced secondary glaucoma include pupillary block, inflammation, iris neovascularization, migration of emulsified and nonemulsified SO into the anterior chamber, and idiopathic open-angle glaucoma [1, 7].

It has been reported that 7.1–10% of patients who underwent vitrectomy and SO injection developed uncontrolled glaucoma despite medical therapy and removal of SO [13]. Eyes with an early postvitrectomy IOP elevation were more likely to have a persistent IOP increase for at least 6 weeks [12]. In this case, we observed an increase of IOP in the first

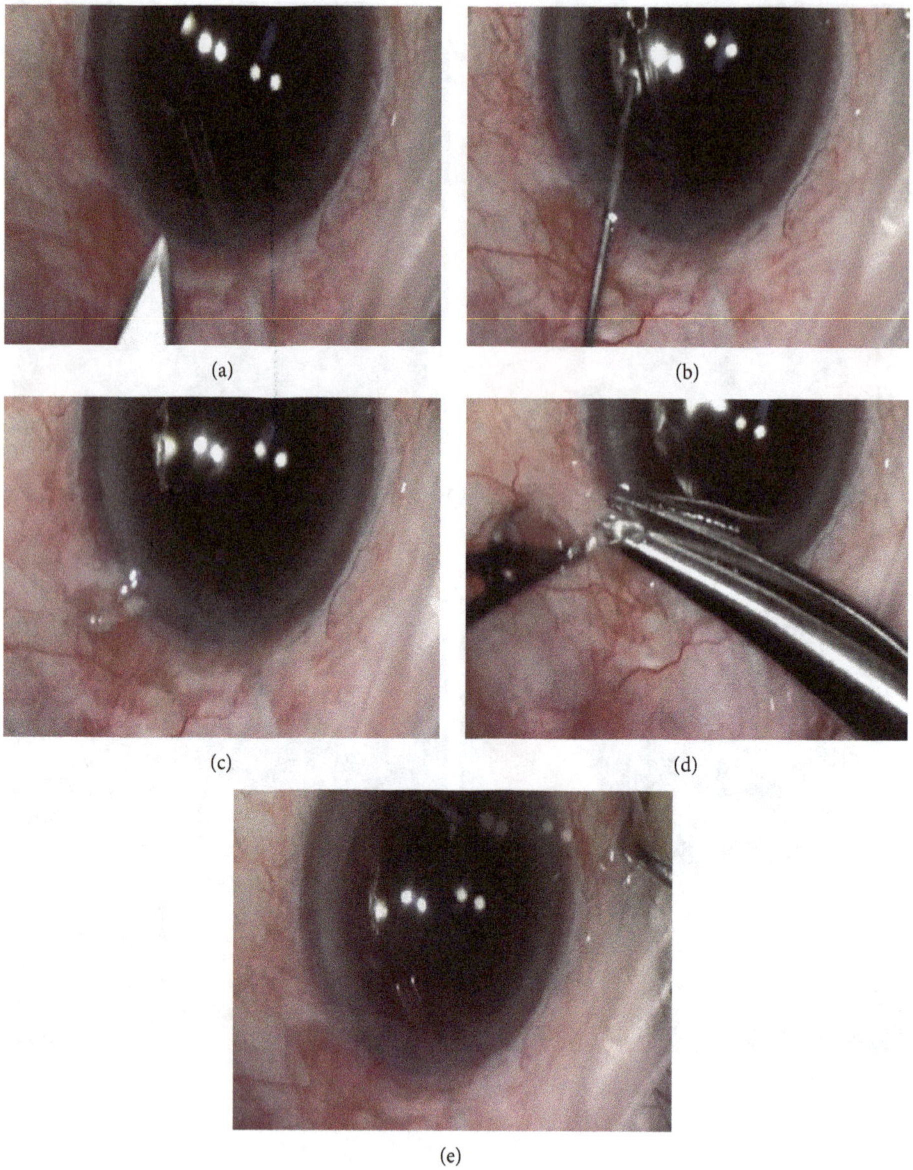

FIGURE 4: The tube trimming technique. (a) A single paracentesis was made approximately 1 clock hour temporally from the tube insertion. (b) Viscoelastic was injected to release the iris tissue blockage from the tip. (c) Through the paracentesis, the tube was pulled out from the anterior chamber using forceps. (d) The tube tip was held steady with forceps and transected with scissors. (e) Then, the tube was inserted back into the anterior chamber.

week after vitrectomy surgery; thus, it was very likely that IOP would remain uncontrolled for longer period as also observed in the previous study.

NVG also played a significant role in this case. Severe PDR is a significant predictor of NVG [14]. In vitrectomized eyes, it is assumed that NVG can be more significant because vasoformative factors in the vitreous cavity could easily diffuse into the anterior chamber [15], although the presence of silicone oil may have a role in inhibiting progressive neovascularization in the anterior segment by preventing the diffusion of angiogenic substances [16]. In the end, the concurrence of NVG along with secondary glaucoma postvitrectomy and silicone oil in this patient contributed to an uncontrolled IOP despite maximum medications.

Refractory glaucoma in this case indicated the need for surgical treatment. Glaucoma implants have become very useful and may be preferred as the primary choice for refractory glaucoma in the eyes with previous vitreoretinal surgery and NVG with either valved or nonvalved implants [7, 8]. In Indonesia, the most commonly used implants are the Ahmed-184 and Baerveldt-350 implant with satisfying results, correlating with the results of studies in other Asian and non-Asian groups [9, 17, 18]. Baerveldt implant was used in a greater number of poor prognosis glaucoma eyes with higher IOP and in the more severe glaucoma cases, including NVG and postvitrectomy surgery [9]. For this rationale, Baerveldt implant was chosen and an anterior chamber tube was placed as pars plana tube placement was not an option due to the presence of silicone oil in the vitreous cavity. Longer tube was placed to anticipate the risk of migration of SO particles through the tube which may cause tube blockage or conjunctival fibrosis.

Complications in tube shunt surgery are not uncommon and may include tube exposure, tube occlusion, endophthalmitis, dysesthesia, uncontrolled IOP, low IOP, and diplopia [9, 10]. In this case, patient had tube blockage by the iris tissue approximately 3 years after the initial BGI surgery which certainly required trimming of the tube. Tube trimming is considered as major surgery and typically involves dissection through a scarred conjunctiva, dissection underneath the scleral patch graft, removal of the tube from the anterior chamber, trimming of the tube, and subsequent reinsertion and suturing. This process can be lengthy and may be fraught with complications.

Asrani et al. [19] demonstrated a case with newer technique for glaucoma tube trimming. In their paper, they explained a technique using two paracentesis, a 30-gauge needle to hold still the distal end of the tube through one paracentesis, a manual membrane peeling and cutting scissors to transect the tube through the second paracentesis, and finally a forceps to grasp and remove the transected part of the tube. Despite being a great technique, it requires multiple paracentesis and instruments. We performed a different approach which we felt easier, more efficient, and effective to perform by pulling the distal end of the tube out of the anterior chamber through a paracentesis, transecting the tube, and inserting it back into the anterior chamber. The tube was trimmed so that it was beveled anteriorly to prevent recurrent blockage by the iris tissue, as also suggested by Wang and Barton [20].

In a series by van Aken et al. [7], the majority of eyes with refractory glaucoma after vitrectomy still required glaucoma medication following BGI, and only 23% did not. Thus, the need of additional medication to control the IOP after surgery was anticipated in this patient.

BGI in combination with FDC glaucoma medication was successful in controlling the IOP in the low teens in this patient with refractory glaucoma. The length and position of the tube in the initial surgery should be tailored case-by-case. If tube trimming is necessary, a simple yet efficient technique described previously may be considered.

References

[1] J. D. Henderer, D. L. Budenz, H. W. Flynn Jr., J. C. Schiffman, W. J. Feuer, and T. G. Murray, "Elevated intraocular pressure and hypotony following silicone oil retinal tamponade for complex retinal detachment: incidence and risk factors," *Archives of Ophthalmology*, vol. 117, no. 2, pp. 189–195, 1999.

[2] Q. H. Nguyen, M. A. Lloyd, D. K. Heuer et al., "Incidence and management of glaucoma after intravitreal silicone oil injection for complicated retinal detachments," *Ophthalmology*, vol. 99, no. 10, pp. 1520–1526, 1992.

[3] S. Chang, "LXII Edward Jackson lecture: open angle glaucoma after vitrectomy," *American Journal of Ophthalmology*, vol. 141, no. 6, pp. 1033–1043.e1, 2006.

[4] C. J. Siegfried, Y. B. Shui, N. M. Holekamp, F. Bai, and D. C. Beebe, "Oxygen distribution in the human eye: relevance to the etiology of open-angle glaucoma after vitrectomy," *Investigative Ophthalmology & Visual Science*, vol. 51, no. 11, pp. 5731–5738, 2010.

[5] M. M. de Vries, R. P. H. M. Müskens, V. W. Renardel de Lavalette, J. M. M. Hooymans, and N. M. Jansonius, "Glaucoma drainage device surgery after vitreoretinal surgery: incidence and risk factors," *Acta Ophthalmologica*, vol. 94, no. 2, pp. 135–139, 2016.

[6] N. M. Holekamp, Y. B. Shui, and D. C. Beebe, "Vitrectomy surgery increases oxygen exposure to the lens: a possible mechanism for nuclear cataract formation," *American Journal of Ophthalmology*, vol. 139, no. 2, pp. 302–310, 2005.

[7] E. Van Aken, H. Lemij, Y. Vander Haeghen, and P. de Waard, "Baerveldt glaucoma implants in the management of refractory glaucoma after vitreous surgery," *Acta Ophthalmologica*, vol. 88, no. 1, pp. 75–79, 2010.

[8] K. S. Schwartz, R. K. Lee, and S. J. Gedde, "Glaucoma drainage implants: a critical comparison of types," *Current Opinion in Ophthalmology*, vol. 17, no. 2, pp. 181–189, 2006.

[9] W. Artini, S. Mustafa, V. D. Octariana, and A. Suryono, "Comparison of Ahmed Versus Baerveldt Implant Outcomes in Malayan Glaucoma Patients," *Makara Journal of Health Research*, vol. 22, no. 3, pp. 115–120, 2018.

[10] S. Weinreb, N. Cardakli, J. Jefferys, and H. Quigley, "Long-term functional outcomes of glaucoma tube shunt revision surgery," *Ophthalmology Glaucoma*, vol. 2, no. 6, pp. 383–391, 2019.

[11] A. Goto, M. Inatani, T. Inoue et al., "Frequency and risk factors for neovascular glaucoma after vitrectomy in eyes with proliferative diabetic retinopathy," *Journal of Glaucoma*, vol. 22, no. 7, pp. 572–576, 2013.

[12] D. P. Han, H. Lewis, F. H. Lambrou Jr., W. F. Mieler, and A. Hartz, "Mechanisms of intraocular pressure elevation after pars plana vitrectomy," *Ophthalmology*, vol. 96, no. 9, pp. 1357–1362, 1989.

[13] D. L. Budenz, K. E. Taba, W. J. Feuer et al., "Surgical management of secondary glaucoma after pars plana vitrectomy and silicone oil injection for complex retinal detachment," *Ophthalmology*, vol. 108, no. 9, pp. 1628–1632, 2001.

[14] X. Liang, Y. Zhang, Y. P. Li, W. R. Huang, J. X. Wang, and X. Li, "Frequency and risk factors for neovascular glaucoma after vitrectomy in eyes with diabetic retinopathy: an observational study," *Diabetes Therapy*, vol. 10, no. 5, pp. 1801–1809, 2019.

[15] T. Inoue, M. Inatani, Y. Takihara, N. Awai-Kasaoka, M. Ogata-Iwao, and H. Tanihara, "Prognostic risk factors for failure of trabeculectomy with mitomycin C after vitrectomy," *Japanese Journal of Ophthalmology*, vol. 56, no. 5, pp. 464–469, 2012.

[16] A. Castellarin, R. Grigorian, N. Bhagat, L. Del Priore, and M. A. Zarbin, "Vitrectomy with silicone oil infusion in severe diabetic retinopathy," *The British Journal of Ophthalmology*, vol. 87, no. 3, pp. 318–321, 2003.

[17] P. G. Christakis, J. W. Kalenak, D. Zurakowski et al., "The Ahmed versus Baerveldt study: one-year treatment outcomes," *Ophthalmology*, vol. 118, no. 11, pp. 2180–2189, 2011.

[18] J. C. Wang, J. L. S. See, and P. T. K. Chew, "Experience with the use of Baerveldt and Ahmed glaucoma drainage implants in an Asian population," *Ophthalmology*, vol. 111, no. 7, pp. 1383–1388, 2004.

[19] S. Asrani, L. Herndon, and R. R. Allingham, "A newer technique for glaucoma tube trimming," *Archives of Ophthalmology*, vol. 121, no. 9, pp. 1324–1326, 2003.

[20] J. Wang and K. Barton, "Aqueous shunt implantation in glaucoma," *Taiwan Journal of Ophthalmology*, vol. 7, no. 3, pp. 130–137, 2017.

38

Management of an Unusual Orbitocranial Penetrating Injury

Han Y. Yin,[1,3] Swetha Dhanireddy,[1] and Alexander E. Braley[2,3]

[1]*SUNY Upstate Medical University, Department of Ophthalmology and Visual Sciences, Syracuse, NY, USA*
[2]*SUNY Upstate Medical University, Department of Neurosurgery, Syracuse, NY, USA*
[3]*Florida International University Herbert Wertheim College of Medicine, Miami, FL, USA*

Correspondence should be addressed to Alexander E. Braley; braleya@upstate.edu

Academic Editor: Irene A. Barbazetto

Background. An intraorbital injury with a blunt penetrating intraorbital foreign body (IOFB) is an unusual cause of penetrating trauma. This type of trauma is considered a surgical emergency given the risk to vision in addition to potential intracranial injuries such as vascular injury, dural laceration, and neurologic injury. A thorough history and physical exam, along with careful radiographic and multidiscipline intervention, is crucial in providing the patient the most appropriate care. *Case Presentation.* A 66-year-old male presented to the emergency room (ER) after falling down the stairs and suffering an orbitocranial penetrating injury. He underwent urgent fluoroscopy-guided foreign body removal with a multidisciplinary team after a workup revealed no significant ocular or intracranial injuries. The foreign body was removed with an anterior approach without any complications. *Conclusion.* In this study, we demonstrated that IOFB in proximity to orbitocranial structures requires a careful multidisciplinary team approach. An interventional radiology- (IR-) guided approach in extracting the foreign body is essential to prevent further injury. A high dose of intravenous steroid was not used due to initial suspicion of intracranial involvement. Prompt removal decreased risk of further vision loss.

1. Background

Penetrating orbitocranial injury carries high mortality and morbidity. Although it is rare, a retained intraorbital foreign body (IOFB) is often a result of high-velocity projectile trauma with a sharp-tipped object. Often, the integrity of orbital contents is violated, resulting in ruptured globe, vascular injury, lid laceration, and orbital bone fractures [1, 2]. Furthermore, deep orbital structures and adjacent intracranial structures are at risk of being injured from a penetrating foreign body. Clearly all intraorbital vascular and neural structures are at risk during intraocular trauma, but trauma that violates the orbital wall makes nearby intracranial structures vulnerable, with potentially catastrophic sequelae. Such structures include but are not limited to the internal carotid artery (ICA), basilar artery, cavernous sinus, pituitary gland, and cranial nerves I-VI, in addition to the frontal lobe, temporal lobe, and the brain stem. Therefore, immediate evaluation and appropriate surgical management are critical. Trauma with IOFB adjacent to the optic nerve is considered an ophthalmologic emergency.

Here, we present a rare and unusual case of facial trauma resulting from a low-velocity injury with a blunt tipped object. This injury led to IOFB with close proximity to adjacent intracranial tissue, therefore warranting an early multidisciplinary surgical intervention to conquer a unique and challenging surgical case.

2. Case Presentation

A 66-year-old right-handed male presented to the emergency room with orbitocranial penetrating injury after falling down the stairs. During the fall, he impacted his face on the coat rack at the bottom of the stairs. One of the coat hooks on the coat rack penetrated into his left orbit and lodged into the posterior orbital wall. The coat hook was cut in the field by the paramedics two to three centimeters from the point of entry. On presentation, he was alert and fully oriented with a Glasgow Coma Scale (GCS) of 15 and his neurological exam was nonfocal. His ophthalmologic exam revealed an edematous left lower eyelid, with a visible large metallic foreign body breached through the lower eyelid bordering the inferior orbital rim (Figure 1). The visual acuity in his left eye (OS) was 20/200 with no improvement on the pinhole, and intraocular pressure (IOP) assessment was deferred in the left eye. There was a left relative afferent pupillary defect (RAPD). Ocular movements were intact in both eyes. The subsequent ophthalmic exam did not suggest an occult globe rupture.

Computed tomography (CT) head was obtained and did not appear to show any significant intracranial injury, although the cast iron hook created a significant metal artifact that limited the quality of the study. CT angiography (CTA) did not show any vascular injury but was also severely limited by the metal streak artifact. He was started on meningitis prophylaxis, and a tetanus booster was administered. He was taken for an urgent diagnostic cerebral angiogram to better investigate the intracranial vascular structures prior to any attempts to remove the hook. This was critical as the metal streak artifact may have obscured an underlying vascular injury that could complicate hook removal. Six-vessel cerebral angiography did not show injury to any intracranial vessels (Figure 2). The majority of the intraorbital vessels appeared uninjured, although the left superior ophthalmic vein was not visualized; this was concluded to be secondary to compression from the foreign object or possibly from thrombosis. A reconstructed 3-dimensional (3D) image confirmed that there was no major violation of vascular structures (Figure 3).

The patient underwent an orbital foreign body removal under fluoroscopic guidance in a multidisciplinary setting with neurosurgery, ophthalmology, and neurointerventional radiology. The neurointerventional radiologist was in the room for immediate support for potential vascular injuries. The groin and the orbit were prepped and draped in the usual sterile fashion. The hook was rotated with ease, but initial resistance to withdrawal of the hook suggested that there may have been a ball-socket interaction with the orbital wall and the ball of the hook, which had to be overcome. The hook then was released successfully from the orbital wall with slightly increased force. The hook was then removed from the orbit under live fluoroscopy by twisting the Kocher in order to allow the hook to exit along the entrance trajectory to prevent iatrogenic injury (Figures 4(a) and 4(b)). No significant hemorrhage was appreciated from the puncture site after removal of the IOFB, and the wound was copiously irrigated with bacitracin-infused saline. Cerebrospinal fluid (CSF) leak was not appreciated.

Postoperatively, he was taken for a conventional CT which showed a displaced comminuted fracture of the greater sphenoid wing, a small amount of retrobulbar hematoma, and a trace left anterior temporal contusion with adjacent subarachnoid hemorrhage (Figure 5). The optic nerve was not suspected to be injured by the fracture fragments as the fractures were lateral to the optic canal. The sphenoid wing fractures were assessed by the neurosurgery service, and no operative repair was indicated given the lack of CSF leak. He was admitted to intensive care unit for blood pressure control and frequent neurologic checks as a result of cerebral contusion and subarachnoid hemorrhage. A repeat CT scan six hours after his surgery was performed to rule out further hemorrhage. The patient underwent ophthalmologic examination daily, without further deterioration of the visual acuity or signs of retrobulbar hematoma or other neurological deficits. Three weeks after the initial injury, the patient had a persistent RAPD and no further improvement in vision. Follow-up vascular imaging two weeks after the incident in the form of CT angiography of the head ruled out delayed vascular injury, pseudoaneurysm, or carotid-cavernous fistula. A formal Humphrey visual field test was performed two weeks after the initial injury which showed a full visual field in the right eye and a central and cecocentral defect with superior and inferior nasal steps in the left eye (Figure 6). At 3 months, the patient's best-corrected Snellen vision improved to 20/30, with persistent RAPD in the left eye.

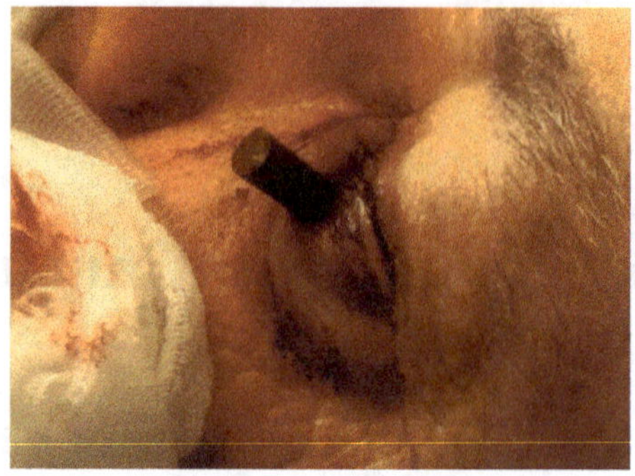

Figure 1: External photograph of the patient's left eye, with a metallic foreign body extruding out from the left lower lid above the inferior orbital rim.

3. Discussion

Penetrating orbital injury with intracranial extension can potentially have a devastating prognosis. Furthermore, when a foreign body is retained in the orbit, management becomes even more complicated. The specific management is dependent on the structures injured as well as the intrinsic material of the foreign body, in addition to the size and the location of the foreign body [1, 3–5].

Most IOFB are categorized into organic or nonorganic material [6]. Organic IOFB warrant aggressive measures to achieve removal due to high risk of intraorbital infection [1, 7]. Nonorganic IOFB do not always require removal, especially if the IOFB is small and comprised of an inert metal. Nonorganic IOFB may be appropriately managed conservatively if they are thought to be in an inaccessible location which would lead to potential serious complications if surgical removal were to be performed. For example, a ferromagnetic metallic foreign body can remain harmless for years; however, they can cause serious ocular injuries when exposed to strong magnetic forces. This serves as a permanent contraindication for the patient to undergo magnetic resonance imaging (MRI) [6].

Strategizing an appropriate surgical approach for removal of an IOFB is incredibly important, as the wrong approach may result in significant morbidity or even mortality. If vascular injury is suspected, an anterior approach

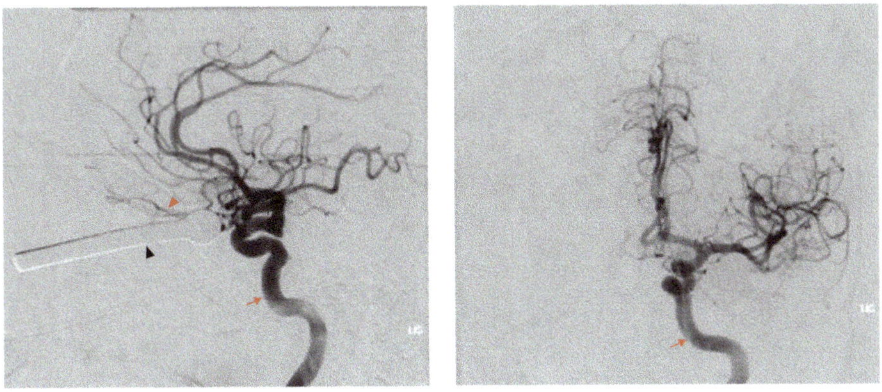

(a) (b)

FIGURE 2: (a) Lateral and (b) Towne's view of an arterial phase digital subtraction angiography showing left internal carotid artery injection demonstrating no major arterial injury. The subtracted silhouette of the foreign object still protruding from the patient's left eye is also visualized.

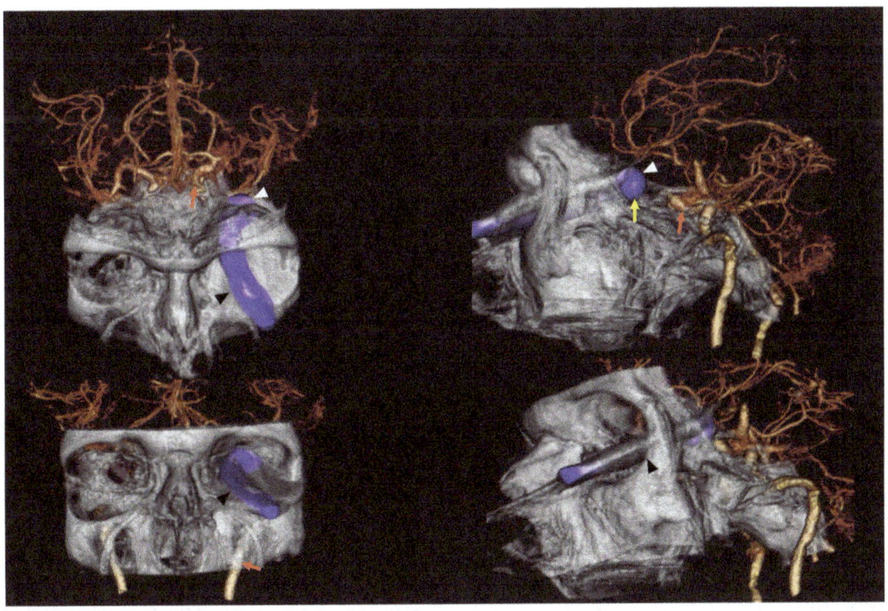

FIGURE 3: CT angiography with a 3D reconstructed image, demonstrating orbitocranial junction and adjacent arterial vasculature with no apparent vascular injury. The black arrowhead depicts IOFB, the white arrowhead shows the blunt tip of IOFB, the red arrow shows the internal carotid artery, and the yellow arrow shows the comminuted sphenoid bone fracture.

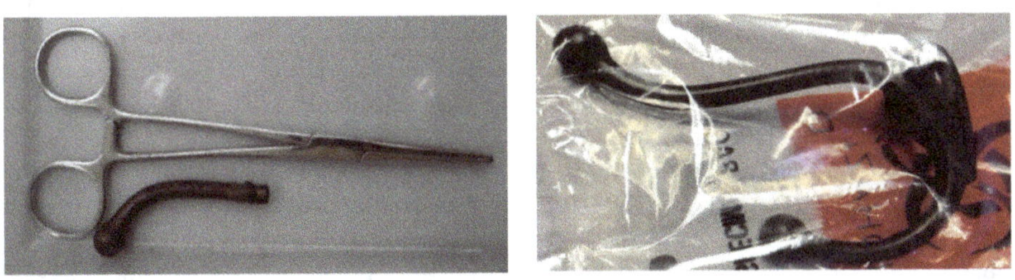

(a) (b)

FIGURE 4: (a) Foreign body after transorbital removal. (b) Another coat hook from the same rack provided to medical personnel by the patient's family.

carries the risk of bleeding and death following removal of the foreign body due to sudden release of the tamponading effect of the foreign body over the injured vasculature [8]. If there is evidence of obvious violation of vasculature, a transcranial approach is often preferred, as it offers better control of the neurovascular anatomy.

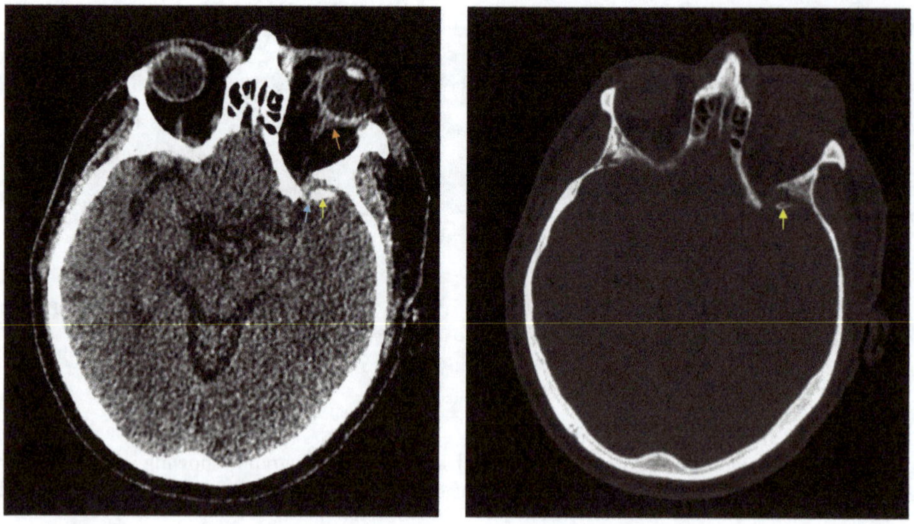

(a) (b)

FIGURE 5: (a) Axial noncontrast CT head brain and (b) bone window obtained after foreign object removal demonstrating a left sphenoid wing comminuted fracture (yellow arrow) and associated small retrobulbar (orange arrow) and subarachnoid hemorrhage (blue arrow).

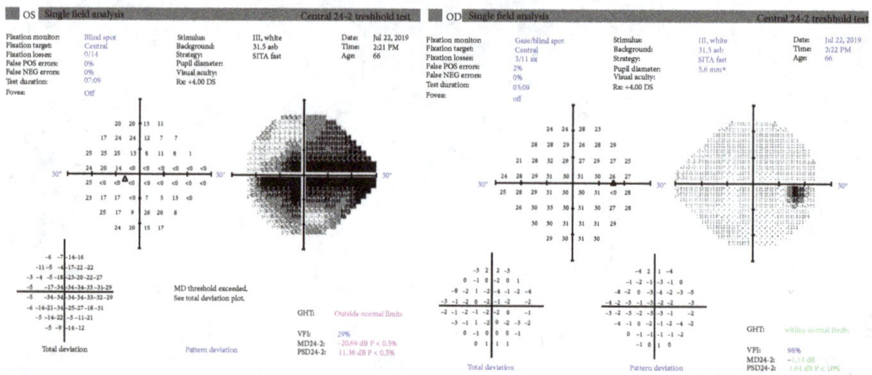

FIGURE 6: Humphrey 24-2 visual field. OD: full with no defect; OS: large central and cecocentral defect with superior and inferior nasal steps.

In our case, performing a craniotomy prior to IOFB removal in order to directly visualize injured structures and to guide removal was considered. However, this was not pursued because the preoperative workup did not show dural laceration and neurologic or intracranial vascular injury. Durotomy would need to be performed in order to visualize the IOFB through the craniotomy which would create more opportunity for infection and CSF leak. A transorbital approach was selected, due to good visualization of neurovascular integrity, the mechanism of injury, the source of IOFB, and the reconstructed 3D image showing no violation of vascular structure. The low-velocity injury and blunt tip of the coat hook (Figure 3) made it less likely to cause dural or vascular laceration.

Visualization of the foreign object is the key to identifying the appropriate management. CT remains the ultimate cranial imaging modality for emergencies. CTs are obtained rapidly and allow for quick identification of hemorrhages and bony injuries with excellent detail. While the quality of soft tissue structures is far inferior to MRI, thin-cut CT does provide vital (and fast) assessment of the orbital integrity and may reveal other intracranial injuries such as hemorrhagic contusions and hematomas. This enabled rapid surgical planning and intervention. With the administration of contrast dye, CTA provides excellent vascular assessment. In fact, advancements in CTA technology are comparable to formal catheter angiography, and such can be performed on a much faster time scale without significant risk of stroke or arterial dissection. Catheter angiography via digital subtraction angiography (DSA) remains the gold standard of vascular integrity; although there is a small risk of stroke or vascular injury during catheterization, the images allow for selective visualization of vessels during the arterial and venous phase. Active hemorrhage or vascular injury can be diagnosed and treated via DSA, creating an incredibly powerful tool. Although MRI has many advantages to CT, it has limited applications in intracranial trauma assessment because of the use of powerful magnets, significant length of data acquisition, and overall limited availability in most hospitals on an emergent basis.

The decision of using high-dose intravenous steroid was deferred due to questionable intracranial involvement initially. Following the removal of IOFB, the decision of high-dose steroid was withheld due to more than eight hours passing since the incident of trauma. In addition, there are no convincing data that steroids provide any additional visual benefit over observation alone [9].

In our case, multidisciplinary careful planning was warranted. IR-guided removal allowed for better intraoperative visualization of orbitocranial structures and the new onset of hemorrhages. After the removal of the IOFB, if a large hemorrhage was appreciated on the open-cone CT scan, neurosurgery was prepared to perform a craniotomy for hemorrhage removal or CSF leak repair if necessary. If there was a sign of arterial injury with massive hemorrhage, IR was available to perform a diagnostic angiogram with possible embolization. Likewise, if there was a pseudoaneurysm or dissection, neurosurgery and/or IR remained available for potential stent, clip, or coil embolization. If there was a secondary globe rupture, ophthalmology was readily available for surgical repair.

Our case report demonstrates a very interesting presentation of an intraorbital foreign body. The management of which required multidisciplinary expertise to achieve the best clinical outcome. The nature of this injury was unusual, and the ball valve implantation of the hook into the orbit was remarkable. The patient was fortunate that the hook did not penetrate further and cause serious intracranial injuries. Good clinical and radiographic workup combined with surgical treatment allowed for a thorough yet expeditious successful management of this unique pathology.

Abbreviations

IOFB: Intraorbital foreign body
ER: Emergency room
IR: Interventional radiology
EMS: Emergency medical service
GCS: Glasgow Coma Scale
OS: Oculus sinister
RAPD: Relative afferent pupillary defect
CT: Computed tomography
CTA: CT angiography
MRI: Magnetic resonance imaging
3D: Three-dimensional
CSF: Cerebrospinal fluid
DSA: Digital subtraction angiography.

Consent

Written informed consent was obtained from the patient for publication of this case report and any accompanying images. A copy of the written consent is available for review by the editor-in-chief of this journal.

Authors' Contributions

H.Y. and A.B. conceived of the presented idea. H.Y. and A.B. diagnosed and provided the management methods. A.B. performed the surgery with supervision of L.C. H.Y. and S.D. contributed to follow-up data acquisition. H.Y., A.B., and S.D. wrote the manuscript. H.Y. formatted the images.

Acknowledgments

L.C. and T.B. were present and supervised the surgery.

References

[1] T. P. Fulcher, A. A. McNab, and T. J. Sullivan, "Clinical features and management of intraorbital foreign bodies," *Ophthalmology*, vol. 109, no. 3, pp. 494–500, 2002.

[2] P. Türkçuoğlu and S. Aydoğan, "Intracranial foreign body in a globe-perforating injury," *Canadian Journal of Ophthalmology*, vol. 41, no. 4, pp. 504-505, 2006.

[3] J. Chen, T. Shen, Y. Wu, and J. Yan, "Clinical characteristics and surgical treatment of intraorbital foreign bodies in a tertiary eye center," *The Journal of Craniofacial Surgery*, vol. 26, no. 6, pp. e486–e489, 2015.

[4] A. D. Bilge, "Intraorbital foreign bodies: clinical features and outcomes of surgical removal," *Turkish Journal of Trauma and Emergency Surgery*, vol. 22, no. 5, pp. 432–436, 2016.

[5] A. Moretti, M. Laus, D. Crescenzi, and A. Croce, "Peri-orbital foreign body: a case report," *Journal of Medical Case Reports*, vol. 6, no. 1, 2012.

[6] A. B. Callahan and M. K. Yoon, "Intraorbital foreign bodies: retrospective chart review and review of literature," *International Ophthalmology Clinics*, vol. 53, no. 4, pp. 157–165, 2013.

[7] A. M. Nasr, B. G. Haik, J. C. Fleming, H. M. Al-Hussain, and Z. A. Karcioglu, "Penetrating orbital injury with organic foreign bodies," *Ophthalmology*, vol. 106, no. 3, pp. 523–532, 1999.

[8] A. Singh, S. I. Sadique, and S. N. Ghosh, "Intraorbital foreign body with intracranial extension: a case series," *International Clinical Neuroscience Journal*, vol. 5, no. 1, pp. 43–45, 2018.

[9] P. Yu-Wai-Man and P. G. Griffiths, "Surgery for traumatic optic neuropathy," *Cochrane Database of Systematic Reviews*, vol. 19, no. 4, 2005.

39

Bilateral Simultaneous Anterior Ischemic Optic Neuropathy following Total Knee Arthroplasty with Epidural Block

Ahmed M. Habib[1,2] **Yousef A. Fouad**[1,2] **and Mahmood O. Mekkawy**[1]

[1] *Al Mashreq Eye Center, Cairo, Egypt*
[2] *Department of Ophthalmology, Ain Shams University Hospitals, Cairo, Egypt*

Correspondence should be addressed to Yousef A. Fouad; yousef.a.fouad@gmail.com

Academic Editor: Takaaki Hayashi

Ischemic optic neuropathy (ION) resulting in perioperative vision loss (POVL) is a rare occurrence following nonocular procedures. Bilateral simultaneous anterior ION (AION) is even rarer, and no cases have been reported after central neuraxial block. We report a case of bilateral simultaneous AION, confirmed by multimodal imaging, in a 66-year-old male patient who underwent total knee arthroplasty under epidural anesthesia in which episodes of hypotension—one intraoperatively and one late postoperatively—had occurred. Hypotension is the most common adverse effect to epidural block, and counseling about POVL should extend beyond general anesthesia to include those undergoing procedures with central neuraxial block.

1. Introduction

Perioperative vision loss (POVL) is a rare but catastrophic complication of nonocular surgical procedures, for which ischemic optic neuropathy (ION)—particularly posterior ION (PION)—is most commonly implicated [1]. The frequency of permanent POVL complicating noncardiac surgery was estimated to be 1 in 118,783 patients in a large retrospective analysis, with all affected cases having undergone general anesthesia and with all ION cases having developed PION [2]. More scarce are reports of POVL with the use of central neuraxial block [3] and POVL due to anterior ION (AION) [4].

Reported risk factors for POVL due to ION are related to perioperative hemodynamic instability, including prolonged surgical duration, anemia, hypotension, and blood transfusion [1]. The most commonly implicated surgeries are cardiothoracic and orthopedic ones, especially spine procedures [2]. The ensuing PION or AION may be unilateral or bilateral [4], and permanent severe visual loss is the final fate in at least 75% of the cases [1].

2. Case Report

A 66-year-old male patient underwent total knee arthroplasty under epidural anesthesia for severe osteoarthritis. The patient had a medical history of controlled hypertension and Type II diabetes mellitus and a stroke in the preceding year that focally involved the right frontal lobe, with minimal residual neurological impairment for which the patient had received the proper urgent management and was maintained on daily clopidogrel (75 mg) and aspirin (75 mg). Ophthalmological examination one month prior to the surgery had shown a corrected distance visual acuity (CDVA) of 20/20 (1.0) in both eyes with a hyperopic refraction of +1.00 D in the right eye and +1.50/−0.75 × 130 in the left eye. No abnormality had been detected on fundus examination except for mild nonproliferative diabetic retinopathy.

The surgery was uneventful with minimal blood loss and a duration of around 90 minutes. There was a brief episode of hypotension (80/50 mmHg) following the introduction of the epidural anesthesia, but the blood pressure returned to normal levels with the aid of vasopressors. The immediate

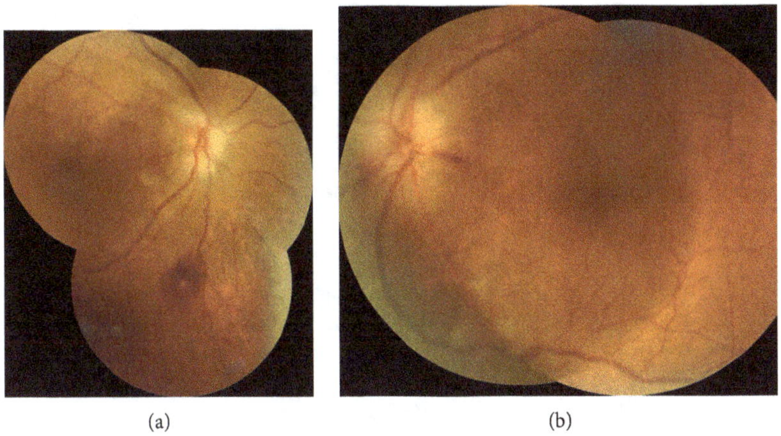

FIGURE 1: Fundus photography of the right (a) and left (b) eyes showing pale, edematous optic discs, cotton wool patches, and intraretinal hemorrhages.

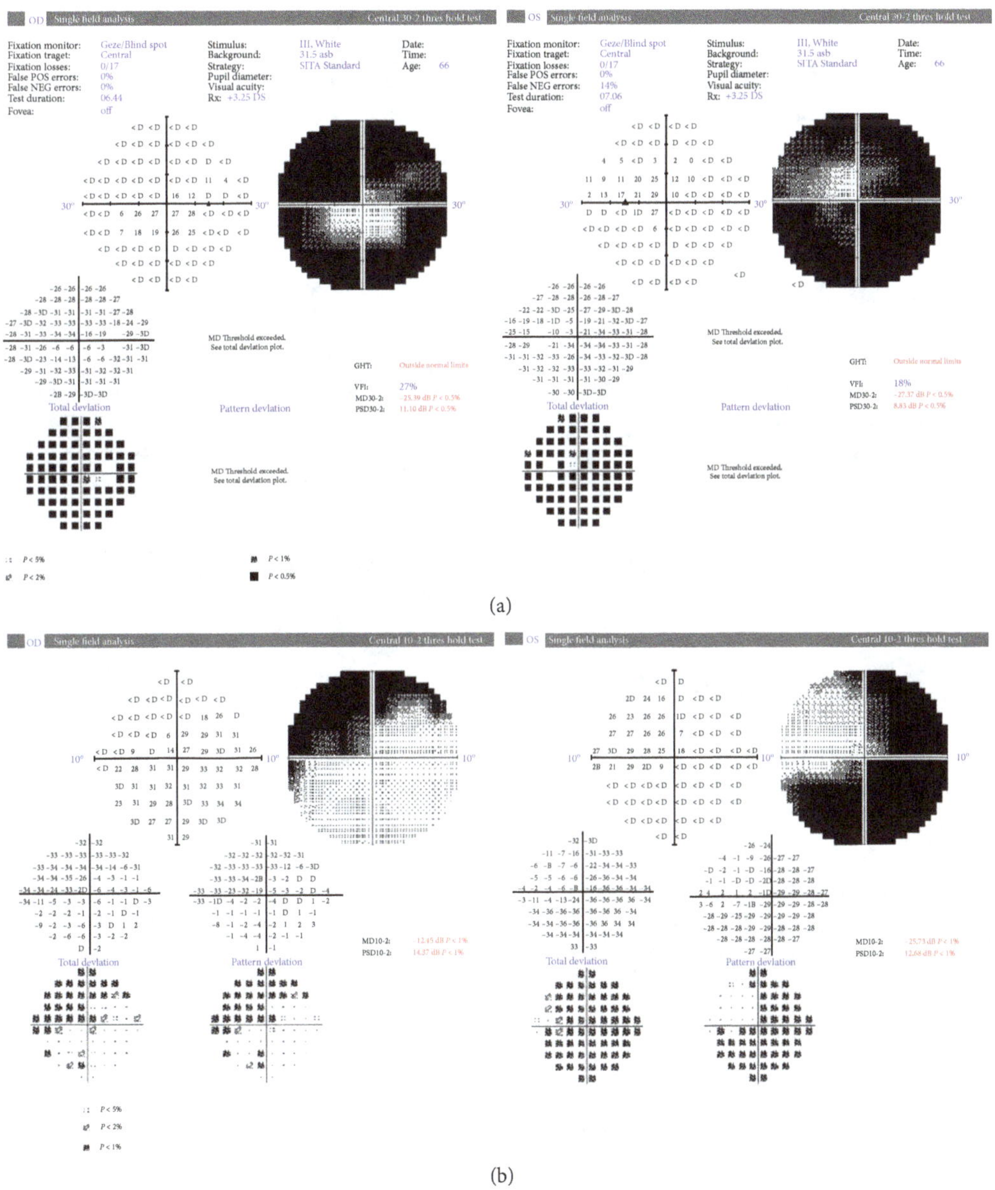

FIGURE 2: 30-2 (a) and central 10-2 (b) visual field plots of both eyes of the patient showing tubular fields with small, central remnant islands of vision.

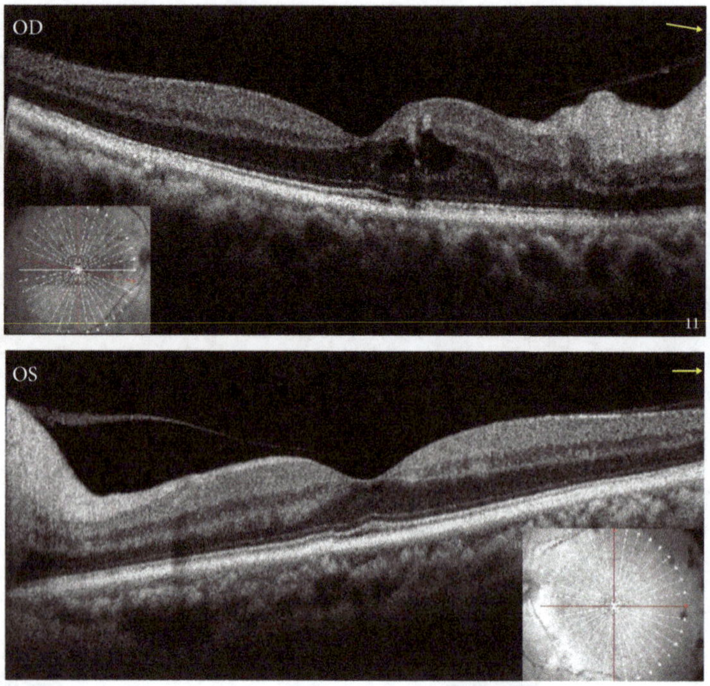

Figure 3: OCT of the right (a) and left (b) maculae showing preserved foveal architecture but distorted and thickened peripapillary nerve fiber layer, more pronounced in the right eye.

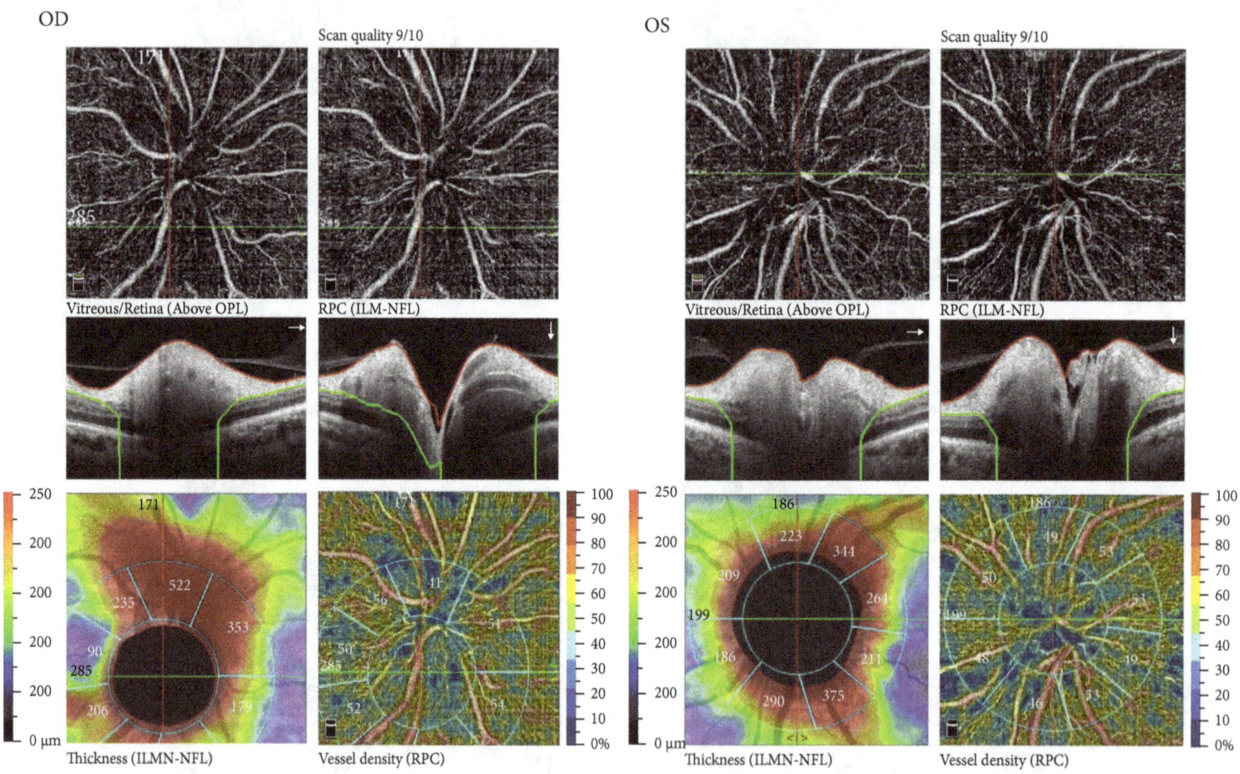

Figure 4: OCT-A of the right and left eyes showing peripapillary distortion of the retinal nerve fiber layer and pronounced loss of the capillary microvascular perfusion.

postoperative period was uneventful. On the first postoperative night, the patient experienced another attack of hypotension with the blood pressure dropping down to 70/40 mmHg; this was successfully managed with the administration of vasopressors and fluids. On the first morning after the surgery, the patient experienced blurring of vision with large blank areas in his field of vision. Magnetic resonance imaging was ordered but revealed no acute cerebral insults.

On ophthalmological examination, the right and left eyes had a CDVA of 20/80 (0.6) and 20/20 (1.0), and an intraocular pressure of 16 mmHg and 21 mmHg, respectively. Both pupils were sluggish to react to light stimuli, but the anterior segments were otherwise free. Fundus examination (Figure 1) revealed bilateral swollen, pale optic discs, with peripapillary cotton wool spots, intraretinal hemorrhages in the right fundus (Figure 1(a)), and retinal nerve fiber layer hemorrhages in the left fundus (splinter hemorrhages, Figure 1(b)). Visual field examination was ordered (Figure 2) and revealed severe constriction in the fields of both eyes (tubular fields) on the 30-2 exams (Figure 2(a)). Central 10 degrees examination (Figure 2(b)) confirmed the presence of small remnant islands in the central fields of both eyes. Optical coherence tomography (OCT) of the macula (Figure 3) revealed preserved foveal anatomy, with thickening and distortion of the peripapillary retinal nerve fiver layer which, in the right eye, was more pronounced and associated with intraretinal edema. OCT-Angiography (OCT-A) of the optic disc (Figure 4) showed diffuse distortion and loss of the peripapillary microvascular cuff in both eyes. No symptoms of arteritis (headache or jaw claudication) were elicited on detailed history taking from the patient, and an ordered erythrocytic sedimentation was within normal values. This led to a diagnosis of bilateral non-arteritic AION. A follow-up of the patient after 1 month did not reveal any change except for mild subjective visual improvement reported by the patient.

3. Discussion

To the best of our knowledge, this is the first report on bilateral simultaneous ION following surgery with central neuraxial block. Only one other report [3] exists in the literature that describes unilateral ION that occurred after epidural block for emergency cesarean section, in which a hypotensive episode had occurred on administration of the anesthetic. Bilateral simultaneous AION has, however, been reported to occur spontaneously [5], after ingestion of sildenafil [6, 7], with hypercoagulability [8] and vasculitis [9], with long-term hemodialysis [10], and after prostatic resection surgery under general anesthesia [11].

In our described case, both intraoperative and delayed postoperative hypotension could be implicated in the development of ION. Perioperative hypotension is recognized as a potential risk for developing POVL due to ION [12] and also as the most common complication of epidural block [12]. Physiological drop in blood pressure often occurs within the initial 30 minutes after introduction of the anesthetic and is thought to majorly be attributed to the sympathetic blockade resulting in arteriolar and venular dilation and an ensuing "functional hypovolemia." This has been reported to respond excellently to vasopressors [12]. On the other hand, the use of vasopressors has been suggested as a—statistical—risk factor for developing POVL [13]. The debate around how significant of a role hemodynamic changes play in POVL is still ongoing [14].

Other risk factors for developing POVL include prolonged surgical procedure, significant blood loss or the need for blood transfusion, anemia, facial edema, pressure on the eyes, and/or prone head positioning intraoperatively [1], none of which had occurred with the case we report. The lack of prospective study design and the reliance on retrospective analysis of large datasets reduce the strength of evidence on risk factors for developing POVL. Nevertheless, the American Society of Anesthesiologists Task Force on Perioperative Visual Loss advises on (1) the continuous intraoperative monitoring of blood pressure with conservation in usage of deliberate hypotensive techniques and vasopressors on a case-by-case basis, (2) use of colloids and crystalloids for patients with substantial blood loss, with continuous monitoring of central venous pressure and hemoglobin/hematocrit values, (3) avoiding eye pressure and maintaining elevated head position whenever possible, and (4) immediate postoperative check on patient's vision after regaining of an alert state and immediate ophthalmological consultation on early suspicion of POVL [15].

Counseling of patients about the minimal risk of developing POVL, especially those with identifiable preoperative medical risk factors, has been recommended for patients scheduled for general anesthesia [1]. Based on the aforementioned case, we conclude that counseling should expand to include those undergoing procedures with central neuraxial block.

References

[1] B. Chwalisz, A. L. Gilbert, and J. W. Gittinger, "Perioperative vision loss after non-ocular surgery," *Seminars in Ophthalmology*, vol. 33, no. 1, pp. 17–22, 2018.

[2] M. E. Warner, M. A. Warner, J. A. Garrity, R. A. MacKenzie, and D. O. Warner, "The frequency of perioperative vision loss," *Anesthesia and Analgesia*, vol. 93, no. 6, pp. 1417–1421, 2001.

[3] M. Gupta, P. Puri, and I. G. Rennie, "Anterior ischemic optic neuropathy after emergency caesarean section under epidural anesthesia," *Acta Anaesthesiologica Scandinavica*, vol. 46, no. 6, pp. 751-752, 2002.

[4] A. Goyal, M. Elminawy, M. A. Alvi et al., "Ischemic optic neuropathy following spine surgery: case control analysis and systematic review of the literature," *Spine (Phila Pa 1976)*, vol. 44, no. 15, pp. 1087–1096, 2019.

[5] M. J. Goff, "Bilateral simultaneous anterior ischemic optic neuropathy in a young, healthy man," *Archives of Ophthalmology*, vol. 121, no. 11, pp. 1652-1653, 2003.

[6] M. M. Moschos and I. Margetis, "Bilateral simultaneous anterior ischemic optic neuropathy associated with sildenafil," *Case Reports in Ophthalmology*, vol. 2, no. 2, pp. 262–265, 2011.

[7] A. Tarantini, A. Faraoni, F. Menchini, and P. Lanzetta, "Bilateral simultaneous nonarteritic anterior ischemic optic neuropathy after ingestion of sildenafil for erectile dysfunction," *Case*

Reports in Medicine, vol. 2012, Article ID 747658, 5 pages, 2012.

[8] M. S. Tönz, V. Rigamonti, and M. E. Iliev, "Simultaneous, bilateral anterior ischemic optic neuropathy (AION) in polycythemia vera: a case report," *Klinische Monatsblätter für Augenheilkunde*, vol. 225, no. 5, pp. 504–506, 2008.

[9] M. Hata, K. Miyamoto, A. Oishi, and N. Yoshimura, "Case of simultaneous bilateral anterior ischemic optic neuropathy associated with Takayasu disease," *Canadian Journal of Ophthalmology*, vol. 48, no. 2, pp. e33–e35, 2013.

[10] U. Limon, B. I. S. Akcay, and E. Akcay, "Bilateral simultaneous non-arteritic anterior ischemic optic neuropathy with occlusion of unilateral cilioretinal artery: a case report," *Journal of Northern Clinics of Istanbul*, vol. 6, no. 4, pp. 407–411, 2019.

[11] L. M. Sadaba, A. Garcia-Layana, M. J. Maldonado, and J. M. Berian, "Bilateral ischemic optic neuropathy after transurethral prostatic resection: a case report," *BMC Ophthalmology*, vol. 6, no. 1, p. 32, 2006.

[12] K. Holte, N. B. Foss, C. Svensén, C. Lund, J. L. Madsen, and H. Kehlet, "Epidural anesthesia, hypotension, and changes in intravascular volume," *Anesthesiology*, vol. 100, no. 2, pp. 281–286, 2004.

[13] M. A. Myers, S. R. Hamilton, A. J. Bogosian, C. H. Smith, and T. A. Wagner, "Visual loss as a complication of spine surgery," *Spine (Phila Pa 1976)*, vol. 22, no. 12, pp. 1325–1329, 1997.

[14] R. Foroozan and K. C. Golnik, "Are anemia and hypotension causally related to perioperative ischemic optic neuropathy?," *Journal of Neuro-Ophthalmology*, vol. 37, no. 1, pp. 81–86, 2017.

[15] American Society of Anesthesiologists Task Force on Perioperative Visual Loss, "Practice advisory for perioperative visual loss associated with spine surgery: an updated report by the American Society of Anesthesiologists Task Force on Perioperative Visual Loss," *Anesthesiology*, vol. 116, no. 2, pp. 274–285, 2012.

Hypopyon after Primary Cryopreserved Amniotic Membrane Transplantation for Sterile Corneal Ulceration: A Case Report and Review of the Literature

Kostas G. Boboridis, Dimitrios G. Mikropoulos, and Nick S. Georgiadis

3rd Ophthalmology Department, Aristotle University of Thessaloniki, Kiriakidi 1, Thessaloniki 546 21, Greece

Correspondence should be addressed to Kostas G. Boboridis; kosbob@otenet.gr

Academic Editor: Hsin Yi Chen

Purpose. To report the acute development of hypopyon after primary cryopreserved amniotic membrane transplantation (AMT) for persistent corneal epithelial defect and sterile ulceration. *Case Presentation.* A selected case report of a 71-year-old male who underwent primary cryopreserved AMT for the management of long-standing corneal epithelial defects and stroma thinning. The patient developed 2 mm sterile hypopyon within 48 hours after AMT for corneal surface reconstruction. He responded well to the intensified routine postoperative topical treatment of steroid and antibiotic eye drops with the hypopyon resolving completely one week later. Five weeks after surgery, the corneal surface was smooth and epithelialized with no anterior chamber reaction or recurrence of hypopyon. *Discussion.* Hypopyon may develop as a rare complication of primary cryopreserved AMT for sterile corneal defects. It may be attributed to immunologic or hypersensitivity reaction and should be differentiated from active ocular infection as it resolves spontaneously with the routine postoperative topical treatment of steroid and antibiotic drops.

1. Introduction

Amniotic membrane transplantation (AMT) has been extensively used for ocular surface reconstruction with a wide range of indications. It provides a biological scaffolding which exhibits distinct antiadhesive, bacteriostatic, and epithelializing properties. The amniotic membrane (AM) and its epithelial cells do not express human leukocyte antigens; it is therefore believed to be immunologically inert and does not initiate an immunologic response of the recipient [1]. AM has been transplanted on to the ocular surface as a patch or a graft for persistent corneal epithelial defects, conjunctival defects, symblepharon, pterygia, chemical burns, and bullous keratopathy [2].

The purpose of this report is to present the acute development of sterile hypopyon into the anterior chamber following primary cryopreserved AMT onto the corneal surface for persistent sterile corneal epithelium defect and stromal thinning. A written informed consent for anonymized patient information and images to be published was provided by the patient.

2. Case Presentation

A 71-year-old male patient with a persistent central corneal epithelial defect and stromal thinning of 5 mm diameter on his right eye with no evidence of infection or corneal neuropathy was intermittently responsive to conservative topical treatment with antibiotic drops and ointment, intensive lubricating drops, and bandage contact lenses. The central cornea had a thinner area of 2 mm diameter with only 1/3 of the stroma remaining before Descemet's membrane and showed no sign of healing with only intermittent epithelialization despite the conservative treatment for over eight weeks from presentation. There was no evidence of corneal hypesthesia, and repeated corneal swabs for microbiology investigation proved the sterility of the lesion. The clinical suspicion of corneal rubbing against the pillow because of

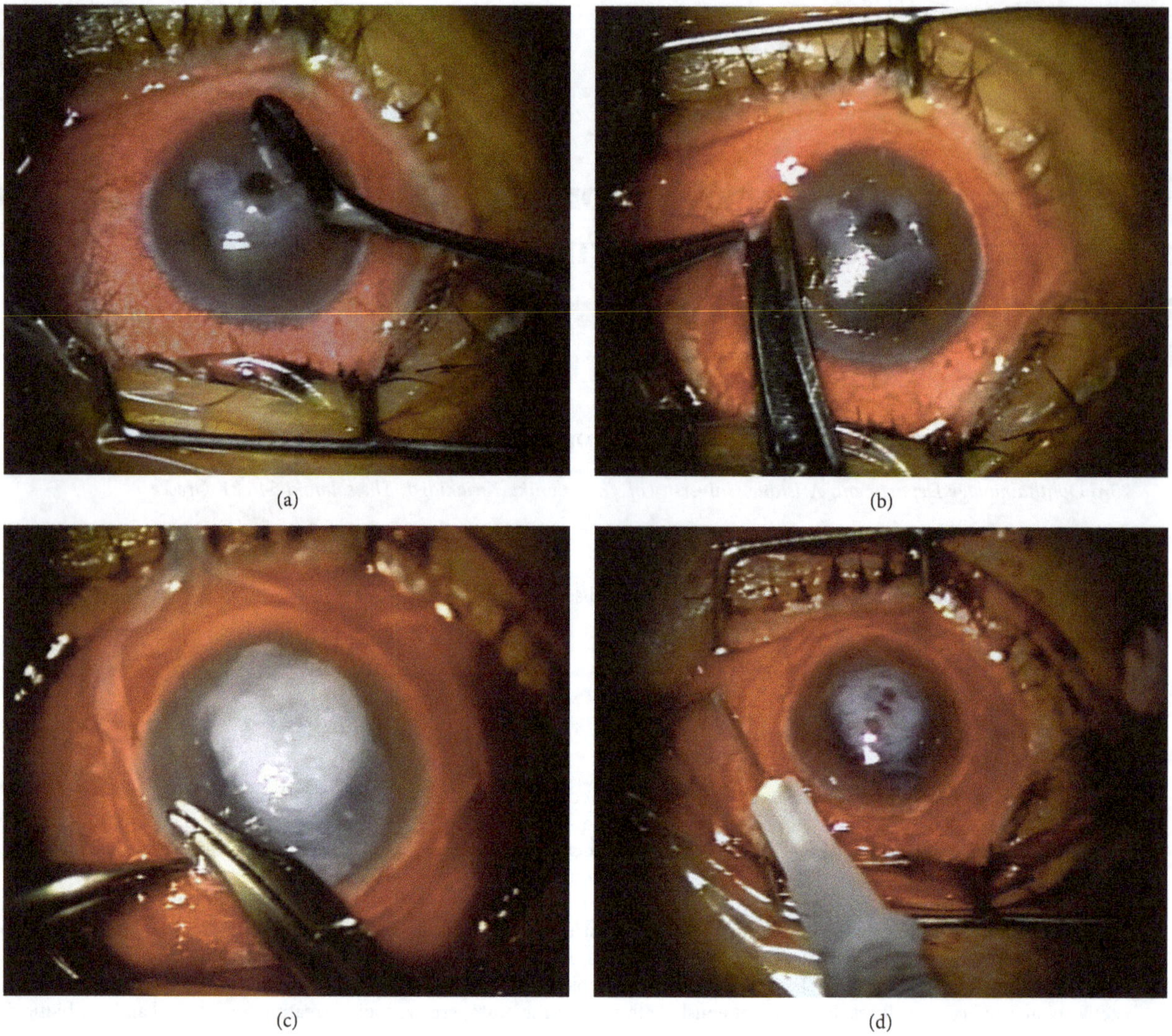

FIGURE 1: (a) The stromal ulceration was debrided, and the corneal epithelium was removed up to the limbal area. (b) 360° conjunctival peritomy is performed adjacent to limbus. (c) The ulcer was filled up to a surface level with multiple pieces of AM, and a larger AM was transferred to the recipient eye with the epithelial side down. The membrane was trimmed to cover the cornea and limbal area and secured with continuous 10-0 nylon sutures to the conjunctival edges. (d) After suturing, we do a subconjunctival injection with a mixture of dexamethasone and gentamycin. Finally, we place a bandage contact lens to cover the transplanted membrane and cornea.

his sleeping preference on his right side was the most probable cause of his condition.

As counselling for his sleep pattern and conservative lubricating treatment had no effect, we proceeded with surgical management of his corneal defect using cryopreserved AM. We followed our previously described standard technique for corneal surface reconstruction with the membrane placed over the whole cornea [2].

Following peribulbar and subconjunctival anaesthesia, we carefully debrided the thinner crater and scraped off the corneal epithelium up to the limbal margin followed by a 360° conjunctival peritomy (Figures 1(a) and 1(b)). Small cut pieces of AM were used to fill the stroma defect level with the surface, and a larger piece was trimmed to cover the whole corneal and limbal area with the epithelial side down used ("sticky" stroma side up) as a patch for a healthy corneal epithelium to grow underneath. We secured the membrane under the conjunctival edges with a continuous 10.0 nylon suture (Figure 1(c)). Finally, we applied a subconjunctival injection of a mixture of dexamethasone and gentamycin and placed a bandage contact lens for 2 to 3 weeks (Figure 1(d)). Our routine postoperative regimen was combined steroid and antibiotic eye drops 6 times daily for two weeks tapering down thereafter.

For deep corneal ulceration, we use small pieces of AM to fill the stroma defect placed as grafts with epithelial side up aiming at subepithelial or transepithelial integration of the membrane in relation to the newly formed epithelium. Following limbal peritomy, a large piece of AM is placed as a patch with the epithelial side down covering the entire cornea and limbal area, aiming at superficial localization (disintegration) of this covering piece of amniotic membrane. In theory, this arrangement will facilitate the growth of a new, healthy corneal epithelium from the intact limbal area under the

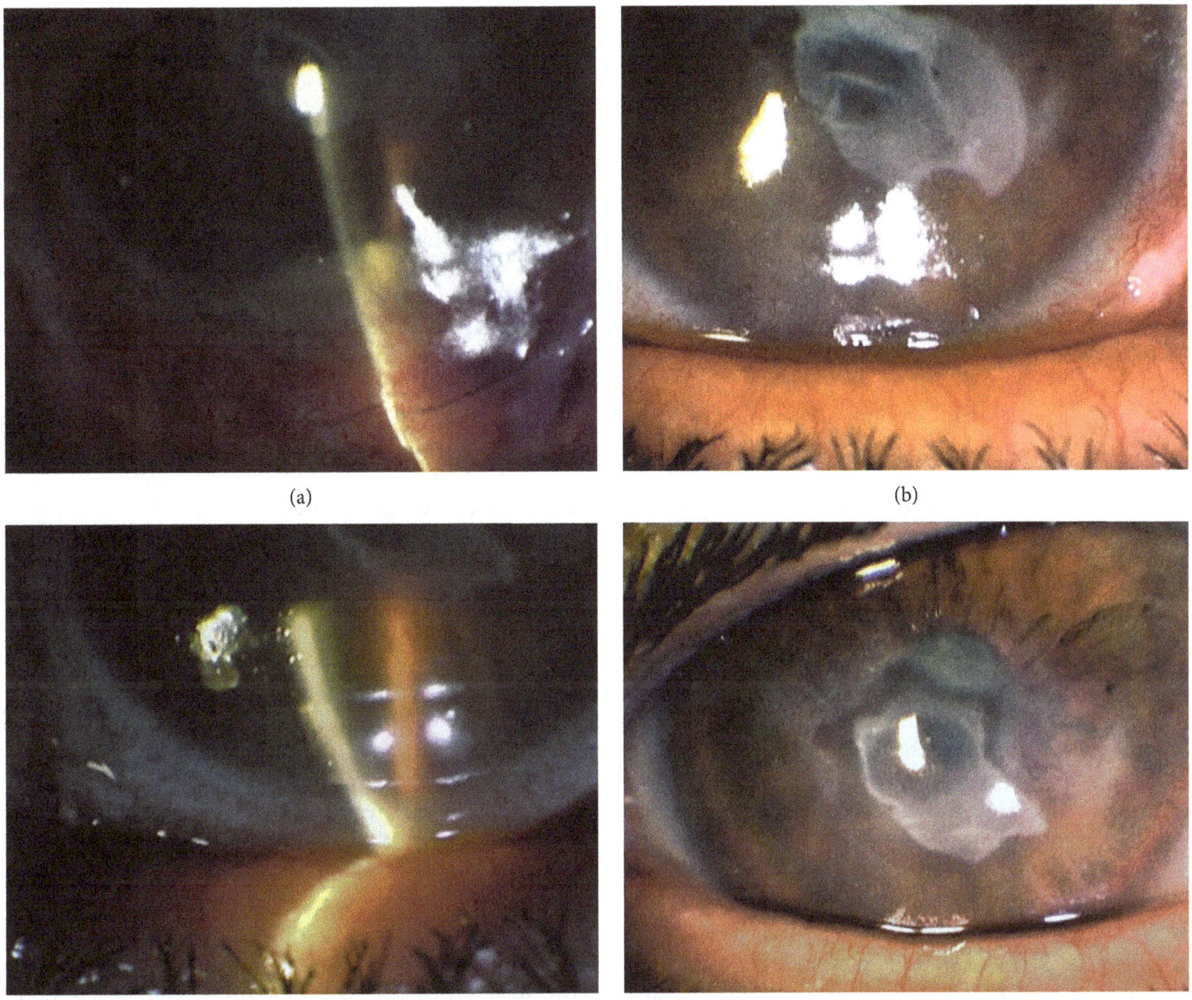

(a) (b) (c) (d)

FIGURE 2: (a) 3 mm hypopyon formation 2 days after cryopreserved AMT. (b) Regression of hypopyon one week later. (c, d) Clear anterior chamber with healed ocular surface and no signs of inflammation 5 weeks after surgery.

superficial layer of AM but over the small pieces of AM covering the stroma defect [3, 4]. We have abandoned the technique of using a smaller than the corneal diameter piece of AM as a graft (epithelium up) which is sutured on to the cornea within the limbus so that the newly formed epithelium will grow over the membrane as less effective and more traumatic for the cornea [5].

The AM graft was prepared and cryopreserved by our local eye bank using the Good Tissue Banking Practice procedures [6]. Despite the tested sterility of the ocular surface, the preoperative antibiotic treatment, and the uneventful perioperative period, he developed a 2 mm hypopyon within 48 hours when we reviewed him after primary AMT (Figure 2(a)). He was using our routine regimen of tobramycin 3 mg/ml and dexamethasone 1 mg/ml eye drops six times daily on a fixed combination.

Despite the alarming clinical presentation, there were no anterior chamber reaction and no signs of active infection; therefore, we considered the hypopyon formation being a sterile toxic or immunologic reaction. To confirm this diagnosis, we took a surface swab from the membrane and performed a full microbiological examination of the residual membrane and its culture medium which we always keep for up to 7 days for quality control which were proven negative.

The patient continued with our standard post-AMT treatment with increased dosage every two hours for three days, followed by 6 times daily for two more weeks tapering down thereafter. The hypopyon resolved completely with the current treatment a week later with no further complications or anterior chamber reaction (Figure 2(b)).

The epithelial defect and corneal thinning healed satisfactorily with smooth epithelium and a visible stromal scar with no recurrence or hypopyon 5 weeks postoperatively (Figures 2(c) and 2(d)).

3. Discussion

We have previously described in detail the standardized method for AM preparation used in our local eye bank since 1999 [2]. The placenta is obtained from an uncomplicated elective caesarean section delivery following all the necessary serologic and microbiology tests for the donor and tissue. After cleaning and rinsing the membrane with antibiotics under sterile conditions (lamellar flow hood), we place it onto a sterile nitrocellulose paper with the epithelial side up which we cut into 3 × 4 cm pieces. These are placed in sterile vials containing Dulbecco's modified Eagle medium and glycerol in a ratio of 1 : 1 for deep freeze (-80°C) storage. The AM is defrosted immediately before surgery and washed in sterile saline at least three times to remove the storage solution completely The process follows all the tissue testing and sterility protocols with quality control and release criteria of tissue adhered to the Good Tissue Practice set by the FDA [6].

Two to five of the stored membranes from each placenta are randomly tested for infection before released for surgery to ensure sterility of the processing and storage method. Similarly, we retain redundant tissue and culture medium after surgery for up to one week for postoperative repeat testing when necessary as it happened in this case.

Infection and toxic or immunologic reaction are the three most possible pathophysiological mechanisms for hypopyon formation in the immediate postoperative period following AMT. Neurotrophic keratopathy which is often requires AMT can present hypopyon in the natural course of the disease, but our case had uncompromised corneal sensation.

We have excluded the possibility of infection on this selected case based on negative microbiology testing and the clinical presentation with no infectious signs. Furthermore, ocular surface toxicity from chemicals may induce anterior chamber reaction but this seems very unlikely because we use a standardized time-tested surgical technique which includes intensive rinsing of the storage medium from the membrane with normal saline before transplantation, and all other cases of AMT had an unremarkable postoperative period.

Thus, we consider an immunologic reaction as the most probable cause for hypopyon formation in this case. There is evidence that the epithelial cells of AM do not express human leukocyte antigens A, B, C, or DR; therefore, AMT onto the ocular surface is considered to be immunologically inert [1, 5]. There is no published evidence of documented immunogenic reaction or graft rejections related to AMT for ocular surface reconstruction in humans although Howell et al. reported histologic evidence of host versus graft reaction after repeated transplantation of bovine AM into cattle with glycogenosis type II [7].

A retrospective review of cryopreserved AMT cases for noninfectious ocular surface reconstruction performed over 15-year period (2005-2015) identified a single case with adequate documentation and imaging out of 525 (0.19%) who developed sterile hypopyon after surgery.

A detailed literature search (Medline, PubMed, and Cochrane database) revealed three reports of sterile hypopyon formation soon after AMT. Gabler et al. reported hypopyon formation possibly due to immunologic reaction after repeated transplantation of amniotic membrane (AM) onto the corneal surface. The reaction occurred after the second and third cryopreserved AMT from the same donor for sterile deep trophic corneal ulceration [8]. Messmer reported two similar cases of hypopyon formation following cryopreserved AMT. However, both reported cases had a significant general medical history with an active atopic dermatitis on the first case in which the hypopyon occurred 4 weeks (rather than a few days) after combined superficial keratectomy, limbal allograft, and AMT in the context of limbal graft rejection. The second case suffered an acute leukaemia treated with full-body irradiation and bone marrow transplantation and developed hypopyon formation 2 days after repeated AMT although a penetrating keratoplasty had been performed between the AMTs [9]. In contrast to our uncomplicated case, both reports had the common feature of prior sensitization and immune reaction by either repeated procedures or allograft tissue. In a similar report, Srinivasan et al. used fresh AM and considered the immunogenicity of the fresh unprocessed tissue as the cause for hypopyon formation [10]. It has been shown that cryopreservation in 50% glycerol preserves the structure of the epithelium of the amniotic membrane but devitalizes cells contributing to reduced immunogenicity compared with fresh membranes which may induce immunologic reaction and explain hypopyon iritis in this case. However, cryopreservation does not exclude the possibility of immune reaction to the remaining antigenic structures [1, 11].

We have used amniotic membrane preparation and surgical techniques comparable to the ones reported in these publications (Figures 1(a)–1(d)) [2]. The presented case developed sterile hypopyon within two days after primary cryopreserved AMT for sterile corneal ulceration with no prior immunological sensitization or other ocular surface disease and resolved with our routine topical treatment for AMT. This report highlights the fact that cryopreserved amniotic membrane, although immunologically inert, when transplanted onto the corneal surface may elicit a localized sterile immune reaction presenting with a transient hypopyon formation. There is a strong need for more investigations into the immunologic implications of AMT and possible complications related to AMT. The uncommon complication of hypopyon formation soon after AMT should be clearly differentiated from surface infection or even endophthalmitis and treated accordingly. The literature suggests that a particular care must be taken for cases of repeated AMT or combined use of allogenic tissue that may stimulate the ocular immune system and more importantly in patients with systemic immunologic disorders.

References

[1] H. S. Dua, J. A. Gomes, A. J. King, and V. S. Maharajan, "The amniotic membrane in ophthalmology," *Survey of Ophthalmology*, vol. 49, no. 1, pp. 51–77, 2004.

[2] N. S. Georgiadis, N. G. Ziakas, K. G. Boboridis, C. Terzidou, and D. G. Mikropoulos, "Cryopreserved amniotic membrane transplantation for the management of symptomatic bullous keratopathy," *Clinical & Experimental Ophthalmology*, vol. 36, no. 2, pp. 130–135, 2008.

[3] M. D. Resch, U. Schlotzer-Schrehardt, C. Hofmann-Rummelt et al., "Integration patterns of cryopreserved amniotic membranes into the human cornea," *Ophthalmology*, vol. 113, no. 11, pp. 1927–1935, 2006.

[4] B. Seitz, M. D. Resch, U. Schlotzer-Schrehardt, C. Hofmann-Rummelt, R. Sauer, and F. E. Kruse, "Histopathology and ultrastructure of human corneas after amniotic membrane transplantation," *Archives of Ophthalmology*, vol. 124, no. 10, pp. 1487–1490, 2006.

[5] V. S. Maharajan, V. Shanmuganathan, A. Currie, A. Hopkinson, A. Powell-Richards, and H. S. Dua, "Amniotic membrane transplantation for ocular surface reconstruction: indications and outcomes," *Clinical & Experimental Ophthalmology*, vol. 35, no. 2, pp. 140–147, 2007.

[6] F. B. Marangon, E. C. Alfonso, D. Miller, N. M. Remonda, M. S. Muallem, and S. C. Tseng, "Incidence of microbial infection after amniotic membrane transplantation," *Cornea*, vol. 23, no. 3, pp. 264–269, 2004.

[7] J. M. C. Howell, P. R. Dorling, P. N. Dimarco, and E. G. Taylor, "Multiple implantation of normal amnion into cattle with generalized glycogenosis type II," *Journal of Inherited Metabolic Disease*, vol. 10, no. 1, pp. 3–10, 1987.

[8] B. Gabler and C. P. Lohmann, "Hypopyon after repeated transplantation of human amniotic membrane onto the corneal surface," *Ophthalmology*, vol. 107, no. 7, pp. 1344–1346, 2000.

[9] E. M. Messmer, "Hypopyon after amniotic membrane transplantation," *Ophthalmology*, vol. 108, no. 10, pp. 1714-1715, 2001.

[10] R. Srinivasan, T. Suchi Smitha, A. Gupta, and S. Kaliaperumal, "Hypopyon iritis after primary fresh amniotic membrane transplantation," *Cornea*, vol. 26, no. 10, pp. 1275-1276, 2007.

[11] M. Nubile, H. S. Dua, T. E. Lanzini et al., "Amniotic membrane transplantation for the management of corneal epithelial defects: an in vivo confocal microscopic study," *The British Journal of Ophthalmology*, vol. 92, no. 1, pp. 54–60, 2008.

Permissions

All chapters in this book were first published by Hindawi Publishing Corporation; hereby published with permission under the Creative Commons Attribution License or equivalent. Every chapter published in this book has been scrutinized by our experts. Their significance has been extensively debated. The topics covered herein carry significant findings which will fuel the growth of the discipline. They may even be implemented as practical applications or may be referred to as a beginning point for another development.

The contributors of this book come from diverse backgrounds, making this book a truly international effort. This book will bring forth new frontiers with its revolutionizing research information and detailed analysis of the nascent developments around the world.

We would like to thank all the contributing authors for lending their expertise to make the book truly unique. They have played a crucial role in the development of this book. Without their invaluable contributions this book wouldn't have been possible. They have made vital efforts to compile up to date information on the varied aspects of this subject to make this book a valuable addition to the collection of many professionals and students.

This book was conceptualized with the vision of imparting up-to-date information and advanced data in this field. To ensure the same, a matchless editorial board was set up. Every individual on the board went through rigorous rounds of assessment to prove their worth. After which they invested a large part of their time researching and compiling the most relevant data for our readers.

The editorial board has been involved in producing this book since its inception. They have spent rigorous hours researching and exploring the diverse topics which have resulted in the successful publishing of this book. They have passed on their knowledge of decades through this book. To expedite this challenging task, the publisher supported the team at every step. A small team of assistant editors was also appointed to further simplify the editing procedure and attain best results for the readers.

Apart from the editorial board, the designing team has also invested a significant amount of their time in understanding the subject and creating the most relevant covers. They scrutinized every image to scout for the most suitable representation of the subject and create an appropriate cover for the book.

The publishing team has been an ardent support to the editorial, designing and production team. Their endless efforts to recruit the best for this project, has resulted in the accomplishment of this book. They are a veteran in the field of academics and their pool of knowledge is as vast as their experience in printing. Their expertise and guidance has proved useful at every step. Their uncompromising quality standards have made this book an exceptional effort. Their encouragement from time to time has been an inspiration for everyone.

The publisher and the editorial board hope that this book will prove to be a valuable piece of knowledge for researchers, students, practitioners and scholars across the globe.

List of Contributors

Elias L. Warrak, Majd S. Haddam, Walid N. Dandan and Fady K. Sammouh
Department of Ophthalmology and Visual Sciences, University of Balamand, Advanced Eye Care Hospital, Lebanon

John E. Warrak
University of Balamand, Faculty of Medicine and Health Sciences, Lebanon

Şükran Bekdemir
Ophthalmology Clinic, Polatlı Duatepe State Hospital, Ankara, Turkey

Ahmet Kaan Gündüz
Department of Ophthalmology, Ankara University Faculty of Medicine, Ankara, Turkey

Ömür Ataoğlu
Private Mikro-Pat Pathology Laboratory, Ankara, Turkey

Josefina A. Mejías Smith, Laura A. Cañola Ramírez, Natalia Agudelo Arbelaez and Bárbara Rubio Lastra
Glaucoma Research Department, Instituto de Ojos Oftalmosalud, Lima, Peru

Juan Carlos Izquierdo Villavicencio
Glaucoma Research Department, Instituto de Ojos Oftalmosalud, Lima, Peru
Glaucoma Department, Instituto de Ojos Oftalmosalud, Lima, Peru

Amrit Banstola, Sweta Singh, Sarita Maharjan and Gyanendra Lamichhane
Lumbini Eye Institute and Research Center, Lumbini, Nepal

Anadi Khatri
Birat Medical College and Teaching Hospital Biratnagar, Nepal
Birat Eye Hospital, Biratnagar, Nepal
Department of Ophthalmology, Birat Medical College and Teaching Hospital, Biratnagar, Nepal

Biljana Kuzmanović Elabjer, Mladen Bušić, Daliborka Miletić, Andrej Pleše and Mirjana Bjeloš
Faculty of Dental Medicine and Health Care Osijek, University Josip Juraj Strossmayer in Osijek, Croatia
Faculty of Medicine Osijek, University Josip Juraj Strossmayer in Osijek, Croatia
University Eye Clinic-WHO Collaborating Center, University Hospital "Sveti Duh", Zagreb, Croatia

Carmen Navarro-Perea, Ignacio Cañas-Zamarra, Enrique Mencía-Gutiérrez, María-Dolores Lago-Llinás, Silvia Pérez-Trigo, Álvaro Bengoa-González, Cristina Calleja-García, Beatriz Alonso-Martín, Bianca-Maria Laslău and Daniela Rojas-Correa
Ophthalmology Department, 12 de Octubre Hospital, Complutense University, 28041 Madrid, Spain

Enrique Revilla-Sánchez
Pathology Department, 12 de Octubre Hospital, Complutense University, 28041 Madrid, Spain

Caroline Casey and Nina Gallo
University of Central Florida College of Medicine, Orlando, FL, USA

Samuel Gallo
Gallo Eye and Facial Plastic Surgery, Dublin, OH, USA

Giancarlo Sborgia, Francesco D'Oria, Alessandra Galeone, Luigi Sborgia and Giovanni Alessio
Department of Medical Science, Neuroscience and Sense Organs, Eye Clinic, University of Bari, Bari, Italy

Alfredo Niro and Alessandra Sborgia
Eye Clinic, Hospital "S. G. MOSCATI, " ASL TA, Taranto, Italy

Francesco Boscia
Department of Surgical, Microsurgical and Medical Sciences, Eye Clinic, University of Sassari, Sassari, Italy

Elena Salvador
Radiology Department, 12 de Octubre Hospital, Complutense University, 28041 Madrid, Spain

Ana-Belén Enguita-Valls
Pathology Department, 12 de Octubre Hospital, Complutense University, 28041 Madrid, Spain

Mojtaba Abrishami, Mehrdad Motamed Shariati, Ali Bolouki and Ghodsieh Zamani
Eye Research Center, Mashhad University of Medical Sciences, Mashhad, Iran

George A. Dumas, Ayesha S. Bryant and Gwendolyn L. Boyd
University of Alabama at Birmingham, Department of Anesthesiology and Perioperative Medicine, Birmingham, Alabama, USA

Saeed Shokoohi-Rad, Samaneh Gholamhoseinpour-Omran, Hamed Hosseinikhah-Manshadi, Mohammad Baghi Yazdi and Hamid-Reza Heidarzadeh
Eye Research Center, Mashhad University of Medical Sciences, Mashhad, Iran

Cevriye Cansız Ersöz
Department of Pathology, Ankara University Faculty of Medicine, Ankara, Turkey

Nikoo Hamzeh and Seyed Mohsen Rafizadeh
Orbital and Oculoplastics Service, Farabi Eye Hospital, Tehran University of Medical Sciences, Tehran, Iran

Mona Safizadeh
Glaucoma Service, Farabi Eye Hospital, Tehran University of Medical Sciences, Tehran, Iran

Zohreh Nozarian
Pathology Department, Farabi Eye Hospital, Tehran University of Medical Sciences, Tehran, Iran

Hiva Saffar
Pathology Department, Shariati Hospital, Tehran University of Medical Sciences, Tehran, Iran

Tatiana Urrea-Victoria, Emiliano Fulda-Graue, Miguel A. Quiroz-Reyes, Felipe Esparza-Correa, Alejandra Nieto-Jordan, Erick A. Quiroz-Gonzalez and Federico Graue-Wiechers
Instituto de Oftalmología Fundacíon Conde de Valenciana (Non-profit Organization), Chimalpopoca 14, Colonia Obrera, Mexico City 06800, Mexico

J. Rios-Nequis Geovanni, J. Abel Ramírez-Estudillo, L. Daniel Gutiérrez-García, Martin Jiménez-Rodríguez and Arthur Levine-Berevichez
Fundación Hospital Nuestra Señora de la Luz IAP, Mexico

Pratap Karki
Department of Ophthalmology, Maharajgunj Medical Campus Tribhuvan University, Institute of Medicine, B. P. Koirala Lions Centre for Ophthalmic Studies, Maharajgunj, Kathmandu, Nepal

Ranju Kharel Sitaula
Department of Ophthalmology, Maharajgunj Medical Campus, Institute of Medicine, Tribhuvan University, B. P. Koirala Lions Centre for Ophthalmic Studies, Maharajgunj, Kathmandu, Nepal

Sagun Narayan Joshi
Dept of Ophthalmology, Maharajgunj Medical Campus, Tribhuvan University, Institute of Medicine, B.P. Koirala Lions Centre for Ophthalmic Studies, Maharajgunj, Kathmandu, Nepal

Haramaya Gurung and Indraman Maharjan
Himalaya Eye Hospital, Pokhara, Nepal

Ananda Kumar Sharma
Department of Ophthalmology, Maharajgunj Medical Campus, Institute of Medicine, B.P. Koirala Lions Center for Ophthalmic Studies, Nepal

Madan Prasad Upadhaya
Ophthalmology, Tribhuvan University, Chair Emeritus B.P Eye Foundation, Children Hospital for Eye, ENT and Rehabilitation (CHEERS), Bhaktapur, Nepal

Yossi Paitan
Sackler School of Medicine, Tel Aviv University, Tel Aviv, Israel
Clinical Microbiology and Virology Laboratories, Meir Medical Center, Kfar Saba, Israel

Anfisa Ayalon, Veronika Yehezkeli and Elad Moisseiev
Department of Ophthalmology, Meir Medical Center, Kfar Saba, Israel
Sackler School of Medicine, Tel Aviv University, Tel Aviv, Israel

Krzysztof Szpila
Department of Ecology and Biogeography, Faculty of Biology and Environmental Protection, Nicolaus Copernicus University, Toruń, Poland

Kosta Y. Mumcuoglu
Parasitology Unit, Department of Microbiology and Molecular Genetics, The Hebrew University-Hadassah Medical School, Jerusalem, Israel

Colin Bacorn and Lily Koo Lin
Department of Ophthalmology and Vision Science, University of California Davis Health, Sacramento, CA, USA

María-C. Garrido
Pathology Department, 12 de Octubre Hospital, Complutense University, 28041 Madrid, Spain

Arif Koytak, Fadime Nuhoglu, Havvanur Bayraktar, Rukiye Ercan and Hakan Ozdemir
Bezmialem Vakif University, Faculty of Medicine, Department of Ophthalmology, Istanbul, Turkey

Pimpiroon Ploysangam
Ross Eye Institute, Department of Ophthalmology, Jacobs School of Medicine and Biomedical Sciences, State University of New York at Buffalo, Buffalo, NY, USA

Sangita P. Patel
Ross Eye Institute, Department of Ophthalmology, Jacobs School of Medicine and Biomedical Sciences, State University of New York at Buffalo, Buffalo, NY, USA
Research and Ophthalmology Services, Veterans Administration of Western New York Healthcare System, Buffalo, NY, USA

Aurelio Hernández-Laín and Justino Jiménez-Almonacid
Neuropathology Department, 12 de Octubre Hospital, Complutense University, 28041 Madrid, Spain

Agustín Martín-Clavijo
Dermatology Department, Queen Elizabeth Hospital, Birmingham University, B15 2TH Birmingham, UK

Stephanie M. Tillit
College of Medicine, University of Florida, Gainesville, FL, USA

Siva S. R. Iyer, Eric J. Grieser and John T. LiVecchi
Department of Ophthalmology, University of Florida, Gainesville, FL, USA

Faisal Ahmed
The Western Eye Hospital, Imperial College Healthcare NHS Trust, 153-173 Marylebone Rd, London, UK
The Imperial College Ophthalmic Research Group (ICORG), Imperial College London, 153-173 Marylebone Rd, London, UK

Nada G. Mohamed
The Ophthalmology Department, Faculty of Medicine, Alexandria University, Champollion Street, Alexandria, Egypt
Whipps Cross Hospital, Barts Health NHS Trust, Whipps Cross Rd, Leytonstone, London, UK

Prema Chendran, Yong Meng Hsien and Wan Haslina Wan Abdul Halim
Department of Ophthalmology, University Kebangsaan Malaysia Medical Centre (UKMMC), Jalan Yaacob Latif, 56 000 Bandar Tun Razak, Kuala Lumpur, Malaysia

J. Minjy Kang, Yen Cheng Hsia and Ying Han
UCSF Department of Ophthalmology, USA

Yu Mizuno, Kazuyuki Hirooka and Yoshiaki Kiuchi
Department of Ophthalmology and Visual Science, Hiroshima University, 1-2-3 Kasumi Minamiku, Hiroshima 734-8551, Japan

Atsushi Hirota
Hirota Eye Clinic, 1-25-1 Shinmachi Shyunanshi, Yamaguchi 745-0017, Japan

Ahmed Alshaikhsalama and Niraj Nathan
Department of Ophthalmology, UT Southwestern Medical Center, Dallas, TX, USA

Hamid Riazi-Esfahani, Arash Mirzaei, Masoud Mirghorbani, Fariba Ghassemi, Mohammad Zarei, Elias Khalili Pour and Nazanin Ebrahimiadib
Retina Service, Farabi Eye Hospital, Tehran University of Medical Sciences, Tehran, Iran

Nima Koosha, Leila Babaei and Mohsen Pourazizi
Isfahan Eye Research Center, Department of Ophthalmology, Isfahan University of Medical Sciences, Isfahan, Iran

Sung Woong Lim, Youngje Sung, Hee Jung Kwon and Won Kyung Song
Department of Ophthalmology, CHA Bundang Medical Center, CHA University College of Medicine, Seoul, Republic of Korea

Ali Kurt
Ahi Evran University Faculty of Medicine, Department of Ophthalmology, Turkey

Ali Hakan Durukan
Health Sciences University Faculty of Medicine, Department of Ophthalmology, Turkey

Murat Küçükevcilioğlu
Gülhane Education and Research Hospital, Department of Ophthalmology, Turkey

Juan Abel Ramirez-Estudillo, Geovanni Rios-Nequis, Martin Jimenez-Rodríguez and Hugo Valdez-Flores
Retina Department, Fundacion Hospital Nuestra Señora De La Luz IAP, Mexico

Ximena Ramirez-Galicia
Research Department, Faculty of Medicine, Universidad La Salle, Mexico

Kinza T. Ahmad, Joseph Chacko, Ahmed B. Sallam, David B. Warner and Sami H. Uwaydat
Jones Eye Institute, University of Arkansas for Medical Sciences, 4301 W. Markham St. Little Rock, AR 72205, USA

Iwan Soebijantoro and Nina Asrini Noor
JEC Eye Hospital Kedoya, Jakarta, Indonesia

Han Y. Yin
SUNY Upstate Medical University, Department of Ophthalmology and Visual Sciences, Syracuse, NY, USA
Florida International University Herbert Wertheim College of Medicine, Miami, FL, USA

Swetha Dhanireddy
SUNY Upstate Medical University, Department of Ophthalmology and Visual Sciences, Syracuse, NY, USA

Alexander E. Braley
SUNY Upstate Medical University, Department of Neurosurgery, Syracuse, NY, USA
Florida International University Herbert Wertheim College of Medicine, Miami, FL, USA

Ahmed M. Habib and Yousef A. Fouad
Al Mashreq Eye Center, Cairo, Egypt
Department of Ophthalmology, Ain Shams University Hospitals, Cairo, Egypt

Mahmood O. Mekkawy
Al Mashreq Eye Center, Cairo, Egypt

Kostas G. Boboridis, Dimitrios G. Mikropoulos and Nick S. Georgiadis
3rd Ophthalmology Department, Aristotle University of Thessaloniki, Kiriakidi 1, Thessaloniki 546 21, Greece

Index

www.ingramcontent.com/pod-product-compliance
Lightning Source LLC
LaVergne TN
LVHW082230200926
848484LV00008B/2330
9798887406497